COPYCAT Recipes

4 Books in 1 Complete Copycat Cookbook to Make the Most Famous Restaurants' Recipes at Home Including the Sirtfood Diet. Step by Step Guide to Learn More than 300 Delicious Recipes

Ashley Gosling

COPYCAT Recipes

2020 Complete Copycat Cookbook to Prepare Your Favorite Restaurants' Recipes at Home on a Budget. Step by Step Guide with Culinary Techniques and Easy and Quick Recipes to Replicate

Ashley Gosling

SPECIAL DISCLAIMER

All the information's included in this book are given for instructive, informational and entertainment purposes, the author can claim to share very good quality recipes but is not headed for the perfect data and uses of the mentioned recipes, in fact the information's are not intent to provide dietary advice without a medical consultancy.

The author does not hold any responsibility for errors, omissions or contrary interpretation of the content in this book.

It is recommended to consult a medical practitioner before to approach any kind of diet, especially if you have a particular health situation, the author isn't headed for the responsibility of these situations and everything is under the responsibility of the reader, the author strongly recommend to preserve the health taking all precautions to ensure ingredients are fully cooked.

All the trademarks and brands used in this book are only mentioned to clarify the sources of the information's and to describe better a topic and all the trademarks and brands mentioned own their copyrights and they are not related in any way to this document and to the author.

This document is written to clarify all the information's of publishing purposes and cover any possible issue.

This document is under copyright and it is not possible to reproduce any part of this content in every kind of digital or printable document. All rights reserved.

© Copyright 2020 Ashley Gosling. All rights reserved.

Table of Contents

INTRODUCTION 19

BREAKFAST COPYCAT RECIPES 22

    SMORREBROD WITH LIVER CHEESE AND CAMEMBERT COPYCAT RECIPE 22

    SMORREBROD WITH MUSHROOM, AVOCADO AND CURRY SPREAD COPYCAT RECIPE 23

    Rack of beef with herb breading, mashed potatoes and sautéed cherry tomatoes 25

    VEGGIE TOSTADAS WITH TOMATO, MOZZARELLA, AVOCADO AND EGG COPYCAT RECIPE 27

    COPYCAT RECIPE TOMATO RICE 28

    COPYCAT RECIPE ZAZIKI 30

    COPYCAT RECIPE VEAL GYROS ON SKEWERS 31

    RICE CRISPY TOADS WITH HERB SALMON, AVOCADO AND BROCCOLI . 32

    COPYCAT RECIPE BURGERS ON A SALAD WITH BRAISED ONIONS AND TOMATO SALSA 34

    Sage lemon vinaigrette 36

    Coleslaw - like in a Greek restaurant 37

    Indian spice rice like in an Indian restaurant 38

    Greek pita bread 39

    Croquettes made from mashed potato 41

    Creamy Aloo Gobi 43

    Insalata dell'amore 45

    SMORREBROD "STRAMMER MAX" COPYCAT RECIPE 46

PORK FILLET IN HERB CRUST ON POTATO GRATIN AND COLORFUL VEGETABLES COPYCAT RECIPE 47

BEEF SALMON WITH WILD GARLIC CROQUETTES, BRAISED TOMATOES AND SALAD WITH AVOCADO YOGURT DRESSING 50

Beef shoulder "Mallorca" COPYCAT RECIPE 53

COPYCAT RECIPE RACK OF BEEF WITH POTATO AND PORCINI PAN AND BABY SPINACH 55

MEATBALL ON FRESH BEET VEGETABLES COPYCAT RECIPE 57

CEVAPCICI À LA ROSIN WITH DJUVEC RICE COPYCAT RECIPE................ 59

COPYCAT RECIPE SEA BREAM ON MEDITERRANEAN VEGETABLES 61

COPYCAT RECIPE PERSIAN-GERMAN OVEN-BAKED CHICKEN ON A COLORFUL VEGETABLE BED... 63

COPYCAT RECIPE Bifteki WITH BEEF 65

ROAST PORK WITH ROASTED VEGETABLE SAUCE AND BOHEMIAN DUMPLINGS 66

ROAST BEEF WITH FRIED POTATOES, FRIED EGG AND VEGETABLE VINAIGRETTE 68

FRIED SEAFOOD SALAD COPYCAT RECIPE.. 71

SUPREME OF CHICKEN WITH TAGLIATELLE COPYCAT RECIPE 73

DESSERTS COPYCAT RECIPES..75

ROSIN'S MEDITERRANEAN BURGER WITH ROASTED VEGETABLES COPYCAT RECIPE... 75

ANDY'S BURGER: COPYCAT RECIPE CHEESEBURGER WITH MUSTARD-MAYO SAUCE 77

COPYCAT RECIPE VEGAN BURGER PATTIES 79

COPYCAT RECIPE Big Mac sauce 81

Goat cheese with dried tomatoes and walnuts on toast COPYCAT RECIPE 82

COPYCAT RECIPE Fried calamari 82

Basic recipe for dark Asia sauce COPYCAT RECIPE.................................. 84

COLORFUL SALAD WITH SHRIMPS COPYCAT RECIPE 85

Spicy cucumber pieces à la Hong Kong COPYCAT RECIPE 87

LUDENSCHEIDER LITTLE CRUST À LA FRANK ROSIN 88

INSALATA Á LA SALVA WITH ROASTED VEGETABLES AND PARMESAN . 90

Potato salad with tomatoes and arugula 92

The tastiest, simplest and yet freshest pizza in the world 93

COPYCAT RECIPE Rasnici 95

COPYCAT RECIPE Macaroni with crab 96

Shiitake mushrooms for sushi COPYCAT RECIPE 97

Carpaccio with a cocktail sauce COPYCAT RECIPE 98

PIZZA WITH ARTICHOKES AND OLIVES 99

MIDIA (MUSSELS) À LA FRANK 101

STUFFED PEPPERS AND TOMATOES COPYCAT RECIPE 102

LANGOS COPYCAT RECIPE 104

COUNTRY POTATO SALAD WITH DRESSED SAUERLAND SAUSAGE 105

SPAGHETTI BOLOGNESE COPYCAT RECIPE 107

POTATO SALAD WITH MEATBALLS COPYCAT RECIPE 109

COD IN MUSTARD SAUCE WITH POTATO HASH BROWNS 111

PASTA WITH SHRIMPS AND HOMEMADE CRUSTACEAN STOCK 113

COPYCAT RECIPE FALSE SLICED BEEF WITH FARMER'S SALAD 115

ROULADES ON A BED OF LETTUCE WITH OSSOBUCO-STYLE VEGETABLE SAUCE 117

BAKED PRESS BAG WITH TOMATO AND CUCUMBER SALAD COPYCAT RECIPE 120

FIRST COURSES COPYCAT RECIPES 121

COPYCAT RECIPE MUSHROOM AND VEGETABLE PAN ON TOASTED BREAD WITH ORGANIC SANDWICH SPREAD 121

COPYCAT RECIPE Italian fish soup 124

COPYCAT RECIPE Chinese fish soup 125

- COPYCAT RECIPE Cognac shrimp cream soup 127
- COPYCAT RECIPE salad dressing 128
- Garlic ajvar sauce COPYCAT RECIPE 129
- COPYCAT RECIPE BURGER SAUCE 130
- HERBED COD FROM THE PAN COPYCAT RECIPE 131
- Savory fry cream – taramosalata COPYCAT RECIPE 132
- Chinese tomato soup COPYCAT RECIPE 133
- RUMP STEAK ON BEAN VEGETABLES WITH FRIED POTATOES COPYCAT RECIPE 134
- Carrot soup with orange juice and mint COPYCAT RECIPE 136
- Potato gratin dauphinois COPYCAT RECIPE 138
- COPYCAT RECIPE CURRYWURST 2.0 140
- COPYCAT RECIPE PEPPER SAUCE 141
- FORESTER SAUCE COPYCAT RECIPE 142
- KAISERSCHMARRN WITH ROASTED ALMONDS COPYCAT RECIPE 144
- GAMBAS IN WHITE WINE STOCK COPYCAT RECIPE 146
- CLASSIC MALLORCAN TRAMPÓ SALAD COPYCAT RECIPE 147
- COPYCAT RECIPE FRIED PULPO 149
- COPYCAT RECIPE BIFTEKI 150
- HOMEMADE MEATBALLS COPYCAT RECIPE 151
- SPICY MANGO AND PEAR CHUTNEY COPYCAT RECIPE 153
- WARM ROMAINE SALAD COPYCAT RECIPE 154
- BEEF CARPACCIO WITH A LIGHT TOMATO AND ROCKET TOPPING COPYCAT RECIPE 156
- TOMAHAWK STEAK WITH MALLORCAN MASHED POTATOES AND TWO TYPES OF VEGETABLES 157
- HOMEMADE GNOCCHI IN A TOMATO AND SALMON SAUCE COPYCAT RECIPE 160

PUFF PASTRY PARCELS WITH SEMOLINA FILLING AND CARAMELIZED FIGS 162

COPYCAT RECIPE MOUSSAKA 164

SPETSOFAI WITH HERB ZAZIKI COPYCAT RECIPE 166

POLPETTONE WITH TOMATO SAUCE COPYCAT RECIPE 168

Roman pot gyros special à la Duchemin COPYCAT RECIPE 170

COPYCAT RECIPE Suflaki marinade 171

Beef with Kritharaki from the oven COPYCAT RECIPE 172

Sicilian caponata COPYCAT RECIPE 173

COPYCAT RECIPE Pork fillet in metaxa sauce 175

DRINKS COPYCAT RECIPES 176

COPYCAT RECIPE Classic iced tea 176

Rhubarb iced tea COPYCAT RECIPE 177

COPYCAT RECIPE Make ginger ale yourself 178

COPYCAT RECIPE Pineapple iced tea 179

CONCLUSION 180

INTRODUCTION 183

REASONS WHY COPYCAT RECIPES ARE BETTER THAN EATING AT RESTAURANTS 184

RESTAURANTS DESSERTS RECIPES 192

LAYERED BERRY DISH 192

BANANA TRIFLE IN THE GLASS 193

BANANA LAYER CREAM IN A GLASS 194

YOGURT MOUSSE WITH POPPY SEEDS 195

FROZEN YOGURT WITH RASPBERRY PUREE 196

GREEK YOGURT WITH HONEY AND PISTACHIOS 197

CLASSIC RED GROATS 198

PANNA COTTA WITH RASPBERRY SAUCE 199

FAST CHOCOLATE PUDDING	200
CREPES SUZETTE WITH ORANGE SYRUP	201
CREPES WITH SALTED CARAMEL APPLES	203
CREPES WITH SOUR CHERRY RAGOUT	204
CREPES WITH ORANGE SAUCE	206
WARM RICE CASSEROLE WITH RASPBERRIES AND PEACHES	207
WARM CHOCOLATE CAKES	208
BAKED BANANA WITH HONEY	209
TYPICAL GERMAN MARBLE CAKE	210
VANILLA PUDDING	211
CHOCOLATE PUDDING WITH SPONGE CAKE	212
WARM SEMOLINA PUDDING	214
VEGAN COCONUT SEMOLINA PUDDING WITH MANGO	215
RICE PUDDING WITH MOCHA SHOT	216
BAKED RICE PUDDING	218
PINEAPPLE AND GINGER RICE PUDDING	219
VEGAN VANILLA TART WITH QUINCE	220
FLORENTINE APPLE PIE	222
ALMOND PANNA COTTA WITH MATCHA POWDER	224
COCONUT PANNA COTTA WITH STRAWBERRY SAUCE	225
MASCARPONE CHOCOLATE CREAM	227
VEGAN PUMPKIN PANNA COTTA WITH WARM CRANBERRY COMPOTE	228
CHIA PUDDING WITH APPLE PULP AND CINNAMON	230
MESQUITE PUDDING	231
POPPY SEED AMARANTH PUDDING WITH A COMPOTE OF PHYSALIS	232
HORSERADISH CREME BRULEE	234
COTTAGE CHEESE PUDDING WITH CHERRY RAGOUT	236
CREME BRULEE WITH VANILLA AND SAFFRON	238

ITALIAN TIRAMISU	239
LEMON TIRAMISU	241
STRAWBERRY TIRAMISU	242
GINGER BREAD TIRAMISU	244
WHITE MOUSSE CAKE	246
MOUSSE-AU-CHOCOLATE SPREAD	247
VEGAN CHOCOLATE NOUGAT MOUSSE WITH MANGO FOAM	248
COTTAGE CHEESE MOUSSE WITH PEACHES	250
ALMOND BUTTERMILK MOUSSE WITH APRICOT COMPOTE	251
ORANGE CURD MOUSSE WITH MIXED BERRY COMPOTE	253
MARZIPAN MOUSSE WITH AMARETTO	254
COTTAGE CHEESE AND POPPY SEED MOUSSE WITH CHERRY WATER	255
GOOD MOOD FRUIT SALAD	256
FRUIT SALAD WITH LEMON FOAM	257
VEGAN AMARANTH PUDDING WITH FRUIT SALAD	258
QUICK FRUIT SALAD WITH SABAYON	259
TROPICAL FRUIT SALAD WITH COCONUT CREAM	260
EXOTIC FRUIT SALAD WITH COCONUT-LIME YOGHURT	261
GINGER FRUIT SALAD WITH VANILLA SAUCE	262
FRUIT SALAD WITH VANILLA SAUCE	263
FRUIT SALAD WITH YOGHURT CREAM	264
Pancakes with apple sauce	265
Back to childhood pancakes	266
Buckwheat pancakes with applesauce	267
Crepes with caramelized pineapple	269
Currant tonka terrine in a crepe coat vegan	270
Lemon crepes with berries	272
Crespelle with raspberries	274

Gâteau des crepes with rose cream 276

Filled espresso crepes 277

Cappuccino and chocolate crepes 279

Iced almond crepes with raspberry sauce 280

Rice pudding with cranberries 281

Cranberry-coconut parfait with chocolate-ginger sauce 282

Sweet onion cake with cranberries 283

Apple cranberry crumble 285

Cranberry baked apple 286

Cranberry-Buchteln 287

Da Capo smoothie 288

Pear and cranberry sauce 289

Yogurt mousse with raspberries and cranberries................................... 290

White choc cranberry cookies 291

Cranberry almond spiral 292

White chocolate bars with poppy seeds and cranberries 293

Apple pancakes with honey curd... 295

Fast apple roses 296

Quinoa parfaits with apple pulp and peanut butter.............................. 297

Baked apple cupcakes.. 298

Hazelnut brownies.. 300

Brownies with pieces of almond.. 301

Pumpkin-coconut brownies.. 302

Blondies with raspberries 303

Nutmeg blondies with Brazil nuts... 304

Blondies with white chocolate 306

Chocolate cube brownies 307

Cheese cream brownies... 308

Baileys brownies with nut crust 309

Apple and cinnamon waffles 310

Basic waffle recipe 311

Chocolate waffles 312

Rice waffles 313

Hearty waffles 315

CONCLUSION 316

Spinach Green Juice 321

Berries Green Juice 322

Broccoli Green Juice 323

Mix Green Juice 324

Celery Green Juice 325

Kale Green Juice 326

Spinach & Apple Juice 327

Cucumber Green Juice 328

Creamy Spinach Juice 329

Parsley Green Juice 330

Apple Porridge 331

Spinach Omelet 332

Tofu & Kale Toast 333

Tofu Scramble 334

Buckwheat Pancakes 335

Waffle Sandwich 336

Buckwheat Porridge 337

Toast with Caramelized Apple 338

Buckwheat Crepe with Apple 339

Buckwheat & Apple Porridge 340

Acai Berry Smoothie Bowl 341

Buckwheat Salad Bowl 342

Spinach Avocado Pomegranate Seeds 343

Beetroot Salad with Spinach 344

Berries Salad with Spinach 345

Pomegranate Salad with Spinach 346

Hot & Spicy Tofu & Broccoli 347

Stir Fried Spinach 348

Kale Stew 349

Stir fry Tofu & Soba Noodles 350

Buckwheat Falafel Bowl 351

Kale Stew 353

Broccoli Soup 354

Buckwheat Noodles Soup 355

Buckwheat Tortilla 356

Sautee Tofu & Kale 357

Stir Fried Green Beans 358

Baked Asparagus 359

Broccoli with Olive Tahini 360

Apple & Walnuts Pie 361

Baked Walnut Bars 362

Coco & Walnuts Milkshake 363

Walnut Butter Cake 364

Walnuts Bits 365

Walnuts Muffins 366

Buckwheat Cinnamon Roll 367

DOUBLE LAYER NO BAKE CAKE 368

Fudgy Brownies 369

Chocolate Pudding With Berries 370

Chocolate Chip Cookies	371
WEEK-1 SIRTFOOD MEAL PLAN	372
WEEK-2 SIRTFOOD MEAL PLAN	374
Green Juice with Lime & parsley	376
Green Juice with Basil & Strawberries	377
Lettuce Green Juice	378
Broccoli & Kiwi Juice	379
Mix Green Juice	380
Basil Juice with Walnuts	381
Kiwi & Cucumber Juice	382
Cucumber & Apple Green Juice	383
Broccoli & Basil Juice	384
Rocket Green Juice	385
Walnuts Porridge	386
Apple Pancakes	387
Morning Parfait	388
Chocolate Pancakes	389
Spinach Muffins	390
Tofu Toast	391
Buckwheat Bread Loaf	392
Broccoli Muffins	393
Buckwheat Waffles	394
Eggless Pudding	395
Turmeric Tea	396
Green Juicy Salad Bowl	397
Green Salad with Flaxseed	399
Beetroot Salad with Spinach	400
Tabbouleh with Lime Dressing	**402**

Salad Wrap with Walnut Cream 404

Buffalo Broccoli Bites 405

Creamy Spinach Curry 406

Broccoli Olives Pizza 407

Spinach Soup 409

Chilli Tofu 411

Spicy Spinach Fillet 412

Broccoli Patties 414

Spinach & Tofu Pizza 416

Broccoli Flatbread Pizza 418

Turmeric Spinach Patties 419

Stir Fried Broccoli & Tofu 421

Wilted Spinach with Onion 422

Broccoli with Garlic sauce 423

Hot & Sour Spinach 424

Spinach & Tofu Curry 426

Easy Walnut Milk 428

Strawberries & Walnut Smoothie 429

Walnut Cream 430

Walnut Butter 431

Dark Chocolate Bites 432

Walnut & Berries Ice-cream 433

Smoothie with Kiwi 434

Blueberries Smoothie 435

Chinese Chocolate Truffles 436

    INTRODUCTION 439

INTRODUCTION OF THE SIRTFOOD DIET 441

    WHAT IS SIRT FOOD? 441

HOW DOES THE SIRT FOOD DIET WORK?	442
The 3 phases of the Sirtfood Diet	442
Sirt food diet: You can eat these foods	443
The Sirt Food: Lean and healthy thanks to proteins	446
HOW SIRTFOOD DIET CAN HELP IN LOSING OF WEIGHT AND BURNING OF FAT	446
THE MOST IMPORTANT SIRT FOODS FOR LOSING WEIGHT	448
HOW TO ACTIVATE YOUR METABOLISM AND YOUR SKINNY GENE	449
EASY EXERCISES TO OPTIMIZE YOUR FAT BURNING	453
WHAT YOU NEED TO KNOW BEFORE TO START (PRO & CONS)	1
WHAT IS IT ABOUT THE SIRT FOOD DIET?	1
CRITICISM OF THE SIRTFOOD DIET	1
CONCLUSION	4
SIRT FOOD RECIPES	5
GREEN TAGLIATELLE WITH PISTACHIO GREMOLATA	6
CHICKEN TAGINE WITH FENNEL AND HARISS CREAM	8
TUNA BALLS ON ZUCCHINI SALAD	10
ZUCCHINI AND BEAN SALAD WITH SPINACH FLAN	12
PAPAYA BOWL WITH TUNA	14
SPICY MUESLI WITH SHEEP'S CHEESE	16
CHICKEN PINEAPPLE SALAD	18
PUMPERNICKEL SANDWICH	20
HAZELNUT PORRIDGE WITH PEAR	22
PORRIDGE WITH PINEAPPLE	24
FLAX SEED CURD WITH APPLE AND CUCUMBER	26
BREAD TOPPED WITH HERRING, EGG AND MUSTARD CREAM	28
STALL WITH PIMENTO CHEESE AND ZUCCHINI	30
FISH BALLS, PAK CHOI AND LEMON KEFIR	32

ARTICHOKE SALAD WITH CAPER AND EGG SAUCE	34
SIRT FOOD SMOOTHIE AFTER GOGGINS AND MATS	36
SIRTFOOD GREEN JUICE	38
SPINACH FLAN WITH TOMATO RAGOUT	40
ENERGY CUTS WITH WALNUT CREAM	42
PUMPKIN SOUP WITH PASTRAMI	44
TORTILLA WITH HERB TOMATOES	46
SALAD WITH LENTILS, PASTRAMI AND PEPPER BANANA	48
GOAT CHEESE OMELET WITH CLEMENTINE	50
TILAPIA FISH STEW WITH SAVOY CABBAGE	52
LIME PASTA WITH SAITHE	54
WHOLE GRAIN PILAF WITH KALE	56
PUMPKIN BOBOTIE	58
PARMESAN CHICORY ZUPPA	60
DEER SHREDS WITH SAVOY CABBAGE	62
TURKEY KEBAB WITH CHAKALAKA	64
FENNEL CREAM CHEESE FRITTATA WITH SALSA	66
CHICKEN AVOCADO TAGLIATA WITH COLORED BEANS	68
STEAMED POTATOES WITH CUCUMBER AND VEGETABLES	70
FETA MEDALLIONS WITH BELL PEPPER SALSA	72
SALAD WITH EGG, RADICCHIO AND POTATO PASTE	74
CUCUMBER AND PINEAPPLE SALAD WITH MACKEREL	76
HUMMUS WITH COLESLAW	78
EGG IN SERRANO HAM CASSEROLE	80
BAKED EGGS OVER AVOCADO WITH GOAT CHEESE OR BACON	82
CHICKEN SALAD WITH AVOCADO	84
TURKEY CURRY	86
CLOUD BREAD	88

FURIOUSLY DELICIOUS CAULIFLOWER SOUP 89

RELAXED MEDALLIONS WITH SWEET AND SPICY SAUCE 91

JERKY LETTUCE WITH LENTILS 93

VEGGIE BOWL WITH FRIED EGG 95

FILLED HOT PEPPER PEPPERS 97

5 SPICES AND READY FILLET WITH PAK CHOI 99

KOHLRABI SCHNITZEL WITH YOGHURT HERB DIP 101

STIR-FRIED FILLET WITH SESAME VEGETABLES 103

SPICY MANGO SALAD WITH SHEEP'S CHEESE 105

TROPICAL FRUIT SALAD WITH COCONUT 107

EXOTIC MUESLI WITH TROPICAL FRUITS 109

INTRODUCTION

COPYCAT RECIPES

Copycat recipes can taste like restaurants recipes. Restaurants recipes are made with readily available recipes which everyone can find in their kitchen. You can duplicate many of your favorite restaurant meal by recreating the recipes at home.

DOES COPYCAT FOOD INDEED POSE A FLAVOR LIKE RESTAURANTS FOOD?

Copycat food can taste fundamentally the same as eatery plans. Frequently eatery plans are made with regular fixings everybody can discover in their kitchen. You can copy a significant number of your preferred eatery suppers by reproducing the formula at home. Some restaurants food truly isn't exceptional or made with mystery fixings. Many of the most well-known dishes are extremely exemplary dishes that we know and love.

REASONS WHY COPYCAT RECIPES ARE BETTER THAN EATING AT RESTAURANTS

Restaurants meal can contain loads of undesirable fixings. There's additionally a ton past what's in the dinner that you pass up when you're eating from a takeout box.

Here are reasons why you ought to think about preparing supper for yourself today around evening time!

1. **It allows you to reconnect**

Cooking together can offer you a chance to reconnect with your accomplice and friends and family. Cooking has different advantages too. It was expressed that trying new things together—like learning another formula—can help keep a couple associated and occupied with their relationship.

2. **It's demonstrated to be more advantageous**

Some studies recommend that individuals, who cook all the more frequently, as opposed to getting takeout, have a general more advantageous eating regimen. These examinations additionally show that eatery dinners normally contain higher measures of sodium, soaked fat, all-out fat, and by and large calories than home-prepared suppers.

When you set up new fixings yourself, or get them transported directly to your entryway with help like Plated, you have all-out command over what is going in your food. That can improve things significantly to your general wellbeing.

3. **It's simpler to watch your calories**

The reasonable inexpensive food request extends between 1,100 to 1,200 calories all out – that is practically the entirety of a lady's suggested every day calorie admission (1,600 to 2,400 calories) and just about 66% of a man's day by day consumption (2,000 to 3,000 calories). Also, if you figured independent eateries and littler chains do any better, reconsider. Those diners siphon in much more calories, with a normal of 1,327 calories for every dinner. Making a supper yourself implies you can ensure the part sizes and carbohydrate contents are the places you need them to be. Plans frequently accompany dietary data and serving size proposals, which makes that much more straightforward.

4. **It's a life hack**

Some portion of requesting takeout methods trusting that the food will show up or heading to get it. Contingent upon where you live, what time you require, and whether the conveyance individual is acceptable with headings, this could take additional time than if you'd mostly made supper at home. Cooking at home doesn't need to take a great deal of time if you don't need it to. By utilizing a help like Plated, you dispose of the need to search for plans or primary food item shop. All you need comes right to your entryway; in the specific pre-divided sums you'll be utilizing.

5. Money saver

Over the long haul, planning dinners at home may set aside your cash. A gathering of fundamental fixings regularly comes in at a lower sticker price than a solitary restaurant dish. Likewise, you can wind up getting more suppers out of a formula you make at home than if you request takeout, or have extras to take to work the following day. After only half a month, you could see perceptible investment funds begin to accumulate.

6. Its customized

Cooking at home offers you the chance to eat the nourishments you love precisely how you appreciate eating them. For instance, with Plated, on the off chance that you like your meat all the more all-around done, or dishes less zesty, the formula incorporates proposed changes.

7. Its good times!

When you're making a supper without preparation, you get the chance to find and analyze various fixings, seasonings, and foods. Plated offers 11 alternatives to browse every week, a considerable lot of which are all-inclusive propelled. Encountering new nourishments on a plated night can be an incredible method to connect with your friends and family or loosen up in the wake of a monotonous day at work.

What's more, similarly, as with any movement, the additional time you spend in the kitchen, the better you become at making excellent meal.

BREAKFAST COPYCAT RECIPES

SMORREBROD WITH LIVER CHEESE AND CAMEMBERT COPYCAT RECIPE

Ingredients for 1 Serving

FOR THE BREAD:

- 1 large slice good Italian white bread
- 1 pc Organic cucumber (3 cm)
- 2nd Roman lettuce leaves
- 1 tsp neutral oil
- 1 slice   Meat cheese
- 1 tbsp   mayonnaise
- 2 thick slices   Camembert
- FOR ONION SALAD:
- 1 small handful arugula
- ¼ pear
- Red onion
- 1 tbsp   White wine vinegar
- 2 tbsp   olive oil
- ½ tsp   mustard
- 1 pinch salt
- 1 pinch pepper from the grinder

Preparation time: 30 minutes

Total: 30 minutes

- For the bread, preheat the oven to 200 ° C top / bottom heat. During this time, wash the rocket for the onion salad, spin dry or pat and roughly chop. Peel and core the pear as desired and cut into fine sticks. Peel, halve and cut the onion into thin rings.
- Whisk vinegar and oil in a bowl. Mix in the onion rings, season with salt and pepper. Fold in pear sticks and chopped rocket. Put aside.
- Bake the bread in a hot oven on a medium rack on the wire rack for a few minutes until crispy. In the meantime, wash the cucumber and cut it into slices. Wash the lettuce leaves and shake or pat dry.
- Heat the oil in a pan and fry the meat cheese on both sides for 2-3 minutes until it starts to brown. Take the bread out of the oven and let it cool down briefly - do not switch off the oven - then brush with the mayonnaise. Spread the cucumber slices and lettuce leaves on top, put the meat cheese on top and arrange the Camembert slices on top.
- Bake the topped bread in a hot oven on a medium rack until the cheese begins to melt. Mix the onion salad again, then top the still hot bread with the salad and serve immediately.

SMORREBROD WITH MUSHROOM, AVOCADO AND CURRY SPREAD COPYCAT RECIPE

Ingredients for 1 Serving

- ½ baguette
- 1 handful Mushrooms
- 2nd Roman lettuce leaves
- ½ small avocado
- ¼ red bell pepper
- ¼ onion
- 2 tbsp olive oil
- 1 shot White wine
- 2 tbsp finely chopped flat-leaf parsley
- 1 pinch salt
- 1 pinch pepper from the grinder
- 2 tbsp Curry spread

- ✓ 4 tbsp coarsely grated, well-matured hard cheese (e.g. Tyrolean eagle; alternatively, Gruyère)

Preparation time: 20 minutes

Total: 20 minutes

- Preheat the oven to 200 ° C top / bottom heat. During this time, clean the mushrooms, rub dry with kitchen paper if necessary and cut in half or quarter, depending on the size. Wash the salad and spin or dab dry. Peel the avocado, remove the core and cut the pulp into strips. Wash the peppers and cut them into small cubes, peel the onions and finely dice them.
- Bake the baguette in the hot oven on the wire rack for a few minutes. In the meantime, heat the oil in a pan and fry the mushrooms in it over high heat. Reduce the temperature, add the onion cubes and sauté until glassy over medium heat. Take the baguette out of the oven and set aside. Do not switch off the oven.
- Sprinkle the pepper cubes in the pan and briefly sweat. Deglaze the contents of the pan with the white wine and let the liquid boil almost completely. Fold in the chopped parsley and season the vegetables with salt and pepper.
- Cut the baguette lengthways. Spread curry spread on one half of the cut surface, put the other half aside and use for a second bread. Place the lettuce leaves on top, cover them with strips of Avocado, spread the vegetable mixture on top and sprinkle with the cheese. Bake the baguette in the hot oven for a few minutes until the cheese begins to melt.
- Take the finished bread out of the oven and serve immediately

Rack of beef with herb breading, mashed potatoes and sautéed cherry tomatoes

Ingredients for 4 Serving

- 2 pieces) Rack of beef (s), whole
- ½ bundle Rosemary, finely chopped
- ½ bundle Thyme, finely chopped
- ½ bundle Parsley, finely chopped
- ½ bundle Mint, finely chopped
- 1 large   Onion (s), finely chopped
- Something butter
- 4 disc / s Toasted bread, without crust, diced finely
- 2 dl milk
- For the puree:
- mashed potatoe
- 8 large ones Potato
- ½ bundle Rosemary, finely chopped
- 150 g   butter
- 2 dl olive oil
- salt and pepper
- For the vegetables: (sautéed cherry tomatoes)
- 2 bowls Cherry tomato (s), halved
- Clove of garlic, cut into fine strips
- 1 stems Rosemary, the needles
- 1 dl olive oil
- salt and pepper

Preparation

- Working time about 30 minutes
- Cooking / baking time approx. 1 hour
- Total time about 1 hour 30 minutes

- Cook whole potatoes on a sheet lined with aluminum foil (so that there is no direct contact) in the oven preheated to 200 ° C for about 1 hour (until they are very soft).

The breading:

- Braise the finely chopped onions with a little butter for a long time, add the toasted bread cubes and add the milk and let it boil gently until you get a nice creamy porridge (add a little more milk if necessary). Let it cool down a bit and then add the herbs. Chill.
- Fry the rack of beef carefully. Brush the breading generously on the top and let it rest at approx. 100 ° C for 15-20 minutes.

The mashed potato:

- Scrape the cooked potatoes from the bowl with a spoon and put them in a saucepan. Crush with the butter and olive oil (do not make a puree from it, pieces are desired). Season with salt and pepper.
- Pull the rosemary in shortly before serving.
- Heat the oven to 180 ° C and give the caries the desired cooking level for another 5-10 minutes.

The tomatoes:

- Meanwhile, fry the cherry tomatoes in a very hot frying pan with olive oil, garlic and rosemary (lightly caramelize). Salt and pepper.
- Then cut the square in half (1/2 karee = 1 portion) and cut again before the last bone (for a nice presentation).
- Arrange and enjoy, possibly pouring on gravy.

VEGGIE TOSTADAS WITH TOMATO, MOZZARELLA, AVOCADO AND EGG COPYCAT RECIPE

Ingredients for 4 Serving

For the receipt:

- ✓ 3rd large vine tomatoes
- ✓ red bell pepper
- ✓ ripe avocado
- ✓ Sprinkle of lemon juice
- ✓ Bunch of arugulas
- ✓ 2nd Balls of creamy mozzarella
- ✓ 2 -3 Pinch of salt
- ✓ 2 -3 Pinch pepper from the mill
- ✓ 4th hard boiled eggs
- ✓ 100 g   spicy Mallorcan sliced cheese (alternatively other sliceable cheese)
- ✓ 1 bunch mixed herbs (e.g. parsley, mint, basil)
- ✓ 1 serving Aïoli (recipe see link in preparation)
- ✓ For the bread:
- ✓ 2nd Garlic cloves
- ✓ 2 -3 EL   olive oil
- ✓ 4th nice slices of fresh rye bread
- ✓ 1 pinch   of salt

Preparation time: 30 minutes

Cooking time: 5 minutes

Total: 35 minutes

- Wash and dry tomatoes and peppers for the topping. Cut the tomatoes into slices without stalks. Cut the peppers into thin rings, core them. Halve the avocado and carefully remove the core. Peel the halves, cut the pulp into thin strips and drizzle with a few drops of lemon juice. Read the

arugula, wash and spin dry. Remove hard stems. Carefully release the seeds from the pomegranate.
- Dab the mozzarella with kitchen paper and pluck it into pieces. Season with 1 pinch of salt and pepper. Peel and slice the eggs. Debark the cheese and cut into small cubes. Wash the herbs, shake dry, chop with the stems and season the aïoli with some of the herbs.
- Peel the garlic for the bread and cut it into fine cubes. Heat the olive oil in a pan and fry the bread slices in it with the garlic until medium crispy. Season with a pinch of salt.
- Place the slices of bread on a plate and brush with a little aïoli. Layer the rocket, tomato, mozzarella, avocado, egg and paprika, adding small blobs of aïoli in between and season with salt and pepper. Sprinkle the turrets with pomegranate seeds and diced cheese, then garnish with the other herbs.

COPYCAT RECIPE TOMATO RICE

Ingredients for 4 Serving

- ✓ 3rd Vine tomatoes
- ✓ red bell pepper
- ✓ 2nd Onions
- ✓ 3rd Garlic cloves
- ✓ 2 branches thyme
- ✓ 2 branches rosemary
- ✓ 0.5 bundle basil
- ✓ 500 ml Tomato juice
- ✓ 2 tbsp Tomato paste
- ✓ 3 tbsp olive oil
- ✓ 1 pinch salt
- ✓ 1 pinch pepper from the grinder
- ✓ 200 g rice
- ✓ 100 ml White wine
- ✓ Sprinkle of lemon juice

Preparation time: 20 minutes

Cooking time: 20 minutes

Total: 40 minutes

- Wash tomatoes and peppers. Cut the tomatoes into cubes without stalks. Halve, core and cut the peppers into pieces. Peel and finely chop onions and garlic. Wash thyme, rosemary and basil and shake dry.
- Puree tomato juice, tomato paste, tomato and paprika cubes in a tall beaker with a hand blender. Heat the olive oil in a pan. Sweat the onion and garlic cubes in it over medium heat. Season with salt and pepper. Add thyme and rosemary to the pan. Stir in the rice and fry with it.
- Deglaze with the white wine and boil the liquid briefly. Pour in the tomato mix, put on a lid and simmer on medium heat until the rice is cooked. In the meantime, always fill up with a little water. During this time, pluck the basil leaves and cut them into strips. Set aside some nice leaves for the garnish.
- When the rice is cooked, remove the rosemary and thyme. Season again with lemon juice, salt and pepper and fold in the basil strips.
- Spread the rice on plates and garnish with the remaining basil leaves. Serve with meat dishes such as bifteki, gyros or fried pulp.

COPYCAT RECIPE ZAZIKI

Ingredients for 7 Serving

- ✓ Organic cucumber
- ✓ Bunch of dill
- ✓ 3rd Garlic cloves
- ✓ 50g feta (Greek brine cheese)
- ✓ 500g Greek yogurt (10% fat)
- ✓ 1 pinch salt
- ✓ 1 pinch pepper from the grinder
- ✓ 1 pinch Sweet paprika powder
- ✓ 1 shot olive oil
- ✓ 1 splash greek vinegar
- ✓ 1 splash Lemon juice

Preparation time: 15 minutes

Total: 15 minutes

- Wash the cucumber thoroughly and grate finely. Lightly salt the pieces and let them stand briefly. In the meantime, wash the dill, shake it dry and finely chop it with the stems. Peel the garlic and cut into the finest cubes. Pat the feta cheese dry with kitchen paper and crumble it.
- Pour off the cucumber water that has settled, additionally squeeze out the cucumber pieces with your hands. Mix the yoghurt, cucumber pieces, garlic and feta in a bowl. Season with paprika powder, salt and pepper.

COPYCAT RECIPE VEAL GYROS ON SKEWERS

Ingredients for 12 Serving

- 2nd kg of veal (e.g. from the top shell)
- large bunch of mixed herbs (flat-leaf parsley, basil, dill)
- 3rd Garlic cloves
- 2nd Tablespoons of olive oil
- 2 Tsp paprika powder sweet
- 1 Tsp salt
- lemon

Preparation time: 30 minutes

Total: 30 minutes

- Remove fat and tendons from the meat, then cut them into slices about 2 cm thick across the grain. Place the slices side by side in a flat baking dish.
- Wash the herbs and shake them dry. Pluck leaves and stems from the stems and chop finely. Peel the garlic, drizzle some olive oil on the work surface and chop finely. Season the meat with paprika, salt and pepper. Spread herbs and garlic over it, then mix everything well with your hands. Finally drizzle the meat with a little lemon juice.
- Place the marinated meat slices on the gyro skewer. Cut off protruding edges on the sides and put them back on the skewer. Put the skewer in the grill and grill the meat for about 15 minutes, then the outer layer is already cooked and nicely browned.
- Cut down the outer layer of meat with a long, sharp knife and arrange. Zaziki and tomato rice go well with this.

RICE CRISPY TOADS WITH HERB SALMON, AVOCADO AND BROCCOLI

Ingredients for 4 Serving

For the rice tourists:

- ✓ 200 g   Rice (alternatively 4 slices of toast as a base)
- ✓ 1 pinch salt
- ✓ 2-3 EL   olive oil

For covering:

- ✓ 300 g very fresh salmon fillet (sushi quality; without skin)
- ✓ 2 pinches salt
- ✓ 1 large bunch   mixed herbs (e.g. parsley, mint, basil, dill, coriander, chives)
- ✓ 250 g   Italian broccoli (Italian cima di rapa or stem cabbage)
- ✓ 2 tbsp   olive oil
- ✓ 1 pinch freshly grated nutmeg
- ✓ 1 pinch pepper from the grinder
- ✓ 100 ml   dry white wine
- ✓ avocado
- ✓ 1 splash Lemon juice
- ✓ Romana salad heart
- ✓ 4 slices spicy Mallorcan sliced cheese (alternatively other sliceable cheese)
- ✓ 1 serving Tomato jam (see recipe for burger on salad)

Preparation time: 40 minutes

Cooking time: 25 minutes

Total: 65 minutes

- For the rice thistle, cook the rice in slightly salted water a little longer than specified, according to the package instructions, soft and sticky. Follow the cooking method in which the liquid is completely absorbed by the rice. Spread the finished rice in a flat baking dish and let it cool.
- In the meantime, wash the salmon for the topping under running cold water and pat dry with kitchen paper. Check the fillet for bones and pull the existing one. Remove the brown trans fat, slice the fish meat diagonally and season with a pinch of salt. Wash the herbs and shake them dry. Pluck and chop the leaves. Turn the salmon slices in the herbs. Set aside covered.
- Clean the broccoli, wash with the stems and dry. Heat the olive oil in a coated pan and fry the broccoli in it. Deglaze with a little white wine and let the liquid boil. Season with 1 pinch of nutmeg, salt and pepper. Keep warm.
- Halve the avocado and carefully remove the core. Peel the halves, cut the pulp into thin strips and drizzle with a few drops of lemon juice. Remove 8 beautiful leaves from the lettuce heart, wash and spin dry.
- Divide the rice into at least 4 equal portions and shape into round thalers. If the rice is particularly sticky, this is best done between two layers of cling film. Heat the olive oil in a coated pan and fry the rice thalers in it slowly and crispy on both sides over medium heat.
- Spread the rice thalers on plates and cover them with the cheese while still hot so that it melts easily. Put on 2 lettuce leaves, spread the avocado strips on top and top with a little tomato jam. Finally, arrange salmon and broccoli on top.

COPYCAT RECIPE BURGERS ON A SALAD WITH BRAISED ONIONS AND TOMATO SALSA

Ingredients for 4 Serving

For the burger patties

- 600 g Ground beef
- 1 pinch salt
- 1 pinch Pepper (best from the mill)
- 2nd Shallots
- 1 large bunch   mixed herbs (e.g. parsley, mint, basil)
- 3rd Onions
- 4 tbsp   olive oil
- 8 slices spicy Mallorcan sliced cheese (alternatively other sliceable cheese)

For the tomato salsa

- 200 g Cherry tomatoes
- 2nd Garlic cloves
- 2 tsp Capers
- 2 tbsp olive oil
- 1 shot   dry white wine
- 1 pinch sugar
- 1 pinch salt
- 1 pinch Pepper (best from the mill)

For the set

- 1red bell pepper
- 1 tbsp   olive oil
- 1 shot   White wine
- 1 pinch salt

- ✓ 1 pinch Pepper (best again from the mill)
- ✓ 2nd large Romana lettuce hearts

Preparation time: 40 minutes

Cooking time: 12 minutes

Total: 52 minutes

- For the patties, season the mince in a bowl with 1 pinch of salt and pepper. Peel the shallots and cut them into fine cubes. Wash the herbs, shake dry and chop with the stems. Set aside 2 tablespoons herbs for the garnish. Mix the shallot cubes and half of the remaining chopped herbs carefully into the minced meat. Form 8 patties of the same size from the mass with slightly damp hands. Peel the onions and cut them into rings or strips.
- Heat two tablespoons of olive oil in two large pans and fry the patties in it. Turn the patties and fry from the second side, pushing them together a little and frying the onions in the open area at a slightly lower heat.
- Wash and halve the cherry tomatoes. Peel the garlic and chop in to fine slithers. Drain the capers. Heat the olive oil in a third pan and fry the tomato halves in it. Add half of the garlic and capers and stir briefly in the pan. Deglaze with the white wine and let the liquid boil almost completely. Season with 1 pinch of sugar, salt and pepper. Pull the pan off the stove and pour the tomatoes into a bowl.
- Cover each patty with 1 slice of cheese and let the cheese melt slightly. Wash the peppers and cut them into rings, removing the seeds. Push the tomatoes together on one side of the pan. Heat the rest in olive oil on the free side and fry the pepper rings in it with the rest of the garlic. Deglaze with a little white wine and loosen the roast set. Season again with 1 pinch of salt and pepper. Finally add the second half of the herbs
- Free the lettuce hearts from withered outer leaves and cut them into 8 beautiful, thumb-thick slices, holding the slices together well so that they do not fall apart into the individual leaves. Place the slices on plates and brush with a little aïoli .

- Remove the patties from the pan and place them on a lettuce leaf. Spread the braised onions over it. Top with tomato salsa and pepper rings. Garnish with the herbs set aside.

Sage lemon vinaigrette

Ingredients for 1 Serving

- ✓ 225 ml olive oil
- ✓ 50 ml   Lemon juice
- ✓ 50 ml   Aceto balsamico, white
- ✓ 3 tbsp Mustard, gritty
- ✓ 3 tbsp honey
- ✓ 5 tbsp Sage (sagebrush, desert sage or mugwort), dried, alternatively normal sage or mugwort
- ✓ salt
- ✓ Lemon pepper

Preparation

Working time about 5 minutes

Total time about 5 minutes

- Mix all the ingredients together and you're done. The amounts of lemon juice, honey, mustard and sage can of course be individually adjusted.
- Since dried "sagas" (mugwort or desert sage) are probably difficult to get here, you can certainly use normal sage or mugwort as an alternative.

Coleslaw - like in a Greek restaurant

Ingredients for 8 Serving

- ✓ White cabbage
- ✓ 2nd Onion (onion)
- ✓ 1 cup Sugar (small)
- ✓ 1 cup Oil (small)
- ✓ 2 tbsp   salt
- ✓ 1 teaspoon pepper
- ✓ ½ bottle Herbal vinegar, e.g. from Kühne, approx. 250 ml - 350 ml
- ✓ 1 bottle Sparkling mineral water, approx. 0.7 liters - 1 liter

Preparation

Working time about 20 minutes

Total time about 1 day 20 minutes

Note: Adjust the amount of water and vinegar to the size of the white cabbage. The brew Is poured off before serving.

- Remove the stalk from the cabbage. Grate the cabbage finely and put In a bowl. Cut the onions Into small cubes and add to the grated cabbage.
- Mix sugar, oil, salt, pepper, herb vinegar and mineral water. The sugar must dissolve well. Be careful, if you add the mineral water, it will foam a little!
- Pour the sauce over the herb. Cover the whole thing with a smaller lid than the bowl and weigh it down with 2-3 cans. Let stand 24 hours.
- Drain and serve the next day.
- Delicious with grilled food, also keeps in the jar in the fridge.

- The coleslaw is a hit with us at many summer festivals. It is very easy to prepare and actually tastes like it does in a Greek restaurant.

Indian spice rice like in an Indian restaurant

Ingredients for 2 Serving

- ✓ 140 g   Basmati rice or other long grain rice
- ✓ 1 tbsp   Clarified butter or oil
- ✓ 2nd Carnation (s), whole
- ✓ 2nd Cardamom capsule (s)
- ✓ Bay leaf
- ✓ ¼ tsp   Turmeric powder
- ✓ Something salt
- ✓ n.B. water

Preparation

Working time about 20 minutes

Cooking / baking time approx. 15 minutes

Total time about 35 minutes

- Crush the cardamom capsules and cloves in a mortar so that they develop their aroma more quickly. Heat the clarified butter in the pan and heat the cloves, cardamom and bay leaf for about 1 minute. Then put the rice in the pan and let it sauté briefly (approx. 2 minutes). Then add 1 - 2 knife tips of turmeric.

- Then pour a little water. Not a lot of water, just so much that the rice doesn't burn. Add a pinch of salt (rather too little than too much). After about 14 - 15 minutes the water should be completely boiled. Possibly. fill up a little in between, because the rice must not burn.
- If you feel like it, you can add crushed pepper afterwards. Don't salt too much!

Greek pita bread

Ingredients for 1 Serving

- ✓ 400 g   Flour
- ✓ ½ cube yeast
- ✓ 1 cup / s Water, lukewarm
- ✓ ½ cup / s milk
- ✓ 2 Tea spoons salt
- ✓ 2 Tea spoons sugar
- ✓ 1 tbsp.   olive oil
- ✓ Oil (sunflower oil)
- ✓ oregano

Preparation

Working time about 30 minutes

Cooking / baking time approx. 20 minutes

Total time approx. 1 day 21 hours 50 minutes

- Mix water and milk. Transfer 1/3 of it into another container - will be needed later.
- Add sugar, crumble yeast and stir.

- Sift the flour into a bowl and press a hollow in the middle. Gradually pour the yeast liquid into the well and knead to a pre-batter. Leave in a warm place, covered, for 15 minutes.
- Mix the remaining milk water with salt and slowly work it into the batter. Knead the dough for about 10 minutes until a loose, homogeneous mass is formed. Add some flour or lukewarm water if necessary. Work in olive oil. Divide the dough into 8 pieces and form into balls. Leave in a warm place covered for 30 minutes.
- Preheat the oven on hot air 160ºc (or top, bottom heat 180ºc).
- Brush the baking sheet with sunflower oil. Roll out balls into flatbreads (approx. 15 cm Ø, thickness 4-5 mm)
- Spread only 4 cakes on the sheet. Please do not put several sheets in the oven at the same time! Bake the flatbreads on the medium shelf for 4-5 minutes. Then turn and bake again. The flatbreads should still be white and soft.
- Wrap in aluminum foil to keep them from getting hard and dry.
- Serve:
- Let some olive oil get hot in a coated pan. Fry the flatbread for 2 minutes on each side. Care with oregano. You can also roast the flatbreads in the toaster on a medium setting. Goes well with gyros, tzaziki, lettuce with tomatoes, cucumber and red onions.

Croquettes made from mashed potato

Ingredients for 4 Serving

- ✓ 82 g Mashed potatoes
- ✓ 75 ml milk
- ✓ 100 ml water
- ✓ 20 g butter
- ✓ 6 g salt
- ✓ 20 g Flour
- ✓ 1 small Egg (er)
- ✓ 1 Msp. nutmeg
- ✓ Fat for deep-frying
- ✓ Breadcrumbs (ready-made breading)

Preparation

Working time about 30 minutes

Total time about 30 minutes

- Proper potato croquettes are difficult to produce, you have to cook potatoes, prepare a puree from them, dry them a bit, and bread the shaped croquettes before baking them in hot fat.
- Therefore, there are ready-made croquettes in the freezer in the supermarket for preparation in the oven or the deep fryer. Unfortunately, they are expensive and do not taste good. So, nothing helps, we have to find out the recipe ourselves.
- The basis is a potato puree powder. In a bag are 82 g, which should be mixed with 375 ml of water, 125 ml of milk, 15 g of butter and 3 g of salt. To make croquettes out of it, only much less liquid is allowed in, I use twice as much salt for this. A tablespoon of flour makes the mass finer. The main trick is a fresh raw egg, which is beaten into the bowl beforehand.

- Beat 1 small raw egg in a bowl. Add 75 ml milk (fresh milk) and 100 ml water (cold tap water). Now add 1 tbsp flour (approx. 20 g 405 wheat flour), 1 tsp butter (approx. 20 g), 1 level tsp salt (approx. 6 g), 1 pinch of nutmeg and 1 bag of mashed potato powder (82 g).
- So, a cold, quite dry mashed potato is prepared, which was also made with 1 egg as a binder. If you only have large eggs or just want to make one serving (1/3 pack), you just take the yolk from the egg and pour the egg white away.
- Mix (it appears very dry, smacking and tearing), let swell for 1 minute. Then knead, it sticks strongly to the fingers.
- First form lumps so that no air is trapped (they should then roll in your hand without sticking), then form a 2 cm thick roll, cut it into 5 cm pieces (or press the mixture through a potato croquette press) and do not store for a long time, but bake in the deep fryer in 180 ° C hot fat (vegetable fat) for about 3 minutes until they turn golden yellow.
- The croquettes are ready in less than 10 minutes as quickly as they are made in the restaurant and without any breading.
- If you want, you can roll the croquettes in breading (ready-made breadcrumbs breadcrumbs) before frying. The croquettes are then a little more granular after baking. I prefer it without breadcrumbs, they even become a little more golden.
- Prepare only a few croquettes at a time in the deep fryer, about 5 pieces, otherwise the temperature of the fat will drop too far and the croquettes will burst open. They also burst if the dough is too watery or the egg is forgotten.
- If you fry too many croquettes at once, they get bright spots if they cannot swim freely, but bake together because they are pressed together due to lack of space.

Creamy Aloo Gobi

Ingredients for 4 Serving

- ✓ 6 m. In size Potato
- ✓ 1 m. Tall cauliflower
- ✓ 2 m. In size Onion (s) or 3 small ones
- ✓ 2 toes   garlic
- ✓ 3 cm Ginger, approx.
- ✓ olive oil
- ✓ 1 can Tomatoes)
- ✓ 1 can Coconut milk
- ✓ 1 teaspoon cumin
- ✓ 1 teaspoon coriander
- ✓ 1 teaspoon turmeric
- ✓ 1 tbsp   Garam Masala
- ✓ 1 teaspoon salt
- ✓ 1 teaspoon Tomato paste
- ✓ n.B. Basmati, cooked as a side dish

Preparation

Working time about 15 minutes

Cooking / baking time approx. 30 minutes

Total time about 45 minutes

- Peel and cut the garlic, onions and ginger. The pieces can be roughly cut because they will be mashed later. In addition, the potatoes must be peeled and diced and the cauliflower divided into small florets.

- Heat the oil in a large pan and fry the onions until translucent over medium heat. After approx. 4 min. Add garlic and ginger. When the onions turn brown, deglaze with coconut milk and canned tomatoes.
- Now add all the spices and puree the sauce with a hand blender. For a particularly fruity taste, I add 1 tsp tomato paste. Don't be surprised if the sauce tastes too seasoned, the vegetables take a few more spices with them when cooking and this makes the sauce taste milder in the end.
- Now bring the sauce to a boil and cook the potatoes in it over a low flame. Stir again and again so that the sauce does not burn. After approx. 15 min. The cauliflower can be added to the cooking time. Don't forget to stir! After another 10 - 15 min. the vegetables should be soft and the dish is ready.
- The Aloo Gobi can be reserved with warm Basmati rice and Naan bread. A few leaves of coriander or parsley could be used as decoration.
- Cooking time can vary due to the size of the potato pieces. So when cutting the vegetables, keep in mind that the larger the pieces, the longer it takes to cook. If you don't have a hand blender, you have to cut the onions, garlic and ginger into small pieces and exchange canned tomatoes for tomatoes that have been passed through.

Insalata dell'amore

Ingredients for 2 Serving

- ¼ head Lettuce, green
- 2 sheets Salad (romaine lettuce)
- 4th Cherry tomato (s)
- 1 tbsp Vinegar (balsamic vinegar)
- ½ tsp Mustard, grainy
- 4 tbsp olive oil
- 1 branch / s rosemary
- ½ disk / n toast
- 1 tbsp Pine nuts
- 150 g Cheese (young soft goat cheese)
- 1 teaspoon Vinegar (raspberry vinegar)
- Salt and pepper, black

Preparation

Working time about 25 minutes

Total time about 25 minutes

- Cut the romaine lettuce into fine strips, cut the lettuce apart. Halve cherry tomatoes, mix everything in a large salad bowl.
- Mix the two types of vinegar as a dressing, add the mustard, salt and black pepper and mix together with 2 tablespoons of oil loosely under the salad.
- Pluck the rosemary leaves and cut the toast into small cubes. Lightly fry both ingredients and the pine nuts in the remaining oil over low heat until the bread is crispy. Then spread over the salad.

- Remove the pan from the hob, cut the goat's cheese into slices about 1 cm thick and add the oil remaining in the pan. Put the pan back on the hob and let the cheese warm up at a low temperature. Warning, cheese should not melt. Place the finished slices on the salad and sprinkle with pepper.
- As a side dish freshly baked bread with aioli or garlic butter.

SMORREBROD "STRAMMER MAX" COPYCAT RECIPE

Ingredients for 1 Serving

- ✓ tomato
- ✓ 1 pc Organic cucumber (3 cm)
- ✓ 1 small handful arugula
- ✓ 2nd Roman lettuce leaves
- ✓ thick slice of farmhouse bread
- ✓ 1 tsp neutral oil
- ✓ egg
- ✓ 2 tbsp Tomato spread
- ✓ 2 slices raw ham (e.g. Parma ham)
- ✓ 1 pinch salt
- ✓ 1 pinch pepper from the grinder

Preparation time: 20 minutes

Total: 20 minutes

- Preheat the oven to 200 ° C top / bottom heat. In the meantime, wash the tomato and cucumber. Slice both. Wash the rocket and lettuce leaves and shake or pat dry. Bake the bread in a hot oven on a medium rack on the wire rack for a few minutes until crispy.

- In the meantime, heat the oil in a small pan, break the egg into the pan and fry in the hot fat to a nice fried egg.
- Meanwhile, take the crispy bread out of the oven and let it cool, then brush with tomato spread. Place the lettuce leaf, ham, tomato and cucumber slices on top of each other and finally put the fried egg on top. Season with salt and pepper and serve directly.

MAIN COURSES COPYCAT RECIPES

PORK FILLET IN HERB CRUST ON POTATO GRATIN AND COLORFUL VEGETABLES COPYCAT RECIPE

Ingredients for 4 Serving

FOR THE GRATIN:

- ✓ 1 kg   predominantly hard-boiled potatoes
- ✓ 1 tbsp   butter
- ✓ Clove of garlic
- ✓ 500 g   cream
- ✓ 1 pinch   freshly grated nutmeg
- ✓ 1 pinch   salt
- ✓ 1 pinch   pepper from the grinder
- ✓ 100 g   grated mountain cheese or parmesan
- ✓ FOR THE VEGETABLES:
- ✓ broccoli
- ✓ large zucchini
- ✓ ¼   Hokkaido pumpkin
- ✓ 2 tbsp   butter
- ✓ 1 pinch   salt
- ✓ 1 pinch   pepper from the grinder

FOR THE MEAT:

- 800 g   pork tenderloin
- 2 pinches salt
- 1 large bunch   mixed   herbs   (e.g.   chives,   parsley, rosemary, coriander)
- 6 tbsp   White   bread   or   bread   crumbs   (alternatively breadcrumbs)
- egg
- 4 tbsp   Flour
- 75 g   butter
- 2 tbsp   neutral oil (e.g. rapeseed oil)

Preparation time: 45 minutes

Cooking time: 45 minutes

Total: 90 minutes

- Preheat the oven to 200 ° C top / bottom heat. Peel the potatoes, cut lengthwise into a fan shape and press lightly with the flat of your hand so that the "compartments" open. Grease a baking dish with 1 tablespoon of butter and spread the potato compartments side by side in the dish.
- Peel the garlic and cut it into fine cubes. Season the cream and garlic vigorously with nutmeg, salt and pepper in a tall beaker, then puree with the hand blender. Pour the cream over the potato fans and bake in the hot oven on a medium rack for 40–45 minutes. In the meantime, wash broccoli, zucchini and pumpkin for the vegetables. Divide the broccoli into florets, halve or quarter the zucchini lengthways depending on the thickness and cut into 2 cm slices. Core the pumpkin and dice the pulp.
- Remove the fat and tendons from the pork fillet for the meat, cut into portions and pat two fingers thick into the shape. Season with salt all around. Wash the herbs and shake them dry. Pluck the rosemary needles from the branches and cut them finely with the other herbs. Mix the white bread crumbs with the herbs in a bowl. Melt the butter in a small

- saucepan and fold it under the breadcrumbs and herb mixture (mis de pain).
- Whisk the eggs in a deep plate for a short while, put the flour on a second plate. First press the pieces of meat into the flour from one side, then pull through the eggs and finally press into the herb-crumb mixture.
- Heat the oil in a pan and fry the pork fillet pieces on the herb crust side over high heat. Carefully turn the meat and also sear it from the other side. Spread the pieces on an oven-proof plate and cook in the hot oven with the potatoes for the last 5 minutes.
- In the meantime, heat the butter in a pan for the vegetables. First, fry the pumpkin for 3-4 minutes, stirring occasionally. Add the broccoli and fry for 4 minutes. Take the finished meat and potatoes out of the oven and let them rest briefly. During this time, add the zucchini and fry everything for another 3-4 minutes until the vegetables are tender but still have a bit of a bite. Season with salt and pepper.
- Spread the gratin and vegetables on a plate, lay the pork fillet with a herb crust and serve.

BEEF SALMON WITH WILD GARLIC CROQUETTES, BRAISED TOMATOES AND SALAD WITH AVOCADO YOGURT DRESSING

Ingredients for 4 Serving

FOR THE CROQUETS:

- 1 kg floury potatoes
- 2nd Pinch of salt
- 250 ml milk
- ½ Bunch of wild garlic
- Pinch pepper from the mill
- egg yolk
- 1-2 tablespoons potato flour
- 50 g butter

FOR SALAD AND DRESSING:

- avocado
- 150 g Whole milk yogurt
- 1-2 tablespoons Vegetable broth
- Sprinkle of lemon juice
- 2 -3 EL White wine vinegar
- 50 ml olive oil
- pinch of salt
- Pinch pepper from the mill
- Head lollo rosso
- red bell pepper
- 2 tbsp finely cut dill tips

FOR THE MEAT:

- 2nd Beef salmon (300 g each)

- ✓ 2nd Garlic cloves
- ✓ 2nd Pinch of salt
- ✓ 3rd Shallots
- ✓ 4th Spring onions
- ✓ Pinch pepper from the mill
- ✓ 2nd Sprigs of thyme
- ✓ 2 tbsp olive oil
- ✓ ½ lemon

FOR THE SAUCE:

- ✓ onion
- ✓ Clove of garlic
- ✓ 2 tbsp butter
- ✓ pinch of sugar
- ✓ 300 ml red wine
- ✓ 400 ml Beef stock
- ✓ pinch of salt
- ✓ Pinch pepper from the mill
- ✓ 2 tbsp chopped basil

FOR THE BRASS TOMATO:

- ✓ 300 g Cherry tomatoes
- ✓ 2nd Shallots
- ✓ Clove of garlic
- ✓ ½ Bunch of basil
- ✓ 3 tbsp Olive oil beef salmon with wild garlic croquettes, braised tomatoes and salad with avocado yogurt dressing
- ✓ 100 ml White wine
- ✓ pinch of sugar
- ✓ pinch of salt
- ✓ Pinch pepper from the mill

Preparation time: 60 minutes

Cooking time: 45 minutes

Total: 105 minutes

- For the croquettes, peel the potatoes and cut them into large pieces. Cover the pieces in a saucepan with water, bring to the boil, season with a pinch of salt and cook gently on medium heat for about 20 minutes.
- Halve the avocado for the salad and remove the core. Scrape the pulp out of the halves and place in a tall beaker with the yoghurt. Add the broth, lemon juice, vinegar, oil, salt and pepper, puree the whole thing. Remove the outer leaves from the lollo rosso. Remove the remaining leaves from the head, wash, spin dry and pluck into bite-size pieces. Wash the peppers, cut them in half, remove the stones and cut them into strips without using a stem. Put aside.
- Drain the soft potatoes and let them evaporate. Warm the milk, wash the wild garlic, dry it, cut it finely and puree it under the milk using a hand blender. Mash the still hot potatoes with the wild garlic milk. Add egg yolk and potato flour and mix. Season with salt and pepper. Cut out small portions of dough with a teaspoon and shape into gnocchi. Put aside
- Preheat the oven to 180 ° C for the meat. Remove fat and tendons from the beef salmon. Peel the garlic and cut into sticks. Cut small pockets into the meat with a sharp, sharp knife and pepper with the garlic sticks. Season with salt and pepper. Peel the shallots and halve lengthways. Wash the spring onions and cut them into coarse rings without root. Wash the thyme and shake it dry. Heat the oil in a pan. Add the beef salmon with the shallots and spring onions and sauté for 3-4 minutes on each side over high heat.
- Lay out 2 strips of aluminum foil on the work surface. Spread the shallots and spring onions, place the meat on top, season with salt and pepper, top with the thyme and drizzle with lemon juice. Seal the aluminum foil loosely and cook the meat pink in the hot oven for 5–8 minutes. In the meantime, peel the onion and garlic for the sauce and cut into fine cubes. Heat the butter in the meat pan, sweat the onion and garlic cubes in it over medium heat. Sprinkle in the sugar and caramelize. Deglaze with half of the red wine and reduce the liquid to half the amount. Pour in the rest of the red wine and bring to the boil again. Pour on the stock and reduce it again by half. Taste the sauce with salt and pepper. Keep warm.
- For the stewed tomatoes, wash and halve the cherry tomatoes. Peel the shallots and garlic and cut into fine cubes. Wash the basil and shake dry.

Pluck the leaves and cut them finely. Heat the olive oil in a pan. Add tomatoes, shallots and garlic and fry over medium heat until the tomatoes melt. Deglaze with the white wine and boil the liquid almost completely. Season with sugar, salt and pepper, then fold in the basil.
- For the croquettes, heat the butter in a pan and fry the gnocchi in it over medium heat. For the salad mix lollo rosso, bell pepper, onion and spring onions in a bowl. Fold in the dressing, dill and basil. Take the beef salmon out of the oven and let it rest briefly, then cut into slices.
- Arrange beef slices and croquettes with the tomatoes and the salad on plates, drizzle with the sauce and serve.

Beef shoulder "Mallorca" COPYCAT RECIPE

Ingredients for 3 Serving

- Beef shoulder, approx. 1,600 g each
- ½ liter   Beer, light
- 0.3 liters water
- 2nd Carrot (s)
- 3rd Bay leaves
- 6 Garlic cloves)
- Lemon (s), organic
- ½ tsp   salt
- Pepper, to taste
- ½ tsp   Pimentón de la Vera, mild
- 50 ml   olive oil
- 3rd Onion (s), white

Preparation

Working time about 30 minutes

Cooking / baking time approx. 3 hours

Total time about 1 day 3 hours 30 minutes

- Peel the carrots, peel the garlic, wash the bio lemon. Now everything is cut into small pieces. If the zest of the lemon is sweet, it can be used. Otherwise only take the pulp. Roughly cut the onions without peeling.
- Have the beef shoulder cut into portions at the butchers. Now place them in a roasting pan with a lid and add all other ingredients. Place in the refrigerator and let marinate for at least 24 hours.
- Put in the oven the next day and cook at 160 degrees for about 3 hours. The meat should come off the bone easily.

COPYCAT RECIPE RACK OF BEEF WITH POTATO AND PORCINI PAN AND BABY SPINACH

Ingredients for 4 Serving

- 2nd Rack of beef approx. 500 g
- 500 g   small waxy potatoes (e.g. triplets)
- 1 tsp   Salt + more to taste
- 400 g   Boletus
- red pointed peppers
- 3rd Shallots
- 2nd Garlic cloves
- ½ Bunch of flat-leaf parsley
- ½ Bunch of basil
- 400 g young spinach
- ½ Bunch of arugula
- 7 tbsp   olive oil
- Pinch pepper from the mill
- 50 g Italian hard cheese (e.g. parmesan or pecorino)

Preparation time: 60 minutes

Cooking time: 30 minutes

Total: 90 minutes

- Remove fat and silver skins from the rack of beef and clean the bones. Wash the potatoes, bring to the boil in a saucepan with sufficient water and a tablespoon of salt and cook gently for about 20 minutes. Preheat the oven to 180 ° C top / bottom heat.
- In the meantime, clean the porcini mushrooms, rub dry with kitchen paper if necessary and cut into pieces. Wash the

peppers, halve lengthways, remove the seeds and cut into strips without a stem. Peel a shallot and the garlic and cut into fine cubes. Wash the parsley and basil and shake dry. Pluck the leaves from the stems and cut them finely. Sort the spinach and arugula, wash and spin dry. Pluck or cut the rocket into small pieces.

- Drain the potatoes, let them evaporate and cut in half. Heat two tablespoons of oil in a pan, sauté potatoes, porcini mushrooms, garlic and pointed peppers all over in a medium to high heat. Season with salt and pepper, fold in the parsley and basil.
- Heat a tablespoon of olive oil in a saucepan and sauté the shallots in it until glassy over medium heat. Add the baby spinach and let the leaves collapse. Refine with arugula and cheese. Heat two tablespoons of olive oil in a coated pan and fry the rack of beef all over it on medium heat for two minutes on each side. Cook the squares in the hot oven on a medium rack for 12–15 minutes.
- In the meantime, peel and halve the remaining two shallots. Heat the remaining olive oil in a separate pan and fry the shallot halves in it over high heat. Deglaze with the red wine and boil the liquid over medium heat for 10 minutes. Season with salt and pepper and let it steep briefly. Take the rack of beef out of the oven and let it rest briefly, then portion it.
- Spread the potato and porcini pan on plates, create the rack of beef, drizzle with the shallot and red wine reduction and serve with the spinach.

MEATBALL ON FRESH BEET VEGETABLES COPYCAT RECIPE

Ingredients for 4 Serving

FOR THE BEET VEGETABLES:

- 1 large turnip
- 300 g   Carrots
- 500 g   floury potatoes
- 400 g   Hokkaido pumpkin
- 2nd Onions
- 1 Clove of garlic
- 2 tbsp   butter
- 2 tsp   sugar
- 100 ml   White wine
- ½ tsp   salt
- 2nd Bay leaves
- 4 tbsp   finely chopped flat-leaf parsley
- 2 tsp mustard
- 1 shot   White wine vinegar
- 1 pinch   freshly grated nutmeg
- 1 pinch   Caraway powder
- 1 pinch   pepper from the grinder

FOR THE MEATBALLS:

- 200 ml   milk
- 2 slices   toast
- 2nd Shallots
- 1 bunch chives
- 5 Sage leaves
- 3 tbsp   Clarified butter
- 100 ml   White wine
- 500 g   mixed minced meat (beef and pork)
- egg

- ✓ ½ tsp Sweet paprika powder
- ✓ 1 tsp salt
- ✓ ½ tsp pepper from the grinder

Preparation time: 45 minutes

Cooking time: 30 minutes

Total: 75 minutes

- For the beet vegetables, peel the beet, carrots and potatoes and cut them into thumb-thick cubes. Wash the pumpkin, remove the seeds and cut it into small pieces. Peel onions and garlic and cut into fine cubes.
- Heat the butter in a saucepan and sauté the onion cubes until translucent. Add the garlic and sweat briefly. Sprinkle in the sugar and caramelise lightly. Add the vegetable cubes and fry briefly. Season with salt, then deglaze with the white wine. Add the bay leaves and cook the vegetables over a medium heat for about 20 minutes, stirring occasionally.
- Meanwhile, heat the milk in a saucepan for the meatballs. During this time, cut the toast into cubes. Put the bread cubes in the warm milk and soak them for 10 minutes.
- Meanwhile, peel the shallots and cut them into fine cubes. Wash chives and sage, shake dry and cut finely. Heat 1 tablespoon of clarified butter in a large pan and sauté the onion cubes until translucent. Deglaze with the white wine and let the liquid boil almost completely.
- Knead minced meat, egg, toasted bread, sweaty onions, chives, sage, paprika powder, salt and pepper in a large bowl. Season the mixture again, then shape it into 8 meatballs of equal size with your hands slightly moistened.
- Heat the remaining clarified butter in the onion pan and sauté the meatballs for 3 minutes on both sides over high heat. Reduce the heat a little and let the meatballs soak for another 2 minutes on each side.
- Fold the meatballs' frying fat and finely chopped parsley under the soft-cooked vegetables, removing the bay leaves. Season the beet with mustard, white wine vinegar, nutmeg, caraway, salt and pepper.
- Spread the beets on plates and put the meatballs on them.

CEVAPCICI À LA ROSIN WITH DJUVEC RICE COPYCAT RECIPE

Ingredients for 2 Serving

- Cevapcici
- 250 g   Ground beef
- 250 g   Minced beef
- 1 strong pinch of salt
- 1 strong pinch of pepper from the mill
- red bell pepper
- 0.5 bundle flat-leaf parsley
- 0.5 bundle dill
- 2nd Shallots
- Clove of garlic
- 2 tbsp   olive oil

Furthermore:

- Djuvec Rice
- 2nd Shallots
- 2nd Garlic cloves
- red chili pepper
- 4 tbsp   olive oil
- 1 pinch sugar
- 2 cups   Long grain rice (200 g)
- 400 ml   Tomato juice
- 2 pinches salt
- 2 pinches pepper from the grinder
- 2nd Vine tomatoes
- red bell pepper
- 0.5 bundle flat-leaf parsley
- 0.5 bundle dill
- 3 tbsp   Ajvar
- 200 g   Peas (frozen goods; thawed)
- 100 ml   White wine

✓ lime

Preparation time: 30 minutes

Cooking time: 20 minutes

Total: 50 minutes

- Season the minced meat in a bowl with salt and pepper. Wash, halve, core and cut the peppers into the finest cubes. Wash the herbs, shake dry and chop finely with the stems. Peel the shallots and garlic and also dice.
- Twist the seasoned meat and the prepared vegetables together again through the meat grinder. Form small rolls out of the mixture with slightly damp hands.
- Heat the olive oil in a pan and fry the meat rolls all around. Reduce the temperature and let the cevapcici steep for a few minutes at a lower temperature.
- Arrange the cevapcici on a plate and serve.
- Djuvec Rice
- Peel the shallots and garlic and cut into fine cubes. Wash the chilli, halve lengthways, core and chop finely. Heat 2 tablespoons of olive oil in a saucepan. Sauté the shallots with half the garlic in them over medium heat, sprinkling with a pinch of sugar. Add the rice and sweat briefly. Add the chilli pepper and also sweat briefly. Pour in the tomato juice, season with a pinch of salt and pepper and cook the rice with the lid on over medium-low heat for 15–20 minutes. If the tomato juice overcooks, add 1 dash of water.
- In the meantime, wash and dry the tomatoes, peppers and herbs. Cut the tomatoes into small cubes without the stalks. Halve the peppers lengthways, core and dice as well. Finely chop the herbs and stems.
- Heat the rest of the oil in a pan and briefly fry the remaining garlic in it. Add tomato cubes, bell pepper, ajvar and peas. Swirl briefly in the pan, then deglaze with the white wine and let the liquid boil. Season with lime juice.
- Stir in the cooked rice - it should now completely absorb the tomato juice and have the consistency of a risotto. Season again with 1 pinch of salt

and pepper. Fold in three quarters of the herbs. Arrange the Djuvec rice on a serving plate and serve garnished with the remaining herbs.

COPYCAT RECIPE SEA BREAM ON MEDITERRANEAN VEGETABLES

Ingredients for 2 Serving

- large sea bream (approx. 350 g; ready to cook)
- 2 -3 pinches salt
- 2 -3 pinches pepper from the grinder
- Organic lemon
- Organic lime
- 1 bunch Mediterranean herbs (e.g. rosemary, thyme, basil)
- onion
- Clove of garlic
- 2nd   Vine tomatoes
- 200 ml   White wine
- red bell pepper
- zucchini
- 0.5 bundle flat-leaf parsley
- 0.5 bundle dill
- 100 g Sheep cheese
- 2 tbsp butter
- 100 g green and black olives

Preparation time: 30 minutes

Cooking time: 15 minutes

Total: 45 minutes

- Wash the sea bream under running cold water and pat dry on the outside and inside with kitchen paper. Season with salt and

pepper. Wash the lemon and lime hot and rub vigorously dry. Slice the lemon, roughly dice the lime. Wash the herbs and shake dry, set aside 1–2 sprigs of rosemary for later. Fill the stomach of the sea bream with lemon wedges and the other sprigs of herbs.
- Peel the onion and garlic and cut into cubes. Wash the tomatoes and roughly dice them without the stem. Dice the sheep cheese.
- Preheat the oven to 150 ° C. Heat the olive oil in a large pan and fry the sea bream in it from both sides. Add onion and garlic and fry briefly, then add rosemary and lime and tomato cubes as well. Deglaze with half of the white wine and pour on the sea bream. Lift the sea bream out of the pan into an ovenproof dish and finish cooking in the hot oven for 8-10 minutes.
- In the meantime, wash the peppers and zucchini. Halve the paprika, remove the seeds and cut into bite-size pieces with the zucchini. Wash the parsley and dill and shake dry, then cut finely with the stems. Cut or crumble the sheep's cheese into small pieces.
- Heat the pan with lime and tomato cubes again, adding the butter. Put the prepared vegetables with the olives in the pan and fry briefly. Deglaze with the rest of the white wine and let the liquid boil almost completely. Add the finely chopped herbs. Season with 1 pinch of salt and pepper. Take the fish out of the oven and fillet.
- Place the vegetables with the sheep's cheese on a large serving plate and arrange the fish fillets on them.

COPYCAT RECIPE PERSIAN-GERMAN OVEN-BAKED CHICKEN ON A COLORFUL VEGETABLE BED

Ingredients for 4 Serving

For the filling:

- 1 bunch Coriander green
- 1 handful Prunes (pitted)
- 1 handful Raisins
- 1 handful Walnut kernels
- 1 strong pinch   salt
- 1 strong pinch   pepper from the grinder

For the meat:

- Corn poulard
- 2nd red pointed peppers
- 4th Carrots
- 0,5 Celeriac
- 2-3 Spring onions
- onion
- 4th Garlic cloves
- 3 branches rosemary
- 5 tbsp   olive oil
- Walnut-sized piece of ginger
- walnut-sized piece of turmeric (alternatively 1 tsp ground turmeric)
- 1 tsp ground coriander + more to taste the vegetables
- 1 tsp ground cumin + more to taste the vegetables
- 1 tsp Sweet paprika powder + more to taste the vegetables
- Juice of 2 limes
- 0,5 tsp Sambal Oelek
- 1 strong pinch   salt

Preparation time: 30 minutes

Cooking time: 60 minutes

Total: 90 minutes

- For the filling, wash the coriander, shake it dry and cut it roughly. Chop plums, raisins and walnut kernels into small pieces and mix with the coriander in a bowl. Season with 1 pinch of salt and pepper.
- Preheat the oven to 160 ° C for the meat. Wash the chicken thoroughly under running cold water and dry it inside and out with kitchen paper. Fill the chicken with the dried fruit mix.
- Wash, halve, core and cut the peppers into pieces. Peel the carrots and celery and cut them into cubes. Clean and wash the spring onions and cut the white to light green part into rings. Peel the onion and cut it into large cubes. Peel and press the garlic. Wash the rosemary and shake it dry.
- Heat 2 tablespoons of olive oil in a pan. Sauté the peppers, carrots, celery, spring onions, onions and garlic in it over medium to high heat. Add the rosemary, peel the ginger and turmeric and rub the ginger with half of the turmeric. Refine the vegetable pan with coriander, cumin and paprika powder as you like.
- Grate the rest of the turmeric in a bowl and mix with 2 sprinkles of lime juice, ground coriander, cumin, paprika powder, sambal oil, remaining olive oil and 1 strong pinch of salt in a bowl to a paste. Rub the chicken generously with it.
- Spread the pan vegetables on a baking sheet or in a large flat baking dish. Place the marinated chicken on the vegetable bed and cook in the hot oven for 60–80 minutes, depending on the size of the poultry.
- Take the crispy, golden brown chicken out of the oven and let it rest briefly, then cut into portions with poultry scissors. Arrange the chicken pieces with the fried vegetables on a large serving plate and serve drizzled with a little lime juice.

COPYCAT RECIPE Bifteki WITH BEEF

Ingredients for 2 Serving

- ✓ 250 g   Ground beef (beef steak)
- ✓ 2 tbsp   low-fat quark
- ✓ 1 pinch (s) Chili powder
- ✓ salt and pepper
- ✓ Feta cheese
- ✓ Olive oil, for frying

Preparation

Working time about 5 minutes

Cooking / baking time approx. 10 minutes

Total time about 15 minutes

- Mix the beef steak, lean quark and spices well.
- Cut the feta into strips and cover with a chop.
- Fry all around in olive oil.

ROAST PORK WITH ROASTED VEGETABLE SAUCE AND BOHEMIAN DUMPLINGS

Ingredients for 5 Serving

For the meat

- ✓ 1½ kg   Roast pork (without rind)
- ✓ 3rd Garlic cloves
- ✓ 3 tbsp   neutral oil (e.g. sunflower oil)
- ✓ 1 pinch salt
- ✓ 1 pinch pepper from the grinder

For the sauce

- ✓ 100 g Carrots
- ✓ 100 g   celery root
- ✓ large onion
- ✓ 1 tsp Caraway seeds
- ✓ 2 pinches sugar
- ✓ 1 tbsp   Tomato paste
- ✓ 100 ml   White wine
- ✓ 400 ml   vegetable stock
- ✓ 1 pinch salt
- ✓ 1 pinch pepper from the grinder
- ✓ 3rd Carnations
- ✓ Bay leaf
- ✓ 2 tsp mustard
- ✓ 150 g   cold pieces of butter

For the dumplings

- ✓ 500 g Flour
- ✓ 2 tsp salt
- ✓ 21 g fresh yeast (½ cube)

- ✓ 150 ml lukewarm milk
- ✓ 1 pinch sugar
- ✓ egg
- ✓ 1 handful Breadcrumbs

Preparation time: 150 minutes

Total: 150 minutes

- Preheat the oven to a temperature of 175 ° C. For the meat, salt and pepper the pork all around, then stab several times evenly with a sharp knife. Peel the garlic, cut it into pieces and push the pieces into the puncture points in the roast pork. Heat the oil in a large roasting pan and sear the pork roast all over in a high heat.
- For the sauce, peel carrots, celery and onions and cut them into large cubes. Place the cubes with the meat in the roasting pan and fry briefly. Sprinkle in caraway seeds and sugar, stir in the tomato paste and also briefly toast. Deglaze with the white wine and reduce the liquid to half the amount. Pour on the stock and so much water that the roaster bottom is covered about 2 cm high. Add cloves and bay leaves, season again with salt and pepper and braise the roast in the hot oven for about 1.5 hours, regularly adding water and turning the roast once after half the cooking time.
- For the dumplings, sift the flour into a large bowl with 1 tsp salt. Press a hollow in the middle, crumble the yeast into it, add the sugar and pour on the lukewarm milk. Cover the bowl with a clean kitchen towel and let the batter rise for 15 minutes.
- Add the eggs and knead everything with your hands or with the kneading hooks of the hand mixer for at least 5 minutes to a homogeneous dough. Finally, add the breadcrumbs and knead the mixture well again by hand. Cover the bowl again with a cloth and let it rest for at least 30 minutes until its volume has increased significantly.
- Knead the dough again vigorously, then divide into 4 equal pieces. Shape each piece into a thick roll, cover again and let it rise for another 30 minutes. Roll the dough rolls again and let them steep in a large saucepan with lightly boiling salted water for 20–25 minutes, depending on their size.

- Take the roast out of the oven and keep warm. Transfer the brew into a saucepan and boil it down a little further if you like. Remove the bay leaves and cloves and season with the mustard, salt and pepper. Pull the pot off the stove and stir in the cold pieces of butter with a whisk to bind the sauce. Lift the dough rolls out of the water, drain and cut into slices with a sharp knife. Also cut the roast pork into slices.

ROAST BEEF WITH FRIED POTATOES, FRIED EGG AND VEGETABLE VINAIGRETTE

Ingredients for 6 Serving

- 1 kg roast beef
- 5 Garlic cloves
- 1 pinch salt
- 1 tbsp medium hot mustard
- 3 branches thyme
- 3 branches rosemary
- 3 tbsp Rapeseed oil
- 1 pinch pepper from the grinder
- 200 ml dry white wine
- 6 Eggs
- 6 stems flat-leaf parsley
- 1 small handful roasted pine nuts
- 1 kg Jacket potatoes (mainly waxy; cooked)
- large white onion
- 3 tbsp Rapeseed oil
- 100 g streaky bacon cubes
- 1 pinch salt
- 1 pinch pepper from the grinder
- 2nd gherkins
- small white onion
- Red onion
- 1 bunch spring onions
- little carrot

- ✓ 1 handful Cherry tomatoes
- ✓ 5 dried tomatoes (in oil)
- ✓ 2 tbsp   Rapeseed oil
- ✓ 1 pinch sugar
- ✓ 5 tbsp   olive oil
- ✓ 2 tbsp   White wine vinegar

Preparation time: 90 minutes

Total: 90 minutes

- Preheat the oven to 160 ° C. The meat from large parts of the fat cover - leave a comb in the middle for the taste - and free the tendons. Peel the cloves of garlic. Use a pointed knife to evenly spread 5 slits into the meat and insert the cloves of garlic. Salt the roast beef all around and brush generously with mustard on the meat side. Wash thyme and rosemary and shake dry.
- Heat 2 tablespoons of rapeseed oil in a cast iron pan and sear the meat on the fat side first. Turn and fry from the other side as well. Season the meat with pepper. Add thyme and rosemary. Deglaze with the wine. Place the meat in an ovenproof dish, pour the broth from the pan, cover with the herbs and cook in the hot oven for 25–30 minutes medium (core temperature 56 ° C - use a meat thermometer is best).
- In the meantime, peel the jacket potatoes for the fried potatoes and cut them into cubes. Peel the onion and cut it into fine cubes. Heat the rapeseed oil in a pan and sear the potato cubes in it over a high heat. When they are lightly browned, push the cubes together on one side of the pan, reduce the temperature and sweat the onion on the free side of the pan over medium-high heat until they also start to brown. Add the bacon and fry briefly. Season with salt and pepper and fry for a further 10 minutes on low heat.
- In the meantime, drain the pickled cucumbers for the vinaigrette and cut them into small cubes. Peel the onions and cut them into fine cubes. Clean and wash the spring onions and cut the white to light green part into rings. Peel and grate the carrot. Wash and halve the cherry tomatoes. Cut the dried tomatoes into fine strips.

- Heat the rapeseed oil in a pan. Sweat the white onion, spring onions, grated carrots, cherry tomatoes and dried tomatoes in it over medium heat. Sprinkle with the sugar. Take the roast beef out of the oven and let it rest briefly on a plate. Deglaze the pan contents for the vinaigrette with the roast beef broth and bring to the boil again. Transfer the vinaigrette to a bowl, stir in the olive oil and vinegar. Fold in the red onion. Season with salt and pepper.
- For the salad, heat the remaining rapeseed oil in a pan and fry the eggs in it to make fried eggs. Cut the roast beef into thin slices. Cut the finished fried eggs into strips as desired. Wash the parsley, shake dry and pluck the leaves.
- Spread the fried potatoes on plates and place a few slices of roast beef on top. Pour the vinaigrette with the vegetables on top, top with 1 fried egg, sprinkle with pine nuts and serve garnished with parsley.

FRIED SEAFOOD SALAD COPYCAT RECIPE

Ingredients for 4 Serving

- ✓ 4th large shrimps (without shell, with head, gutted)
- ✓ 100 g Monkfish fillet
- ✓ Kalmartube (ready to cook)
- ✓ 150 g mixed seafood
- ✓ Perch of celery
- ✓ 4th Sprigs of oregano
- ✓ 2nd Sprigs of rosemary
- ✓ 200 g White bread from the previous day
- ✓ onion
- ✓ 2nd Garlic cloves
- ✓ 4 tbsp   Olive oil + a little more to drizzle
- ✓ pinch of salt
- ✓ Bay leaf
- ✓ 150 ml   White wine
- ✓ lemon

Preparation time: 30 minutes

Cooking time: 40 minutes

Total: 70 minutes

Clean the shrimp. Cut the anglerfish into cubes and the squid tube into thin rings. Wash and slice the celery. Wash oregano and rosemary and shake dry. Also dice the white bread. Peel the onion and the garlic. Cut a clove of garlic into fine cubes. Press on the second toe.

Heat two tablespoons of olive oil in a pan. Fry the white bread cubes in it with the pressed garlic over medium heat until golden brown. Remove and drain on kitchen paper. Heat the rest of the oil in the pan. Fry fish and seafood in it, then add the garlic and fry briefly. Season with salt, add celery, bay leaf, rosemary and oregano. Deglaze with the white wine and let everything simmer for about 5 minutes. Remove the bay leaf again and season the salad with a dash of lemon juice, salt and pepper.

Spread the seafood salad on plates, garnish with the croutons and serve drizzled with olive oil (see tip). Tip: The dish can also be served on a bed of lettuce, but it also tastes great when tomatoes with some melted cherry tomatoes as a sauce with pasta or as a soup. For sauce or soup with fish and seafood, sweat two tablespoons of tomato paste. For a soup, pour a can of peeled tomatoes (à 400 g) as well as hot vegetable broth or fish stock as you like.

SUPREME OF CHICKEN WITH TAGLIATELLE COPYCAT RECIPE

Ingredients for 4 Serving

FOR THE MEAT

- 4th Corn Chicken Suprêmes (breast with skin and wing club)
- ½ Bunch of rosemary
- Shallot
- Clove of garlic
- 2 tbsp olive oil
- pinch of salt
- 100 ml White wine
- 2 tbsp butter
- Organic lime
- FOR THE NOODLES
- 300 g Cherry tomatoes
- 2nd Shallots
- 2nd Garlic cloves
- Bunch of mixed herbs (e.g. parsley, basil, chives)
- 2 tsp Salt + more to taste
- 400 g Ribbon pasta (e.g. tagliatelle)
- 2 tbsp olive oil
- pinch of salt
- pinch of sugar
- 100 ml White wine
- 125 g finely grated mozzarella
- Pinch pepper from the mill

Preparation time: 30 minutes

Cooking time: 20 minutes

Total: 50 minutes

Preheat the oven to 120 ° C. For the meat, wash the chicken suprêmes under cold running water and pat dry with kitchen paper. Wash the rosemary and shake it dry. Peel the shallot and garlic and dice finely. Cut a pocket into the meat in the chicken breasts from the side below the skin and add 1 sprig of rosemary.

Wash and halve the cherry tomatoes for the pasta. Peel the shallots and garlic and dice finely. Wash the herbs, pluck the leaves and cut them roughly. Bring plenty of water with 2 teaspoons of salt to a boil in a large pot.

For the meat, heat the olive oil in an ovenproof pan and first fry the chicken parts on the skin side until they are crispy and golden brown. Turn the suprêmes, add shallot and garlic cubes with a few sprigs of rosemary and fry briefly. Deglaze with the white wine, add the butter and pour the broth from the pan over the meat. Cook the meat in the hot oven for about 10 minutes.

Meanwhile, cook the tagliatelle bite-proof in boiling salted water according to the package instructions. Heat the olive oil in a pan, then fry the shallots and garlic in it. Add the tomato halves, lightly salt and swirl in the pan. Sprinkle with sugar, deglaze with white wine and melt the tomatoes over a medium heat for 2-3 minutes. Season with salt and pepper.

Drain the finished pasta, let it drain briefly and add to the melted tomatoes. Sprinkle in herbs and mozzarella, stir well. Take the corn chicken out of the oven and let it rest briefly, then cut it into beautiful slices. Meanwhile, wash the lime hot and rub vigorously dry.

To serve, spread the tomato noodles on plates, create the chicken slices and finely grate a lime peel.

DESSERTS COPYCAT RECIPES

ROSIN'S MEDITERRANEAN BURGER WITH ROASTED VEGETABLES COPYCAT RECIPE

Ingredients for 4 Serving

- 1 handful Cherry tomatoes
- 1 red pointed pepper
- ½ thick zucchini
- ½ thick eggplant
- 1 Fennel bulb
- 1 onion
- 1 Clove of garlic
- 600 g   mixed minced meat (beef and pork)
- 4 tbsp   Parmesan shavings
- 4 tbsp   roughly chopped basil leaves
- 2 pinches salt
- 2 pinches pepper from the grinder
- 2 balls   Mozzarella
- 4 tbsp   olive oil
- 200 g   sieved tomatos
- 2 tbsp   neutral oil
- 4th Burger buns
- 4 tbsp spicy mayonnaise

Preparation time: 30 minutes

Cooking time: 30 minutes

Total: 60 minutes

Wash and dry cherry tomatoes, peppers, zucchini, eggplant and fennel. Halve or quarter the cherry tomatoes depending on their size. Cut the peppers lengthways into narrow strips without using the stem. Cut the zucchini, aubergine and fennel lengthways in about 5 mm thin slices. Peel onion and garlic and chop finely.

Knead the minced meat thoroughly in a bowl with parmesan shavings and basil. Season the mixture with salt and pepper, then divide into 4 equal portions and form flat, round patties. Dab the mozzarella with kitchen paper and cut 6 slices each.

Heat 2 tablespoons of olive oil in a pan and sauté the onion and garlic cubes until translucent. Add the cherry tomatoes and sweat until they collapse. Pour on the strained tomatoes, season the sauce with salt and pepper and boil down for about 15 minutes like a jam. In the meantime, brush the vegetable slices with the remaining olive oil and fry them in a hot pan or on the grill.

Heat the neutral oil in a second pan and briefly fry the patties on both sides over high heat. Reduce the heat, cover the patties with 3 slices of mozzarella and let them cook for another 2-3 minutes until the cheese begins to melt.

During this time, briefly bake the buns in a hot oven at 200 ° C top / bottom heat or on the toaster.

Brush the bottom half of the burger buns with mayo and top with the fried vegetables. Put on 1 patty each, top with 1 dab of tomato jam and put on the top half of the bun.

ANDY'S BURGER: COPYCAT RECIPE CHEESEBURGER WITH MUSTARD-MAYO SAUCE

Ingredients for 4 Serving

FOR THE BURGERS

- large onion
- 2nd tomatoes
- 4 sheets Iceberg lettuce
- 2nd Pickles
- 600 g Ground beef
- 1 level tsp salt
- ½ tsp pepper from the grinder
- 6 slices Cheddar cheese
- 4 tbsp neutral oil
- 4th Burger buns
- 4 tsp brown butter (at will)

FOR THE SAUCE

- 4 tbsp mayonnaise
- 1 tsp Dijon mustard
- 1 tbsp Vinegar (from pickled gherkins)
- 1 tbsp Chive rolls
- 4 tbsp tomato ketchup
- 2 splashes Chili sauce (e.g. sriracha)

Preparation time: 30 minutes

Cooking time: 10 minutes

Total: 40 minutes

For the burgers, preheat the oven to 200 ° C top / bottom heat. Peel, halve and cut the onion into strips. Wash tomatoes and lettuce. Cut the tomatoes in slices without the stalks, the lettuce in strips. Slice the pickles lengthways.

Season the minced meat in a bowl with salt and pepper, knead thoroughly, divide into 4 equal portions and shape into flat patties. Cut the cheddar cheese into strips.

Heat 2 tablespoons of oil in a small pan and fry the onion strips in it slowly over a low heat until golden brown. Heat the rest of the oil in a second pan and briefly fry the patties on both sides in high heat.

Reduce the heat, cover the patties with the cheddar strips and let them soak for another 2-3 minutes until the cheese begins to melt.

In the meantime, cut the buns in half lengthways, lightly brush the interfaces with brown butter and roast on the tin in the hot oven for a few minutes until golden brown. For the sauces, stir the mayonnaise, mustard, vinegar and chive rolls in a small bowl. Mix the tomato ketchup and chili sauce in a second bowl.

Take the halves of the bread out of the oven. Brush the inside with 1 tablespoon of spicy mayo, the top half with the tomato-chilli sauce. Top each bottom with 1 patty, followed by cucumber and tomato slices, roasted onion and lettuce strips. Place the top of the bun on top and serve the burgers.

COPYCAT RECIPE VEGAN BURGER PATTIES

Ingredients for 4 Serving

- 100 g   carrot
- 100 g   celery root
- ½ bundle flat-leaf parsley
- medium onion
- Clove of garlic
- Organic lemon
- 50 g   dried tomato fillets (in oil)
- 240 g   Canned chickpeas (drained weight)
- 150 g   canned white beans
- 100 g   Kidney beans (drained weight)
- 2 tbsp   olive oil
- 2 tsp   Tahina (oriental. Sesame paste)
- ½ tsp   Garam Masala
- 2 Msp.   Cinnamon powder
- 1 level tsp salt
- ½ tsp   pepper from the grinder
- 4 tsp   Wheat flour (at will)
- 2 tbsp   neutral oil

Preparation time: 30 minutes

Cooking time: 15 minutes

Total: 45 minutes

Peel the carrot and celery and grate medium-fine. Wash the parsley, shake dry and chop finely with the stems. Peel the onion and garlic and cut into fine cubes. Wash the lemon hot, rub vigorously dry and finely grate the peel. Drain the tomato fillets thoroughly on kitchen paper. Drain the chickpeas and white beans in a sieve and transfer to a bowl. Now drain the kidney beans and chop them roughly with the tomato fillets. Heat the olive oil in a pan and sauté the onion and garlic cubes until translucent. Add chopped tomatoes and kidney beans and sweat for 3-4 minutes. In the meantime, puree the chickpeas and white beans in the bowl with the hand blender. Pull the pan off the heat and let the onion and bean mixture cool slightly.

Add the grated carrots and celery, parsley, lemon zest, tahina, garam masala, cinnamon, salt, pepper and the onion-bean mixture from the pan to the chickpea and bean puree in the bowl. Knead everything thoroughly into a handy, not too moist mass. Season again with salt and pepper. Divide the mass into 4 large or 6 smaller portions with slightly damp hands and shape into patties. Heat the neutral oil in a pan, dust the patties lightly with flour as desired and fry in hot fat on both sides until golden brown. Assemble the patties as you like with buns and other components into burgers.

COPYCAT RECIPE Big Mac sauce

Ingredients for 4 Serving

- ¼ Onion
- ½ Garlic cloves
- 125 ml   mayonnaise
- 4 tsp Relish
- 1 splash White wine vinegar
- ½ tsp Paprika powder
- ½ tsp   Ketchup
- 1 tbsp   mustard
- 3 pinches pepper
- 2 pinches salt

Preparation

Working time about 10 minutes

Total time about 10 minutes

Cut the onion and the garlic into fine cubes and mix together with the remaining ingredients to a homogeneous mass.

Season with salt and pepper. The sauce tastes great with classic burgers, but as a dip with grilled meat.

Goat cheese with dried tomatoes and walnuts on toast COPYCAT RECIPE

Ingredients for 1 Serving

- 2 disc / s Toasted bread (whole grain)
- 2nd Tomato (s), dried, pickled in oil
- 4th Walnuts, halves
- 3 tsp Goat cream cheese

Preparation

Working time about 10 minutes

Total time about 10 minutes

Toast the whole grain toast in the toaster. Roughly chop the walnuts and lightly roast them in a small pan without oil. Chop the tomatoes.

Spread the goat cheese on a toast and spread the tomatoes and walnuts on top. Place the second slice of toast on top and eat warm.

COPYCAT RECIPE Fried calamari

Ingredients for 4 Serving

- 1 kg   Squid tube (s)
- Lemon juice
- salt
- 2nd   Egg (er)
- 300 ml milk
- 2 tbsp dill

- ✓ Flour
- ✓ Oil or fat, for deep-frying

Preparation

Working time about 15 minutes

Cooking / baking time approx. 10 minutes

Total time about 25 minutes

Wash the squid tubes and pat them dry. Cut the calamari into thick rings. Drizzle with lemon juice, lightly salt and season with the dill.

Let oil or fat get hot (deep fryer or saucepan).

Mix eggs and milk. Prepare the egg milk mixture and the flour in separate bowls. Now briefly pull the calamari through the egg-milk mixture and then flour. Bake in hot fat and drain on kitchen paper.

We prefer to eat paprika rice, tzatziki and coleslaw. Of course, fresh lemon should not be missing.

Basic recipe for dark Asia sauce COPYCAT RECIPE

Ingredients for 4 Serving

- 250 ml   Vegetable broth
- 2 tbsp   Soy sauce, dark
- 1 tbsp   Soy sauce, light
- 1 teaspoon sugar
- chili
- pepper
- 2 tbsp   Sauce binders
- Oyster sauce

Preparation

Working time about 2 minutes

Cooking / baking time approx. 3 minutes

Total time about 5 minutes

Mix all the ingredients in the saucepan and let simmer until the sauce thickens. Season with oyster sauce.

Then process the sauce with the desired wok content (vegetables, chicken, etc.) according to your taste.

COLORFUL SALAD WITH SHRIMPS COPYCAT RECIPE

Ingredients for 4 Serving

FOR THE SALAD

- Romana salad heart
- Bunch of arugula
- 250 g   Cherry tomatoes
- 2nd red or orange pointed peppers
- Fennel bulb
- mild chili pepper
- Bunch of basil
- ½ bunch of chives
- 3 tbsp   olive oil
- 1-2 tablespoons white balsamic vinegar
- 20th King prawns (without head and shell; gutted)
- 3rd Shallots
- asian garlic
- 3 tbsp   olive oil
- 60 g Pine nuts
- Dash of white wine
- 4 tbsp   chunky tomatoes (canned)
- pinch of sugar
- pinch of salt
- Pinch pepper from the mill
- 100 g   Parmesan shavings

Preparation time: 30 minutes

Cooking time: 5 minutes

Total: 35 minutes

Remove the outer withered leaves from the lettuce. Cut or pluck the remaining leaves into bite-size pieces. Read the arugula and remove long stems. Wash the leaves with the Romaine lettuce and spin dry. Wash tomatoes, peppers, fennel and chilli. Halve the tomatoes. Halve the bell pepper and chilli lengthways and remove the stones. Cut the paprika halves into thin strips and the chilli halves into fine cubes. Wash the fennel, cut out the stalk and cut the tuber diagonally into thin slices. Wash the basil and shake dry. Pluck the leaves into pieces. Wash the chives, shake dry and cut into rolls.

Wash the shrimp under running cold water and pat dry with kitchen paper. Peel the shallots and garlic and cut into fine cubes. Heat 2 tablespoons of olive oil in a pan and fry the pine nuts in it until medium brown. Transfer to a bowl.

Heat another 1 tablespoon of olive oil in the pan and fry the prawns briefly and spicy with the shallots over high heat. Add the garlic and fry briefly. Deglaze with the white wine and let the liquid boil almost completely. Stir in the chunky tomatoes with half of the basil and pine nuts and briefly swirl everything in the pan again.

Mix Romaine lettuce, arugula, tomatoes, bell pepper, fennel, chilli and the rest of the basil in a bowl. Season the salad with white balsamic vinegar and olive oil, season with sugar, salt and pepper.

Spread the lettuce on plates, arrange the shrimp with the remaining basil, sprinkle with chives and serve garnished with parmesan shavings.

Spicy cucumber pieces à la Hong Kong COPYCAT RECIPE

Ingredients for 12 Serving

- 2nd Cucumber
- 1 m Carrot (s)
- 1 small Chili pepper (s), red
- 2 tbsp Vinegar essence, 25%
- 2 tbsp Vinegar, darker, milder, Chinese, alternatively balsamic vinegar
- 1 tbsp Lime juice
- 10 tbsp water
- 5 tbsp Sugar, whiter
- 10 g salt
- 1 tbsp Glutamate
- n.B. salt
- n.B. sugar
- n.B. Vinegar, 5%
- n.B. Lime juice

Preparation

Working time about 15 minutes

Total time about 4 hours 15 minutes

Wash the cucumbers, cut both ends, peel, halve lengthways and remove the seeds. Halve the halves lengthways again. Cut diagonally into approx. 5 mm thick slices. Wash the carrot, cut both ends, peel and cut into thin sticks.

Wash the chilli and cut it into fine rings. Place in a larger bowl with the remaining ingredients, mix well and season to taste. Let it steep for at least 3 to 4 hours, mixing occasionally. Season again with salt, sugar, vinegar and lime juice.

Do not remove the vinegar-salt water. Keeps in the fridge for about a week.

LUDENSCHEIDER LITTLE CRUST À LA FRANK ROSIN

Ingredients for 4 Serving

FOR THE MEAT

- ✓ 800 g Beef fillet
- ✓ 2nd red pointed peppers
- ✓ 250 g brown mushrooms
- ✓ 2nd Shallots and red onions
- ✓ 2nd Stalks of flat-leaf parsley
- ✓ 3rd Stems of coriander green
- ✓ 3rd Sprigs of thyme
- ✓ 3rd Sprigs of rosemary
- ✓ 4 tbsp   olive oil
- ✓ pinch of salt
- ✓ Pinch pepper from the mill
- ✓ 100 ml   White wine
- ✓ 4th Slices of Gruyère (Gruyère cheese)
- ✓ 2 tbsp   butter
- ✓ 4th Slices of white bread
- ✓ 4 tbsp   Chives rolls for sprinkling

FOR THE SAUCE HOLLANDAISE

- ✓ 200 g   butter
- ✓ 4th egg yolk
- ✓ 100 ml   White wine
- ✓ pinch of sugar
- ✓ pinch of salt
- ✓ Pinch pepper from the mill
- ✓ ½ Organic lemon zest and juice

Preparation time: 45 minutes

Cooking time: 20 minutes

Total: 65 minutes

Preheat the oven to 100 ° C top / bottom heat. Remove fat and tendons from the fillet of beef, then cut into 4 equal portions. Wash the peppers, halve lengthways, core and cut into cubes. Clean the mushrooms, rub dry with kitchen paper if necessary and quarter or eighth depending on the size. Peel the shallots and cut them into fine cubes. Wash the herbs and shake them dry.

Heat 2 tablespoons of olive oil in a pan and briefly sear the meat all around. Heat the remaining olive oil in a second pan and fry the vegetables in it as well. Season the meat and vegetables with salt and pepper, then deglaze with half of the white wine. Add the parsley, coriander, thyme and rosemary to the broth. Boil down the liquid almost completely.

Cover the meat with the vegetables, top with 1 Gruyère slice each and cook in a hot oven on the oven rack, depending on the thickness, for 10–15 minutes to a core temperature of 58–60 ° C (for medium-cooked meat, measure with the meat thermometer) until pink to let.

In the meantime, heat the remaining olive oil in the meat pan and fry the prepared vegetables in it over medium heat until soft but still firm.

For the sauce, heat the butter in a saucepan and simmer over medium-high heat until it starts to smell slightly brown and nutty. Line a fine sieve with kitchen paper and pour the butter through to clarify and keep warm in a second saucepan.

Put on a water bath. To do this, heat sufficient water to 70-80 ° C in a large saucepan. Whisk egg yolks, white wine and 1 tablespoon of water in a metal bowl over the hot water bath with the whisk of the hand mixer. Season with sugar, salt and pepper. Allow the clarified butter to run in in a fine stream, stirring constantly until the sauce becomes light and creamy. Season with 1 pinch of lemon peel and 1 dash of lemon juice.

Heat the remaining olive oil with the butter in a pan and fry the bread slices in it over medium heat until golden and crispy. Season with salt.

Spread the bread slices on plates. Place the baked meat and vegetables on top and serve drizzled with hollandaise sauce.

INSALATA Á LA SALVA WITH ROASTED VEGETABLES AND PARMESAN

Ingredients for 4 Serving

- 200 g brown mushrooms
- 200 g Cocktail tomatoes
- aubergine
- 2nd small red pointed peppers
- small clove of garlic
- 7 tbsp olive oil
- 2 pinches sugar
- 3 pinches salt
- 3 pinches pepper from the grinder
- 200 ml White wine
- 4 tbsp Tomato Sugo
- 3 stems basil
- 2nd Romana lettuce hearts
- 1 bunch arugula
- 1 bunch mixed herbs (e.g. parsley, chives, chervil)
- 2 tbsp white balsamic vinegar
- 1 pinch sugar
- 1 handful green olives (without stone)
- 1 glass Artichoke hearts (310 g), drained
- 125 g Mini mozzarella balls, drained
- 1 handful roughly shaved parmesan shavings

Preparation time: 45 minutes

Cooking time: 15 minutes

Total: 60 minutes

Clean the mushrooms, rub dry with kitchen paper if necessary and cut into quarters. Wash and dry the cocktail tomatoes, eggplant and pointed peppers. Halve the tomatoes, roughly dice the eggplant and cut the pointed peppers into rings, core them if necessary. Peel the garlic and chop in to fine slithers.

Heat 2 tablespoons of olive oil in a pan and sauté the mushrooms in it over high heat. Add the garlic over a slightly reduced heat and fry briefly. Season the mushrooms with 1 pinch of sugar, salt and pepper. Deglaze with half of the white wine and let the liquid boil. Add the halved cocktail tomatoes and swirl in the pan. Pull the pan off the stove.

Heat 2 tablespoons of olive oil in a second pan and fry the eggplant cubes in it over high heat. Season with 1 pinch of salt and pepper. Deglaze with the rest of the white wine, add the tomato sauce. Pluck the basil leaves from the stems, wash, dry and pluck into the eggplants. Also pull the pan off the stove.

Cut the Romana lettuce hearts and stalk into strips, wash and spin dry. Read the rocket, wash with the herbs, shake dry and cut roughly. Whisk the remaining olive oil in a large bowl with the balsamic vinegar. Season with 1 pinch of sugar, salt and pepper. Add Romaine lettuce, rocket and herbs and mix with the vinaigrette. Add pointed pepper rings, olives and artichoke hearts and mix thoroughly again.

Spread the salad on deep plates, arrange the mozzarella balls, fried aubergine cubes and mushroom and tomato mixture on it and serve the Insalata Salva sprinkled with parmesan shavings

Potato salad with tomatoes and arugula

Ingredients for 4 Serving

- ✓ 1 kg — Potato (s), small (triplets)
- ✓ ½ kg — Beef tomato (s)
- ✓ 125 g — arugula
- ✓ 100 ml — White wine vinegar
- ✓ 150 ml — olive oil
- ✓ Salt and pepper from the mill

Preparation

Working time about 30 minutes

Total time about 30 minutes

Cook the triplets as jacket potatoes. In the meantime, scald, peel and core the beef tomatoes and cut the flesh into pieces the size of a thumbnail. Wash and read the arugula, remove thick stalks.

Make a salad dressing out of vinegar, oil, pepper and salt, using salt and pepper generously.

Peel the cooked potatoes and cut them hot into thumbnail-sized pieces. Mix with the tomatoes and rocket. Pour the salad dressing over the mixture and serve the salad immediately.

We had this salad in Croatia with steaks with green pepper sauce, but it also tastes great with fish and grilled meat.

The tastiest, simplest and yet freshest pizza in the world

Ingredients for 2 Serving

- ✓ 300 g   Flour
- ✓ salt
- ✓ 6 tbsp   olive oil
- ✓ 1 pack   Dry yeast
- ✓ 1 kg Tomato (s), ripe

For the sauce:

- ✓ Onion (onion)
- ✓ 1 large   Garlic cloves)
- ✓ 2 pack   Mozzarella
- ✓ Pepper, freshly ground black
- ✓ 3 tbsp   Oregano, (dried)
- ✓ Oil, for the baking sheet

Preparation

Working time about 30 minutes

Total time about 1 hour 30 minutes

First stir in the flour, approx. 2 teaspoons of salt and the olive oil in a bowl with a dough hook.

Now dissolve the dry yeast in 1/8 l of lukewarm water with stirring, add to the flour and knead until a smooth dough is formed.

Leave it covered for about 45 minutes.

For the sauce:

Pour boiling water over the tomatoes and let them soak. Then put in a colander and quench with cold water. This way they can be easily peeled.

These are then cut into small pieces (remove the stalk).

Now heat 2 tablespoons of oil in a small saucepan and braise the onion and garlic until translucent. Add the small tomatoes and simmer for about 1/2 hour. Then season with pepper and salt and, if necessary, puree if the sauce is too coarse.

After the 45 minutes have passed, knead the dough vigorously again by hand and divide it in half. Then roll them out in suitable pizza trays to a diameter of approx. 32 cm and spread the pizza sauce on them.

For a pizza margerita,

Simply slice the mozzarella, place on top, sprinkle with a little oregano and bake in the oven at 170 ° for about 15 minutes.

If you want a pizza salami, just add the salami.

Note: In the case of smaller forms, the ingredients would also be sufficient for 4 servings, but the ingredients for the sauce must be doubled.

COPYCAT RECIPE Rasnici

Ingredients for 2 Serving

- ✓ 6 thin   Pork steak (s), from the salmon piece, without fat edge
- ✓ 500 ml   Vegetable oil
- ✓ Paprika powder
- ✓ Curry powder
- ✓ salt and pepper
- ✓ Herbs, Italian, dried
- ✓ Onion (s), also red

Preparation

Working time about 10 minutes

Total time about 1 day 10 minutes

Sprinkle the pork steaks vigorously with the spices and massage in or press firmly. Place the seasoned meat slices in a sealable container in the oil and leave in the fridge overnight.

The next day, heat a coated pan, let the meat slices drip off briefly and fry briefly on both sides.

Garnish with fresh onion rings.

This goes very well with fried potatoes or French fries and a curry mayonnaise or rasnici sauce. Mix the mayonnaise, crème fraîche, yoghurt, salt, pepper and curry powder and let it steep for a day.

COPYCAT RECIPE Macaroni with crab
Ingredients for 2 Serving

- 250 g   Macaroni (Bucatini)
- 10th   Cherry tomato (s)
- Chili pepper (s)
- 150 g   Crab
- 3rd Garlic cloves)
- ½ Onion (onion)
- n.B. olive oil
- 50 g arugula
- 12 Basil leaves
- Lemons
- salt

Preparation

Working time about 10 minutes

Cooking / baking time approx. 10 minutes

Total time about 20 minutes

Cook the pasta in salted water according to the package instructions.

Dice the onion. Halve the cherry tomatoes. Cut the garlic into small, fine slices. Finely chop the chili pepper. Roughly cut the basil leaves.

Heat plenty of olive oil in the pan, not too hot! Lightly fry the onions, garlic and the chilli pepper. 2 min. Before the noodles are cooked, add the crabs to the pan. Thaw frozen crabs beforehand or fry them right at the start.

Fold in a little (approx. 10 g) arugula and the basil and season with a dash of lemon juice and a pinch of salt.

Mix the rest of the rocket (40 g) with lemon juice, olive oil and salt in a small bowl and mix briefly.

Put the pasta on the plates and serve with rocket salad as a crown.

Shiitake mushrooms for sushi COPYCAT RECIPE

Ingredients for 2 Serving

- ✓ 10th Shiitake mushroom (s), dried
- ✓ 2 tbsp   soy sauce
- ✓ 2 tbsp. sugar
- ✓ 2 Tea spoons   Mirin

Preparation

Working time about 5 minutes

Cooking / baking time approx. 10 minutes

Total time about 30 minutes

The shiitake mushrooms are ideal for vegetarian sushi, e.g. shiitake cream cheese maki.

Cover the dried shiitake mushrooms with boiling water and soak for 15 minutes. Alternatively, you can also take cold water and soak it for an hour (this will make the mushroom aroma even more intense).

Drain the mushrooms and collect the soaking water. If necessary, remove the hard stem ends. If the mushrooms are used for sushi, it is advisable to cut them into strips at this point.

Cover the mushrooms in a saucepan with the soaking water and bring to a boil, then reduce the heat and simmer for 2 minutes. Add the sugar and soy sauce and simmer, stirring occasionally, until the liquid has completely evaporated.

Finally add the mirin and stir. The last step is not absolutely necessary, but the mirin gives the mushrooms the finishing touch.

Carpaccio with a cocktail sauce COPYCAT RECIPE

Ingredients for 4 Serving

- 500 g   Beef fillet (s), thinly sliced
- 1 big   Bread (caviar bread)
- 3 pack   Grissini
- For the sauce:
- 125 ml   Salad Cream (Miracel Whip)
- 2 tbsp   Ketchup
- 1 teaspoon   Worcester sauce
- 1 tbsp   Mustard medium hot
- 1 small Glass   Cognac, alternatively good brandy
- 1 tbsp   Paprika powder, spicy
- 1 tbsp   Chili sauce

Preparation

Working time about 5 minutes

Total time about 5 minutes

Arrange the fillet slices decoratively on four plates.

Mix the ingredients for the sauce well with a blender and spread the sauce evenly over the meat.

I also serve caviar bread or breadsticks.

PIZZA WITH ARTICHOKES AND OLIVES

Ingredients for 4 Serving

FOR THE DOUGH

- ✓ 500 g Pizza flour, plus a little more for the work surface
- ✓ 2 tsp   salt
- ✓ ⅛ dice   fresh yeast (approx. 2.5 g)
- ✓ 1 tbsp   olive oil
- ✓ FOR THE SUGO
- ✓ 500 g   sieved tomatos
- ✓ 2 tbsp   olive oil
- ✓ 1 pinch sugar
- ✓ 1 tsp salt
- ✓ ½ tsp pepper from the grinder
- ✓ 1 handful Basil leaves

FOR COVERING

- ✓ 250 g   Mini mozzarella balls, drained
- ✓ 1 glass   Artichoke hearts (310 g), drained
- ✓ 1 handful green olives (without stone)
- ✓ ½ bundle arugula
- ✓ 2 tbsp   olive oil
- ✓ 1 Pizza stone (optional)

Preparation time: 180 minutes

Cooking time: 15 minutes

Total: 195 minutes

    Mix half of the flour and salt in a bowl for the dough. Crumble in the yeast, add 300 ml of lukewarm water and use the whisk of a hand mixer or food processor to make the liquid dough. Cover the bowl with a kitchen towel and let the dough rest for 30 minutes.

    Mix the remaining flour with the dough hook or hands under the dough and continue to knead vigorously for 3 minutes. Shape the dough into a ball or roll and divide into four equal pieces. Leave each piece in a bowl with cling film tightly closed in a warm place for another 2 hours.

    In the meantime, stir the tomatoes in a bowl with the olive oil for the sugo and season with sugar, salt and pepper. Wash the basil leaves, dry thoroughly, pluck into small pieces and fold under the sugo. Preheat the oven and baking sheet to 220 ° C in a fan oven. When using a pizza stone, preheat the stone according to the instructions for use.

    Roll out the dough pieces on the floured work surface into millimeter-thin pies, turning over and over again. Place the dough on baking paper, brush with tomato sauce, top with mozzarella balls, artichoke hearts and olives. Place the pizza with the baking paper on the hot pizza stone or hot plate and bake in the oven until crispy for 12–15 minutes. Bake the pizzas simultaneously or one after the other, depending on the size of the oven.

    During this time, read out the arugula, wash, shake dry and roughly cut or pluck. Take the finished pizza out of the oven, sprinkle with arugula and serve drizzled with a little olive oil.

    Tip:

    The dough is prepared with Italian flour. Alternatively, you can also use Type 405 wheat flour. You can also prepare the dough the day before and extend the second walking time accordingly. In this case, keep the portioned dough in the refrigerator.

MIDIA (MUSSELS) À LA FRANK

Ingredients for 4 Serving

- ✓ 2 kg fresh mussels (e.g. mussels)
- ✓ 2nd Romana lettuce hearts
- ✓ ½ red pointed pepper
- ✓ ½ yellow pointed pepper
- ✓ 200 g Cherry tomatoes
- ✓ ½ Bunch of dill
- ✓ 2nd Shallots
- ✓ 2nd Garlic cloves
- ✓ 4 tbsp   olive oil
- ✓ 2 pinches sugar
- ✓ 400 g   chunky tomatoes (canned)
- ✓ 2nd Shot of Greek anise schnapps (e.g. ouzo)
- ✓ 1 pinch salt
- ✓ 1 pinch pepper from the grinder

Preparation time: 45 minutes

Total: 45 minutes

Water the mussels to remove the sand, then clean and sort out any specimens that are already open. Remove the outside leaves of the Romaine lettuce. Wash the heads whole and dry them carefully. Wash, core and cut the peppers into cubes. Wash the cherry tomatoes and halve lengthways. Wash the dill, shake dry and chop finely. Peel the onion and garlic and cut into fine cubes.

Heat 2 tablespoons of olive oil in a pan and sauté the onion cubes until golden brown over medium to high heat. Add half of the garlic with the tomato halves and fry briefly. Sprinkle in a pinch of sugar and lightly caramelize.

Add the pepper cubes and fry briefly. Add chopped tomatoes, bring to the boil, then season with salt and pepper. Mix in the mussels and bring to the boil again. Deglaze with 1 shot of ouzo and add the dill. Taste again.

Heat the rest of the olive oil in a second pan and stir in the remaining garlic. Halve the lettuce hearts lengthways and fry on the cut side. Deglaze with ouzo and let the liquid boil almost completely.

Arrange the Romaine lettuce on a plate and drizzle with olive oil and garlic from the pan. Season with salt and pepper and arrange the mussels.

STUFFED PEPPERS AND TOMATOES COPYCAT RECIPE

Ingredients for 8 Serving

- ✓ 4th Beef tomatoes
- ✓ 4th green peppers
- ✓ 4th Stem oregano
- ✓ 4th Stalks of parsley
- ✓ ½ Bunch of dill
- ✓ onion
- ✓ 5 tbsp   Olive oil plus more to taste
- ✓ pinch of sugar
- ✓ pinch of salt
- ✓ 500 g   mixed minced meat (beef and pork)
- ✓ 200 g   rice pudding
- ✓ 400 g   chunky tomatoes (canned)
- ✓ 1 pinch pepper from the grinder

Preparation time: 35 minutes

Cooking time: 60 minutes

Total: 95 minutes

Preheat the oven to 200 ° C top / bottom heat. Wash and dry the tomatoes and peppers. Cut the lid off the tomatoes and peppers and hollow out the vegetables. Chop the removed pulp of the tomatoes and set aside for filling.

Wash oregano, parsley and dill and shake dry. Pluck the leaves of mint and parsley and chop them finely. Finely cut the dill tips. Peel the onion and cut it into fine cubes. Heat 2 tablespoons of olive oil in a pan and sauté the onion cubes until golden brown over medium heat. Sprinkle with 1 pinch of sugar and salt and lightly caramelize the sugar. Add the minced meat and fry vigorously at a slightly higher temperature. Wash the milk rice, fold it into the onion and minced meat mixture and fry briefly. Mix in the pulp of the tomatoes and the canned tomatoes. Season with a dash of olive oil, salt and pepper. Fold in the herbs and bring to the boil again briefly.

Pour the minced meat and rice mixture into peppers and tomatoes. Put the lids on, put the vegetables in a baking dish and drizzle with the remaining olive oil. Cook the stuffed vegetables in the hot oven on a medium rack for 45 minutes until the rice is tender.

Serve the filled peppers and tomatoes in the tin. Go with rice or baguette.

LANGOS COPYCAT RECIPE

Ingredients for 4 Serving

- 10 g fresh yeast (1/4 cube)
- 250 g   Wheat flour type 550
- 1 pinch sugar
- 1 kg Deep frying fat or 500 ml of neutral oil (e.g. sunflower oil) for baking
- 150 g   Cocktail tomatoes
- Clove of garlic
- 1 bunch chives
- 200 g   sour cream
- 1 pinch salt
- 1 pinch pepper from the grinder
- 200 g   grated cheese (e.g. gratin cheese)

Preparation time: 40 minutes

Total: 40 minutes

For the dough, put 150 ml of lukewarm water in a bowl, crumble in the yeast and dissolve in it. Mix in half the flour and sugar. Cover the bowl with a clean kitchen towel and let the batter rise for 15 minutes.

Add the remaining flour and salt. Knead the dough with the kneading hooks of the hand mixer for about 5 minutes. Cover the bowl again with a cloth and let the dough rise for 1 hour until it has visibly increased in volume.

In the meantime, wash the cocktail tomatoes for the topping and halve or quarter them, depending on the size. Peel the garlic and press through the press. Wash the chives, shake dry and cut into rolls. Mix the sour cream until creamy. Season with salt and pepper.

Heat the frying fat in a high-walled saucepan to 160 ° C. The fat is at the right temperature when bubbles rise up on a wooden spoon or wooden skewer. Divide the dough into 4 equal pieces and roll each out to 15 cm in diameter. Carefully slide a dough into the fat and bake for about 4 minutes, turning over and over again.

Lift out the finished làngos and let them drain briefly on kitchen paper, then brush a quarter of the sour cream and the pressed garlic, top with tomatoes, sprinkle with cheese and garnish with chive rolls. Do the same with the rest of the dough.

COUNTRY POTATO SALAD WITH DRESSED SAUERLAND SAUSAGE

Ingredients for 4 Serving

- 750 g   stuck potatoes
- 2nd Pinch of salt
- Roll brawn
- 2nd red pointed peppers
- 2nd Red onions
- white onion
- asian garlic
- Bunch of flat-leaf parsley
- 4 tbsp   Rapeseed oil
- 4 tbsp   white balsamic
- Pinch pepper from the mill
- 15 radish
- 10th Gherkins
- 4 tbsp olive oil
- 50 ml   beef broth
- 2 tsp medium hot mustard
- Shot of pickle water
- pinch of sugar

Preparation time: 35 minutes

Cooking time: 20 minutes

Total: 55 minutes

Wash the potatoes and cook gently in a bowl in salted water for about 20 minutes. In the meantime, cut the brawn into bite-size cubes. Wash the peppers, halve lengthways, remove the seeds and cut into cubes without using the stem. Peel onions and garlic and dice finely.

Mix the brawn, bell pepper, half of the red onions, garlic and parsley in a large bowl. Marinate the salad with 1 tablespoon of rapeseed oil and 1 tablespoon of vinegar, season with salt and pepper. Set aside and let go.

Wash the fennel, cut out the stalk and cut the tuber diagonally into thin slices. Clean and wash the radishes, cut them in half without stalks and roots and cut the halves into thin slices. Drain and throw the gherkins.

Drain the potatoes and let them steam briefly, then peel them hot. Cut the slightly cooled potatoes into cubes. Whisk remaining rapeseed oil, olive oil and other vinegar with the beef broth and mustard.

Mix potatoes, remaining onions, fennel, radishes and gherkins and marinate with the dressing. Season the salad with cucumber water, sugar, salt and pepper.

To serve, pour some potato salad into small glasses, then spread 1-2 tablespoons of brawn on top.

SPAGHETTI BOLOGNESE COPYCAT RECIPE

Ingredients for 4 Serving

- ✓ carrot
- ✓ 100 g elery
- ✓ Pointed peppers
- ✓ onion
- ✓ Clove of garlic
- ✓ 4 tbsp   olive oil
- ✓ 2 pinches salt
- ✓ 1 pinch freshly ground pepper
- ✓ 1 pinch Chilli flakes
- ✓ 300 ml Red wine to wipe off
- ✓ 400 g   mixed minced meat
- ✓ 1 tbsp   Tomato paste
- ✓ 400 g   sieved tomatos
- ✓ 1 tbsp   dried oregano
- ✓ 500 g   spaghetti
- ✓ 4 tbsp   fresh parmesan shavings to serve
- ✓ 4th Stems of basil for garnish

Preparation time: 20 minutes

Cooking time: 30 minutes

Total: 50 minutes

Peel the carrot and celery. Wash, halve and core the peppers. Cut the vegetables into small cubes. Peel the onion and the garlic and also finely dice.

Heat 2 tablespoons of olive oil in a pan and fry the carrot, celery, bell pepper, onion and garlic in it over medium heat for about 4 minutes. Season with 1 pinch of salt, pepper and chilli. Deglaze with half of the red wine and use it to loosen the roast set.

Heat the remaining oil in a saucepan and fry the minced meat in it over high heat. Stir in the tomato paste and fry briefly. Add the pan vegetables, pour in the remaining red wine and the tomatoes, sprinkle the oregano and cook the sauce over medium heat for about 20 minutes.

In the meantime, cook the spaghetti bite-proof in plenty of boiling salted water according to the package instructions. Drain the pasta and drain. Season the Bolognese sauce again with salt and pepper.

Spread the spaghetti on deep plates, pour the Bolognese sauce on top, sprinkle with Parmesan and serve garnished with basil.

POTATO SALAD WITH MEATBALLS COPYCAT RECIPE

Ingredients for 4 Serving

FOR THE SALAD:

- 1 kg stuck potatoes
- 2½ tsp   salt
- 3rd Eggs
- 2nd Carrots
- 150 g   Peas
- 2 -3 EL   mayonnaise
- 1 tbsp   mustard
- 2nd medium sized pickles
- 1 prs.   salt
- 1 prs   pepper from the grinder
- 4th Stalks of parsley
- 8th Cherry tomatoes

FOR THE MEATBALLS:

- Bread from the previous day
- 200 ml   milk
- 600 g mixed minced meat (pork and beef)
- egg
- 1 tbsp Dijon mustard
- 1 prs. salt
- 1 prs. pepper from the grinder
- 4 tbsp   Sunflower oil

Preparation time: 45 minutes

Cooking time: 30 minutes

Total: 75 minutes

For the salad, wash the potatoes thoroughly and cover them with water in a saucepan. Season the water with 2 teaspoons of salt, bring to the boil and cook the potatoes gently in the medium heat for 20–25 minutes. Meanwhile, cook the eggs hard. Peel the carrots and cut them into fine slices. Blanch peas and carrots in boiling water for 4–5 minutes, frozen and thawed peas take less time. Drain the vegetables, quench in ice water and drain. Quench the eggs with cold water and let them cool.

For the meatballs, pour the milk in a small bowl and soak in it. Squeeze the soft roll well, pluck into small pieces and knead in a large bowl with minced meat, egg, mustard and 1 strong pinch of salt and pepper.

Drain the finished potatoes, let them evaporate briefly, peel while hot and cut into slices. Peel the eggs and cut them into slices with the cucumber. In a bowl, carefully mix the potatoes, eggs, cucumber, peas and carrots with the mayonnaise and mustard. Season with salt and pepper. Set aside and let go.

Form meatballs from the minced meat mixture. Heat the oil in a pan and fry the meatballs in it over high heat until it is golden brown and crispy. Season the salad again. Wash the parsley, shake dry and pluck the leaves. Wash and halve or quarter the cherry tomatoes.

Arrange potato salad and meatballs on plates and serve garnished with parsley and tomatoes.

COD IN MUSTARD SAUCE WITH POTATO HASH BROWNS

Ingredients for 4 Serving

- 800 g floury potatoes
- onion
- 2 prs salt
- bunch of chives
- egg yolk
- 1 prs pepper from the grinder

For fish and sauce

- 600 g   Cod fillet
- 2 prs   salt
- 2 tbsp   Sunflower oil
- lemon
- 2 prs pepper from the grinder
- onion
- 3 tbsp   butter
- 100 ml   White wine
- 250 ml   vegetable stock
- 100 g   cream
- Bay leaf
- Dijon mustard
- Bunch of mixed herbs (e.g. flat-leaf parsley, basil, dill)
- 4th Cherry tomatoes

Preparation time: 45 minutes

Cooking time: 15 minutes

Total: 60 minutes

For the Rösti peel the potatoes and onions, grate them coarsely, lightly season with a pinch of salt and let them rest for 10 minutes. In the meantime, wash the chives, shake them dry and cut them into rolls. Drain the liquid that has settled from the potatoes, gently squeezing out the mixture. Mix the potatoes in a bowl with the egg yolk, the chive rolls and 1 pinch of salt and pepper.

Preheat the oven to 100 ° C for the fish. Rinse the cod under running cold water and pat dry with kitchen paper. Check the fillet for bones and pull the existing one. Season with a pinch of salt. Heat the oil in an ovenproof pan and fry the fish in it over high heat, drizzling with 1 dash of lemon juice. Season the fillets with a pinch of pepper and finish cooking in the hot oven for about 10 minutes.

In the meantime, heat a little oil for the Rösti in 2 large pans, add small portions of potato mass with a tablespoon, press flat with the back of the spoon and fry on both sides until golden and crispy on medium to high heat. Add more oil to the pan if necessary. Drain the finished hash browns on kitchen paper and keep warm in the oven.

Peel the onion for the sauce and cut into fine cubes. Heat 1 tablespoon of butter in a pan and sauté the onion cubes until translucent. Deglaze with the white wine and reduce the liquid to half the amount. Pour in the vegetable stock and cream, add the bay leaf and 1 dash of lemon juice and reduce the liquid again a little. Stir in the remaining butter and mustard and remove the bay leaf. Mix the sauce with the hand blender, then season again with salt and pepper. Keep warm. Wash the herbs, shake dry, pluck the leaves from the stems and cut roughly. Wash and quarter the cherry tomatoes.

Spread the potato rösti on plates, place the fish, drizzle with sauce, top with the herbs and serve garnished with the tomato quarters.

PASTA WITH SHRIMPS AND HOMEMADE CRUSTACEAN STOCK

Ingredients for 4 Serving

- 20th medium-sized shrimp (with head and shell)
- 200 g Cherry tomatoes
- Bunch of spring onions
- red chili pepper
- 2nd Sprigs of rosemary
- 2nd Sprigs of thyme
- 3rd Garlic cloves
- 4 tbsp   olive oil
- 2 prs salt
- 2 prs pepper from the grinder
- 2 cl Brandy
- 100 ml   White wine
- 400 ml   Vegetable broth
- 700 -800 g fresh ribbon pasta
- Tin of white beans (400 g; drained)
- 100 g   Parmesan shavings
- small can of tomato paste (70 g)
- Handful of basil leaves

Preparation time: 20 minutes

Cooking time: 20 minutes

Total: 40 minutes

Twist off the heads of the shrimp, remove the shells and set aside. Carve the prawns along the back, gut, wash and dry. Wash cherry tomatoes, spring onions and chilli pepper. Halve or quarter the tomatoes depending on their size. Cut the spring onions into rings without root. Cut the chilli into cubes with or without seeds. Wash the rosemary and thyme and shake dry. Peel and slice the garlic.

For the sauce mix, heat 2 tablespoons of olive oil in a pan and fry the shrimp shells with half of the garlic. Add rosemary and thyme, season with 1 pinch of salt and pepper. Add half of the spring onions and sweat briefly. Deglaze first with the brandy, then with the white wine. Reduce the liquid to half the amount. Pour in the vegetable broth and simmer over medium heat.

Cook the pasta bite-proof in boiling salted water according to the package instructions. In the meantime, heat the remaining oil in a second pan. Fry the prawns and remaining garlic in it over medium to high heat. Add tomatoes, chilli and other spring onions. Season with 1 pinch of salt and pepper.

Add the beans and pour the sauce into the pan through a fine sieve. Mix in the tomato paste and half of the parmesan shavings. Drain and drain the pasta, then add to the pan and swirl.

Spread the pasta with the shrimps on plates, sprinkle with the remaining parmesan and serve garnished with basil.

COPYCAT RECIPE FALSE SLICED BEEF WITH FARMER'S SALAD

Ingredients for 4 Serving

- ✓ 4th Rump steaks (180 g each)
- ✓ 400 g   Mushrooms
- ✓ red pointed pepper
- ✓ yellow bell pepper
- ✓ 200 g   Cherry tomatoes
- ✓ 2nd Carrots
- ✓ 1-2 Romana lettuce hearts
- ✓ large white onion
- ✓ Red onion
- ✓ Bunch of mixed herbs (e.g. flat-leaf parsley, basil, mint)
- ✓ 75 ml olive oil
- ✓ 3 prs salt
- ✓ 3 prs   pepper from the grinder
- ✓ 50 g butter
- ✓ 100 ml   White wine
- ✓ 300 ml   Beef jus
- ✓ 2 tbsp   Lemon juice

Preparation time: 40 minutes

Cooking time: 15 minutes

Total: 55 minutes

Preheat the oven to 160 ° C. Dab the rump steaks with kitchen paper. Clean the mushrooms, dry with kitchen paper if necessary and quarter them. Wash the peppers and tomatoes. Halve the peppers lengthways, remove the stones and cut into strips. Halve or quarter the cherry tomatoes depending on their size. Peel the carrots, quarter them lengthways and cut the quarters into thin slices. Remove the outer leaves of the lettuce hearts, pluck or cut the remaining leaves into bite-sized pieces, wash and spin dry. Peel both onions. Cut the white onion into fine cubes and the red onion into strips. Wash the herbs, shake dry and pluck the leaves from the stems.

Heat 2 tablespoons of olive oil in a pan and fry the meat on both sides for 2-3 minutes, depending on the thickness. Season the steaks with 1 pinch of salt and pepper, put them in a flat baking dish and let them cook in the hot oven for 5–10 minutes, depending on the desired degree of cooking (medium or well done)

Fry the carrots in the meat pan, adding the butter. Mix in the mushrooms and fry. Finally, add the white onion cubes to the pan and also briefly fry. Season with 1 pinch of salt and pepper. Deglaze the vegetables with the white wine and reduce the liquid to a third of the amount. Pour the beef jus and bring to a boil slightly.

Mix the peppers, tomatoes, Romaine lettuce, red onion strips and herb leaves in a salad bowl. Whisk 50 ml of olive oil with the lemon juice and season with 1 pinch of salt and pepper. Marinate the salad with the dressing. Take the steaks out of the oven, let them rest briefly and cut them into slices.

To serve, arrange the steak slices on plates and spread the sauce over them. Hand in the farmer's salad separately.

ROULADES ON A BED OF LETTUCE WITH OSSOBUCO-STYLE VEGETABLE SAUCE

Ingredients for 4 Serving

FOR THE MEAT:

- 4th Slices of beef roulades
- 4 tsp mustard
- 1 tsp Marjoram grated
- 4 pinches salt
- 4 pinches pepper from the grinder
- 2 -3 gherkins
- 100 g   thin slices of bacon
- onion
- 1 pinch sugar
- 100 ml   Vegetable broth
- 2 tbsp   neutral oil
- FOR THE SAUCE:
- 2nd Carrots
- 100 g   celery root
- Leek stick
- onion
- Clove of garlic
- 2 pinches sugar
- 50 g butter
- Bay leaf
- 4th Juniper berries
- 1 heaped tablespoon   Tomato paste
- 400 ml   red wine
- 300 ml   Beef stock
- red bell pepper
- 1 pinch salt
- 1 pinch pepper from the grinder

FOR THE SALAD:

- ✓ 4th large handful of green mixed salad (e.g. green salad, lollo rosso, arugula)
- ✓ red bell pepper
- ✓ onion
- ✓ 3 tbsp   White wine vinegar
- ✓ Sprinkle of lemon juice
- ✓ 100 ml   neutral oil
- ✓ 1 pinch sugar
- ✓ 1 pinch salt
- ✓ 1 pinch pepper from the grinder
- ✓ small handful of basil leaves
- ✓ small handful of parsley leaves

FOR TOPPING:

- ✓ 150 g   Creme fraiche Cheese
- ✓ 2 tbsp   Chive rolls
- ✓ wooden skewers to attach

Preparation time: 45 minutes

Cooking time: 90 minutes

Total: 135 minutes

For the meat, pat the roulades thinly between 2 layers of cling film. Brush with mustard, then season with marjoram, salt and pepper. Cut the pickled cucumbers into thin strips. Briefly fry the bacon slices in a coated pan without fat, then spread them with the cucumber strips on the roulades. Peel the onion and cut it into thin slices. Heat the bacon pan again and fry the onion strips in it. Sprinkle with the sugar and caramelise lightly. Deglaze with the broth and let the liquid boil. Spread the onion over the meat as well.

Fold the sides of the roulades inwards and roll up the slices from bottom to top, then fix them with a wooden skewer. For the sauce, peel carrots and celery and cut them into small cubes. Clean, wash and cut the leek into rings. Peel and dice the onion and garlic.

For the meat, preheat the oven to 160 ° C top / bottom heat. Heat the oil in the onion pan and fry the roulades in it all over a high heat. Add carrots, celery, leeks, onions and garlic for the sauce and sweat briefly. Remove the meat from the pan and set aside. Sprinkle the vegetables with a pinch of sugar. Add butter, laurel and pressed juniper. Stir in the tomato paste and sweat briefly. Deglaze with a third of the red wine and boil down the liquid almost completely. Repeat the process with the rest of the wine two more times. Pour in the beef stock and bring to a boil until the sauce is nice and strong. In the meantime, wash the peppers, halve, core and cut into small cubes without using the stem.

Place the roulades in an ovenproof dish, pour the sauce over them and cook in the hot oven for 1 hour 20 minutes. During this time, read out the lettuce, wash, spin dry and pluck into bite-size pieces. Wash, halve, remove the seeds and cut the strips into strips without using the stem. Peel the onion and cut it into fine rings. Mix the paprika and onion in a bowl with the salad. Whisk the vinegar, lemon juice, oil, 1 pinch of sugar, salt and pepper and season to the salad.

Take the stew pan out of the oven, lift out the roulades and keep warm. Add the pepper cubes to the sauce in the braising pan and continue to boil down the sauce. Season with sugar, salt and pepper.

Arrange a serving of salad on each plate and garnish with basil and parsley. Remove the roulades from the oven, cut them in half and arrange on the salad. Season the sauce again and drizzle with the vegetable cubes over the meat. Add 1 dollop of crème fraîche each and serve sprinkled with chive rolls.

BAKED PRESS BAG WITH TOMATO AND CUCUMBER SALAD COPYCAT RECIPE

Ingredients for 4 Serving

- ✓ 2 handfuls Cocktail tomatoes
- ✓ ½ Organic cucumber
- ✓ Red onion
- ✓ 1 tbsp   mild white wine vinegar
- ✓ 2 tbsp   olive oil
- ✓ 1 pinch sugar
- ✓ 2 pinches salt
- ✓ 2 pinches pepper from the grinder
- ✓ 2nd   Eggs
- ✓ 100 g   Flour
- ✓ 100 g   breadcrumbs
- ✓ 4 slices fine red press bag
- ✓ 200 ml   neutral oil for deep frying
- ✓ 1 handful mixed herb leaves (e.g. parsley, chervil, basil)

Preparation time: 15 minutes

Cooking time: 3 minutes

Total: 18 minutes

Wash cocktail tomatoes and cucumber. Halve the tomatoes, cut the cucumber into thin slices.

Peel the onions and cut them into thin rings. Whisk the vinegar and oil in a bowl and season with 1 pinch of sugar, salt and pepper. Marinate the tomatoes, cucumber and onions in the dressing.

Whisk the eggs in a deep plate and season with 1 pinch of salt and pepper. Put the flour and breadcrumbs on another plate.

First turn the press sack in the flour, then pull it through the egg and finally bread in the breadcrumbs. Heat the neutral oil in a pan to around 180 ° C and bake the press sack slices in it until it is golden yellow, always letting hot oil run over the pieces. Lift out and drain on kitchen paper.

Arrange a bed of lettuce on each plate. Put on the breaded press bag slices and serve garnished with herbs.

FIRST COURSES COPYCAT RECIPES
COPYCAT RECIPE MUSHROOM AND VEGETABLE PAN ON TOASTED BREAD WITH ORGANIC SANDWICH SPREAD

Ingredients for 4 Serving

FOR THE ROASTED BREAD WITH SANDWICH SPREAD

- ✓ great avocado
- ✓ ½ yellow bell pepper
- ✓ 1 splash Lime juice
- ✓ ½ small bunch of chives
- ✓ 2 pinches salt
- ✓ 2 pinches pepper from the grinder
- ✓ 5 tsp olive oil
- ✓ 4 slices farmers bread
- ✓ Clove of garlic
- ✓ 1 shot White wine

FOR THE MUSHROOM VEGETABLE PAN

- ✓ Handful of mixed mushrooms (butter mushrooms, mushrooms)
- ✓ ¼ cauliflower
- ✓ 1 handful Brussels sprouts
- ✓ 2 sticks Celery
- ✓ 2nd large vine tomatoes

- ✓ ½ pear
- ✓ 2nd Onions
- ✓ Clove of garlic
- ✓ 3 tbsp   olive oil
- ✓ 3 pinches salt
- ✓ 3 pinches pepper from the grinder
- ✓ 1 shot   White wine
- ✓ 1 handful Basil leaves

Preparation time: 30 minutes

Cooking time: 15 minutes

Total: 45 minutes

Halve the avocado for the sandwich bread and remove the stone. Peel the pulp and cut it into small cubes. Wash and core the peppers and also finely dice them.

Mix the avocado and paprika cubes in a bowl with 1 dash of lime juice, gently pressing the avocado. Wash the chives, shake dry, cut into rolls and fold in. Season with 1 pinch of salt and pepper.

Peel the garlic and chop in to fine slithers.

Heat 1 teaspoon of olive oil in a coated pan. Rub the bread slices with 1 teaspoon of olive oil and toast with the garlic in the hot pan over medium heat until golden brown, being careful not to burn the garlic. Lift the bread out of the pan and drain on kitchen paper.

Deglaze the garlic in the pan with the white wine and stir into the sandwich spread.

For the mushroom and vegetable pan, clean the mushrooms, rub dry with kitchen paper if necessary and cut into slices.

Wash cauliflower, Brussels sprouts, celery, tomatoes and pear. Roughly chop the cauliflower. Remove the outer leaves from the Brussels sprouts and slice the heads with the celery. Remove the stem from the tomatoes and cut them into at least 8 beautiful, slightly thicker slices.

Divide the bulb into columns without a core. Peel the onions and finely dice them.

Heat 2 tablespoons of olive oil in a pan. Sauté the onions, garlic and cauliflower in it over a medium heat for 3-4 minutes. At the same time, heat the remaining oil in a second pan and briefly fry the tomato slices on both sides.

Season with 1 pinch of salt and pepper, then pull the pan off the heat.

Fold the Brussels sprouts and mushrooms under the onion and cauliflower mixture and fry for 2–3 minutes. Add celery and pear and also briefly fry. Season with 1 pinch of salt and pepper. Deglaze with the white wine and let the liquid boil almost completely.

Pull the pan off the stove and season the vegetables again with 1 pinch of salt and pepper.

Spread the bread slices on plates and spread the sandwich spread. Place the tomato slices on top, then arrange the vegetables on top. Serve garnished with basil leaves.

COPYCAT RECIPE Italian fish soup

Ingredients for 2 Serving

- 200 g Salmon fillet (s)
- 200 g Cod fillet (s)
- 4th Gambas
- 1 m Shallot (s)
- ¼ Bell pepper (s), red
- 1 m Carrot (s)
- 1 bar / s Celery
- 1 handful Rosemary and
- Thyme, fresh
- 2nd Bay leaves
- salt and pepper
- 1 pinch (s) Sweetener (stevioside) or sugar
- 1 liter water
- 1 tbsp olive oil

Preparation

Working time about 1 hour

Total time about 1 hour

Dice the shallot and bell pepper. Fry in a coated saucepan with olive oil. When the shallots are brown, add the finely chopped tomato and some of the water. Cook with the lid on for about 5 - 10 minutes over medium heat.

Then add the rest of the water, the sliced carrot, the chopped celery and the fresh spices (only the leaves of the thyme and rosemary). Then season to taste with salt, pepper and stevioside or sugar. Cook with the lid closed until the vegetables are done (about half an hour on medium heat).

Only then put the diced fish fillets and prawns in the pot and only let them cook for a short time. It is best to take the pan off the stove when the fish is medium, as it will follow and otherwise taste dry.

COPYCAT RECIPE Chinese fish soup

Ingredients for 6 Serving

- ✓ 600 g   Fish fillet (s), white, e.g. pollack, frozen
- ✓ 250 g   Tuna, fillet, frozen
- ✓ 250 g   King prawns, frozen
- ✓ 1 bunch Spring onions)
- ✓ 1 can   Pineapple, approx. 8-10 slices, depending on taste and size
- ✓ 5 Mushrooms, brown, small
- ✓ 1,200 ml fish stock
- ✓ 400 ml   Chicken broth, light
- ✓ 1 glass   White wine, dry
- ✓ Chili pepper (s), red
- ✓ 1 teaspoon Vegetable oil, e.g. rapeseed oil
- ✓ 3rd Tomatoes)
- ✓ 1 glass   Mung bean seedlings, approx. 175 g drained weight
- ✓ 3 tbsp   Balsamic, white
- ✓ 1 teaspoon Sambal Oelek
- ✓ salt

Preparation

Working time about 20 minutes

Cooking / baking time approx. 30 minutes

Total time about 50 minutes

Allow the fish and the king prawns to defrost for a sufficient time. Then cut the fish into cubes and halve the shrimp lengthways.

Drain the pineapple, catch the juice and cut the rings into small pieces.

Wash the tomatoes, remove the stems, remove the seeds and cut them into cubes. Clean the mushrooms, cut the bottom piece off the stem and cut into fine slices.

Pour the mung beans through a sieve, rinse them and let them drain. Wash the chilli, halve lengthways, core and cut into fine strips. Clean and wash the spring onions and cut the white into fine rings.

Put the really nice green pieces aside.

Heat the oil in a soup pot and gently fry the white rings of the spring onions in it over low heat. Deglaze with the white wine and reduce it to about 1/4 of its amount. Add the fish stock and the chicken stock as well as the chopped chilli, bring to the boil and cover and simmer gently for about 5 minutes. Meanwhile, cut the green of the spring onions diagonally into fine rings.

Then add the pineapple, mung beans and mushrooms to the soup, salt well, add about half of the pineapple juice and 2 tablespoons of vinegar. Bring to the boil once, put the stove on the smallest setting, add the fish and the shrimp to the soup and let it sit for 10 minutes with the lid closed.

Finally, add the tomato cubes and the green spring onion rings to the soup and season them spicy with Sambal Oelek, if necessary with 1 tablespoon of vinegar, salt and some more of the pineapple juice. I use about 3/4 of the juice collected. If necessary, warm it up a bit, but never bring it to a boil again or let it simmer.

COPYCAT RECIPE Cognac shrimp cream soup

Ingredients for 2 Serving

- 1 point Lobster paste
- 300 ml water
- 2 pts. Shrimp (s), (party shrimp)
- 1 tbsp Dill, finely chopped
- 1 stick Dill, for garnish
- 2 tbsp Whipped cream
- 2 cl Cognac, (possibly also brandy or calvados)
- 1 glass White wine, for the soup
- 1 glass White wine, for the cook
- salt and pepper
- Lemon juice
- Something Cream, liquid

Preparation

Working time about 15 minutes

Total time about 15 minutes

First pour the glass of white wine for the cook - nice and cool.

Then - unless you cook the stock yourself - boil the lobster paste in the water and let it simmer for a while. Cut the party shrimp into smaller pieces. Put the glass of white wine for the soup in the saucepan, add the liquid cream, season with dill, salt, pepper and lemon juice and bring to the boil again. Add the party prawns, season with the cognac, leave for 5 minutes.

Divide the soup into two cups and garnish with a dollop of cream and dill.

Alternative: Cover with puff pastry circles and gratin, also looks very nice.

You can, of course, also take unshelled shrimps, or take lobster tails, release them and boil the carcasses and then mutate them to the stock with white wine, water and spices. I just don't think that is always so timely, I'm very happy with the pastes.

COPYCAT RECIPE salad dressing

Ingredients for 10 Serving

- ✓ 500 g   Mayonnaise, (salad mayonnaise) neutral taste
- ✓ 250 g   cream
- ✓ 10 g   oil
- ✓ 10 g   vinegar
- ✓ Something Sweetener, (diet sweetness)

Preparation

Working time about 15 minutes

Total time about 15 minutes

Put the salad mayonnaise in a bowl. Add the cream and oil, stir everything until the desired consistency is achieved.

Add a dash, an estimated 3 tablespoons, of vinegar and season with diet sweetness.

The sauce is kept in a Tupper jar in the refrigerator for up to four weeks.

Garlic ajvar sauce COPYCAT RECIPE

Ingredients for 2 Serving

- ✓ 200 ml   Whipped cream
- ✓ 2 tbsp   Ajvar, mild or spicy (depending on taste)
- ✓ 1 shot   White wine
- ✓ ½ tsp   Beef broth, instant
- ✓ Pepper, freshly ground from the mill
- ✓ 2 toes   Garlic, amount to taste
- ✓ 1 teaspoon Sunflower oil
- ✓ Chili flakes, (who likes)

Preparation

Working time about 15 minutes

Cooking / baking time approx. 10 minutes

Total time about 25 minutes

Peel the garlic and press it out with a garlic press or cut it into very fine cubes. Put some oil in a pan and briefly roast the garlic in it. Deglaze with cream and white wine. Season with pepper and the broth. Then stir in Ajvar and let everything boil down briefly. Season to taste, season if necessary. If you like it spicier, you can add some chilli flakes from the mill.

Chicken breast and fried potatoes, rice or chips go well with this.

COPYCAT RECIPE BURGER SAUCE
Ingredients for 4 Serving

- ✓ small pickle
- ✓ 1 tsp Capers
- ✓ 1 tbsp   finely chopped mixed herbs (e.g. chives, dill, basil)
- ✓ 4 tbsp   mayonnaise
- ✓ 1 tsp   medium hot mustard
- ✓ 1 pinch salt
- ✓ 1 pinch pepper from the grinder

Preparation time: 15 minutes

Total: 15 minutes

Peel the onion. Drain the pickle and capers, then chop finely with the onion.

Stir the chopped ingredients with the herbs and mustard into the mayonnaise. Season the burger sauce with 1 pinch of salt and pepper.

HERBED COD FROM THE PAN COPYCAT RECIPE

Ingredients for 4 Serving

- ✓ 4th Portion pieces of cod fillet (150–180 g each)
- ✓ 2nd Shallots
- ✓ 1 -2 Garlic cloves
- ✓ ½ Bunch of dill
- ✓ small bunch of parsley
- ✓ ½ Organic orange
- ✓ ½ Organic lemon (juice)
- ✓ 2 tbsp   olive oil
- ✓ pinch of salt
- ✓ 1 tbsp   butter
- ✓ 150 ml   White wine
- ✓ Pinch pepper from the mill

Preparation time: 15 minutes

Cooking time: 7 minutes

Total: 22 minutes

Rinse the fish under running cold water and pat dry with kitchen paper. Check the fillets for bones and pull existing ones. Peel the shallots and garlic and cut into fine cubes. Wash the parsley and dill and shake dry. Pluck the parsley leaves and chop finely with the dill. Wash the orange hot and rub dry vigorously. Rub your bowl finely and set aside. Reuse the orange yourself. Squeeze the lemon juice.

Heat the olive oil in a pan and fry the cod, seasoning with a little salt. Push the fish together on one side in the pan. Spread the shallot and garlic cubes on the free side of the pan and fry. Add the butter and let it melt. Deglaze with the white wine, add herbs and 1 pinch of orange zest. Drizzle the fish with lemon juice. Briefly swirl everything through and let the stock run over the fish again and again with a spoon.

Spread the cod on plates and season with pepper. Pour the herbs over it and serve the fish drizzled with the broth. Add a slice of baguette, a salad or a Risoni risotto.

Savory fry cream – taramosalata COPYCAT RECIPE

Ingredients for 6 Serving

- 250 g   Potato
- Onion (onion)
- 5 tbsp   milk
- 100 g   Roe (tarama or trout caviar)
- 200 ml   olive oil
- ½ Lemon (s), the juice of it

Preparation

Working time about 30 minutes

Cooking / baking time approx. 20 minutes

Total time about 50 minutes

Peel the potatoes, roughly dice them. Cook in salted water for about 20 minutes.

Peel the onion, dice finely. Drain the potatoes.

Add milk, onion, roe and oil, puree. Season with salt and lemon juice. Refrigerate.

Chinese tomato soup COPYCAT RECIPE

Ingredients for 4 Serving

- ✓ 1 big Egg (er)
- ✓ salt and pepper
- ✓ ½ tbsp oil
- ✓ 1 bar / s leek
- ✓ 500 g   Tomato puree
- ✓ 1 large Onion (onion)
- ✓ 1 tbsp   oil
- ✓ 1 liter   chicken broth
- ✓ 3 tbsp   soy sauce
- ✓ 1 tbsp   vinegar
- ✓ 2 tbsp. sugar
- ✓ 1 tsp. Ginger powder
- ✓ 4 tbsp   applesauce
- ✓ 1 tbsp   food starch
- ✓ 1 teaspoon Sambal Oelek

Preparation

Working time about 30 minutes

Total time about 30 minutes

The first thing to do is make an omelette. Whisk the egg with salt and pepper. Heat the oil in a pan and, as soon as the oil is hot, spread it out with kitchen paper. Add the egg and spread well. Close with a lid and switch off the stove. Turn over after a while and when the omelette is ready, take it out, roll it in and let it cool.

Clean the leek and cut into rings. Release the rings with your fingers. Finely chop the onion and sauté until translucent in the oil. Add the tomato puree and bring to the boil briefly while stirring. Now fill up with the chicken broth, keep stirring and now add soy sauce, vinegar, sugar, ginger and apple sauce. Bring to the boil and then reduce the heat.

In the meantime, cut the rolled omelet into "rings". Halve these rings again.

Mix the cornstarch and 2 - 3 tablespoons of the soup until it is smooth and add to the soup. Stir until the soup is well cooked and turn off the stove.

Now add the sambal while stirring and either distribute the leek rings and cut omelette strips in the soup or add them to the portions in the plate.

RUMP STEAK ON BEAN VEGETABLES WITH FRIED POTATOES COPYCAT RECIPE

Ingredients for 4 Serving

- 600 g   stuck potatoes
- 2 pinches salt
- 300 g   green princess beans
- 100 g   Cocktail tomatoes
- 3rd medium-sized onions
- 2nd Garlic cloves
- 2 tbsp   olive oil
- 4 tbsp   neutral oil (e.g. rapeseed oil)
- 4th Rump steaks (200-250 g each)
- 75 g cold butter
- 100 ml   White wine
- 1 branch rosemary
- 2 tsp green peppercorns (in lake)
- 4 cl Brandy

- ✓ 100 ml   red port wine
- ✓ 200 ml   Beef jus (alternatively 400 ml beef stock)

Preparation time: 30 minutes

Cooking time: 45 minutes

Total: 75 minutes

Wash the potatoes thoroughly, bring to the boil in a saucepan with plenty of water and a pinch of salt and cook gently on medium heat for about 20 minutes. Meanwhile preheat the oven to 150 ° C top / bottom heat.

Clean, wash, unthread and halve the beans if necessary. Wash and cut the cocktail tomatoes in half. Peel the onion and garlic and cut into fine cubes. Drain the soft potatoes, peel them while hot and cut them into rough cubes.

Season the rump steaks with 1 pinch of salt. Heat 2 tablespoons of neutral oil in a pan and sear the meat on both sides. Remove from the pan, season again in an ovenproof dish with a pinch of salt and pepper and cook in the hot oven for 8-10 minutes, depending on the thickness of the steaks.

During this time, heat the olive oil in a pan. Add the beans, season with a pinch of salt and fry over medium-high heat for 2-3 minutes. In a second pan, heat 2 tablespoons of neutral oil and fry the potato pieces all over it over high heat. Push the pieces together a little and reduce the temperature a little, then fry a third of the onion cubes and half of the garlic on the free surface, taking care not to burn the garlic. Reduce the temperature further if necessary.

Also push the beans together on one side of the pan, fry cocktail tomatoes, another third of the onion cubes and the remaining garlic on the free surface until the tomatoes start to release liquid. Deglaze with the white wine and boil down the liquid. Meanwhile, keep swirling the fried potatoes in the pan.

For the sauce heat 1 tablespoon butter in the meat pan and sauté the remaining onion cubes in it over medium heat. Add the peppercorns, then deglaze with brandy and port to loosen the pan set. Add the washed sprig of rosemary and bring the liquid to the boil. Pour on the jus or the stock and bring everything to the boil again. If you use a stock, boil the liquid quickly over a third of the amount over high heat. Strain the sauce through a fine sieve, return to the pan and bring to the boil again. Pull the pan off the stove and stir in the remaining (cold) butter in pieces. Season the potatoes, vegetables and sauce again with salt and pepper to taste. Take the rump steaks out of the oven and let them rest briefly, then cut them into slices.

Divide the bean vegetables on four plates and put on the rump steak slices. Drizzle some sauce all around on the plates. Serve the fried potatoes separately.

Carrot soup with orange juice and mint COPYCAT RECIPE

Ingredients for 4 Serving

- 5 large ones, Carrot (s)
- 1 m Onion (onion)
- 1 glass   orange juice
- 1 pinch (s) Chili powder
- 1 tbsp   oil
- 1 tsp, heaped   butter
- Lemon juice
- salt and pepper
- coriander
- 1 tbsp   broth
- ⅛ liter   milk
- ¾ liter   water
- Curry powder
- 1 pinch (s) Mint, dried

Preparation

Working time about 15 minutes

Total time about 15 minutes

Peel the carrots and cut them into pieces. Peel and chop the onion and sauté in the butter-oil mixture. Add the carrot pieces and fry everything for about 10 minutes.

Add the broth, add the chilli powder and curry and deglaze with the water. The carrots should be well covered. Simmer the carrots for about 20 minutes until they are tender.

Use a hand blender to make a cream. If the mass is too solid, add a little water.

Put the pot back on the stove, very little flame, and add the orange juice and lemon juice. Refine with milk. Under no circumstances should the soup cook, otherwise it will curdle! You can also use cream instead of milk. Then less accordingly, otherwise the soup becomes too substantial.

Season with spices. The soup is ideal as a starter or, if served with toasted bread, as a delicious main course.

Potato gratin dauphinois COPYCAT RECIPE

Ingredients for 6 Serving

- ✓ 1 kg Potato (s), mostly waxy
- ✓ Clove of garlic, in wafer-thin slices
- ✓ 500 ml   cream
- ✓ 1 tbsp   butter
- ✓ Salt and pepper
- ✓ Nutmeg, grated

Preparation

Working time about 30 minutes

Cooking / baking time approx. 1 hour

Total time about 1 hour 30 minutes

Wash the potatoes with their skins only, no more after peeling. The strength is important for the binding and it should not be washed off. That is one difference, many even wash the potato slices. Then plan the tubers into very fine slices so that you can almost see through them.

Grease a gratin dish that is a good size or grease two small ones with some of the butter and place a few slices of garlic on the ground. Then pour in enough of the cream to cover the bottom. Salt and pepper the cream a little and season with nutmeg.

Preheat the oven to 150 ° C. With recirculated air, it is not yet necessary here.

Now put in potato slices, but if possible separately, not sticking together, so that the cream can go anywhere. Make 2 to 3 layers of the thin slices, then add salt and nutmeg, a little garlic, a little pepper and cream. Then press the slices into the cream so that they are really covered everywhere. Now comes the next layer, keep pressing it into the cream. If the cream is not enough, you can fill up with a little milk. If everything is in shape, the cream should be just over the potato slices, if it is a little more, it does not matter if it is too little.

Now put the butter in small flakes and spread it out a little bit more, because then the crust tastes particularly good.

Place the gratin in the oven on the lower rail at 150 ° C for one hour with forced air. Depending on the stove, it can also be a little longer. The casserole is ready, if there is very little resistance when piercing, the potatoes are nice and soft and creamy.

In France, this gratin is the classic accompaniment to all types of meat. Whether steak, roast veal or beef, there is almost always this gratin in the restaurant, which is never dry, even if you have little sauce or jus.

COPYCAT RECIPE CURRYWURST 2.0
Ingredients for 4 Serving

- red bell pepper
- 4th large vine tomatoes
- 8th Shallots
- 2 tbsp   olive oil
- 1 tbsp   sugar
- 2 tbsp   Tomato paste
- 1 tbsp   mild curry powder
- ½ tsp   salt
- 2nd Pinch pepper from the mill
- 150 ml   White wine
- 300 ml   Vegetable broth
- 3 tbsp   neutral oil for frying
- 4th neutral butcher sausages

Preparation time: 30 minutes

Cooking time: 30 minutes

Total: 60 minutes

Wash the peppers and tomatoes and remove the stalks. Halve the peppers, remove the stones and cut into cubes with the tomatoes. Peel 2 shallots and cut into rings.

Heat the olive oil in a saucepan and sauté the shallot rings in it until glassy over medium heat. Sprinkle in the sugar and caramelise lightly. Add the peppers and tomatoes and sweat briefly. Stir in the tomato paste and briefly sweat. Sprinkle in the curry powder and season with salt and pepper. Deglaze with the white wine and dissolve the roast with the liquid.

Pour in the vegetable broth and simmer the sauce over medium heat for 20 minutes. In the meantime, peel the remaining shallots and cut them into fine rings. Heat 2 tablespoons of neutral oil in a pan and fry the shallot rings in it over a low heat, slowly glazing, then browning.

During this time, heat the remaining neutral oil in a second pan and fry the sausages all around. Puree the boiled sauce with a hand blender. If the sauce is not yet thick enough, continue to boil down. If it is too viscous, mix in a little more vegetable broth. Season the sauce again with sugar, salt and pepper.

Cut the finished sausage into slices and spread it on small bowls. Pour a small ladle of curry sauce over each and serve the currywurst sprinkled with the homemade fried onions.

COPYCAT RECIPE PEPPER SAUCE

Ingredients for 4 Serving

- red pointed pepper
- yellow pointed pepper
- orange pointed pepper
- 2nd Carrots
- 2nd Onions
- big clove of garlic
- 2 tbsp olive oil
- 1 tbsp green peppercorns i (n Lake; drained)
- 1 tbsp Tomato paste
- 200 g Ajvar mild (paprika paste)
- 100 ml White wine
- 200 ml Vegetable broth
- 400 g sieved tomatoes
- 2 pinches salt
- 2 pinches Pepper from the mill (at will)
- 2 tbsp finely chopped flat-leaf parsley

Preparation time: 15 minutes

Cooking time: 15 minutes

Total: 30 minutes

Wash the peppers, remove the stalks and remove the seeds. Cut the pods into fine rings or strips. Peel the carrots, onions and garlic. Roughly grate the carrots on the vegetable grater. Halve the onions and cut them into rings. Roughly chop the garlic.

Heat the oil in a pan and briefly swirl the peppers in it. Push the vegetables together on one side of the pan, add onions and garlic on the free side and sauté briefly on medium heat. Add the grated carrots and green peppercorns and fry briefly.

Stir in the tomato paste and ajvar. Deglaze with white wine and broth. Stir in the strained tomatoes and salt the whole thing. Bring the sauce to a boil over low heat. Season again with salt and pepper to taste and sprinkle with the parsley to serve. Go with schnitzel.

FORESTER SAUCE COPYCAT RECIPE

Ingredients for 4 Serving

- 250 g Mushrooms
- 2nd Shallots
- 2 tbsp olive oil
- 2 tbsp butter
- 1 tbsp green peppercorns (in brine; drained)
- 1 pinch salt
- 4 cl cognac
- 100 ml White wine
- 250 ml Vegetable broth
- 200 g cream
- carrot
- 75 g mixed smoked bacon cubes
- 1 bunch Herbs of your choice (e.g. parsley, thyme, chives)

- ✓ 1 pinch pepper from the grinder

Preparation time: 15 minutes

Cooking time: 15 minutes

Total: 30 minutes

Clean the mushrooms, rub dry with kitchen paper if necessary and roughly dice. Peel the shallots and cut them into fine cubes. Heat the oil in a pan, sweat the shallots and mushrooms in it. Add 1 tablespoon butter and melt. Sprinkle in the green peppercorns and season with a pinch of salt.

Deglaze the contents of the pan with the cognac and fbeefé briefly. Pour in white wine and 200 ml of vegetable broth, bring to the boil and reduce the liquid to half the amount over medium heat. Stir in the cream and let the sauce continue to simmer.

In the meantime, peel the carrot and grate it roughly on the vegetable grater. Heat a coated pan without fat and let the bacon cubes in it over medium heat. Add the grated carrots to the bacon and fry, adding the remaining butter. Deglaze with the remaining vegetable stock and stir the pan contents into the mushroom sauce.

Wash the herbs, shake dry and chop finely. Pull the pan off the stove and fold the chopped herbs under the sauce. Season with 1 pinch of salt and pepper. Go with schnitzel.

KAISERSCHMARRN WITH ROASTED ALMONDS COPYCAT RECIPE

Ingredients for 4 Serving

For the dough

- 4th Eggs
- Vanilla bean
- 3 tbsp sugar
- 2 Msp. Organic lemon zest
- 40 g liquid butter
- 1 pinch salt
- 150 g Flour
- 250 ml milk

Other ingredients:

- 50g roughly chopped almond kernels (alternatively almond sticks)
- 1 tbsp sugar
- 50 g Raisins
- 2 Msp. Organic lemon zest
- 100 ml orange juice
- 4 cl rum
- 4 tbsp butter
- 3 tbsp powdered sugar
- 4 balls vanilla icecream

Preparation time: 15 minutes

Cooking time: 20 minutes

Total: 35 minutes

Separate the eggs for the dough. Carve the length of the vanilla pod and scrape out the pulp with a sharp knife. Set the vanilla pod aside for later. Whisk the egg whites in a mixing bowl with the whisk of the hand mixer or in the food processor, adding 1 teaspoon of sugar.

Whisk egg yolks, vanilla pulp, 2 tablespoons sugar, lemon zest, butter and salt in a second mixing bowl with a hand mixer or in a food processor. Alternately stir in flour and milk. Carefully lift the egg whites under the dough with a spatula (see tip). Set aside and let the dough rest briefly.

In the meantime, preheat the oven to 50 ° C. Spread the almonds and the sugar from the remaining ingredients in a coated pan and roast over a medium heat until the sugar melts. Swing the almonds in the sugar. Transfer to a bowl and let cool.

In a second pan, bring the raisins with lemon zest, orange juice and 2 cl rum to the boil and bring the liquid to a boil almost completely.

In a large coated pan (ø 28 cm), melt 1 tablespoon butter over medium heat. Pour in half of the dough. As soon as the bottom is golden brown after 4-5 minutes, turn the Kaiserschmarrn carefully and fry for another 3-4 minutes until golden brown, adding 1 tablespoon of butter in flakes to the pan.

Use the spatula to pluck the Kaiserschmarrn into pieces. Deglaze and fbeefé with the rest of the rum as desired. Finally sprinkle well with 1 tbsp icing sugar and swirl the pieces again in the pan until the icing sugar caramelizes. Transfer to a baking dish and keep warm in the oven. Put 1 tablespoon of butter in the pan again and fry the rest of the dough into Kaiserschmarrn as described above.

Spread the finished Kaiserschmarrn on a large or 4 small plates and sprinkle again with the remaining icing sugar. Sprinkle the toasted almonds and the flavored raisins on top and arrange the pancakes with 1 scoop of vanilla ice cream.

GAMBAS IN WHITE WINE STOCK COPYCAT RECIPE
Ingredients for 3 Serving

- 300 g   King prawns (without head and shell; gutted)
- 1 -2 Vine tomatoes
- 3rd spring onions
- 2nd Garlic cloves
- 2nd Shallots
- 5 stems parsley
- 3 branches thyme
- 3 tbsp   olive oil
- 100 ml   White wine
- 1 splash White wine vinegar
- 1 splash Lemon juice
- 1 pinch salt
- 1 pinch pepper from the grinder

Preparation time: 20 minutes

Cooking time: 5 minutes

Total: 25 minutes

Wash the shrimp under running cold water and pat dry with kitchen paper. Wash, quarter, core the tomatoes and cut them into cubes without using the stem. Clean, wash and cut the spring onions into rings. Peel the shallots and garlic and dice finely. Wash parsley and thyme and shake dry. Pluck the parsley leaves and chop them finely.

Heat the olive oil in a pan. Add shrimps, shallots and garlic with the thyme and fry everything for 2 minutes. Alternatively, preheat the oven to 200 ° C in circulating air and push the (oven-proof) pan into the hot oven for 2-3 minutes.

Deglaze with the white wine. Add the tomatoes, spring onions and parsley to the pan. Drizzle the prawns with white wine vinegar and lemon juice. Briefly swirl everything through again, then season with salt and pepper.

Transfer the prawns with the broth into a large bowl or distribute several small bowls. Remove the thyme and let it cool down lukewarm before serving.

CLASSIC MALLORCAN TRAMPÓ SALAD COPYCAT RECIPE

Ingredients for 3 Serving

- 4th   Beef tomatoes
- 2nd red pointed peppers
- large white onion
- 1 -2 Garlic cloves
- 0 , 5 Teaspoons of sugar
- 1 , 5 Tsp salt
- 5 tbsp olive oil
- 2 tbsp White wine vinegar
- 0 , 5 tsp pepper from the grinder
- 1 small handful Parsley leaves for garnish

Preparation time: 15 minutes

Total: 15 minutes

Peel the tomatoes and pointed peppers with a peeler, quarter them lengthways and core them. Cut the quarters into small cubes without the stem. Peel the onions and garlic and also dice finely, optionally press the garlic through the press.

Place the prepared ingredients in a fine sieve and place the sieve in the drip tray. Season the ingredients with 1 pinch of sugar and salt, then drizzle with 2–3 olive oil. Mix everything well, set aside and let it rest for about 30 minutes.

Season the vegetable juice that has collected in the drip tray with white wine vinegar and pepper, add a little salt if desired and refine with olive oil.

Arrange the tomato and pepper salad in deep plates and pour the dressing over them and serve garnished with parsley.

COPYCAT RECIPE FRIED PULPO

Ingredients for 5 Serving

- Pulpo, pre-cooked
- red bell pepper
- onion
- 2nd Garlic cloves
- 2nd Sprigs of thyme
- 2nd Sprigs of rosemary
- 3rd Stems of basil
- 4 -5 EL   olive oil
- 1 pinch salt
- 1 pinch pepper from the grinder
- 100 ml   White wine
- 1 splash Lemon juice

Preparation time: 20 minutes

Cooking time: 10 minutes

Total: 30 minutes

Cut the pulpo into pieces by first separating the arms from the body and, depending on the length, leave them whole or cut them into pieces. Wash, halve, core and cut the peppers into cubes or strips. Peel the onion and garlic and cut into fine cubes. Wash thyme, rosemary and basil and shake dry.

Heat 3 tablespoons of olive oil in a pan and sear the pulpo in it over high heat. Season with salt and pepper. Turn the pulpo, add onion and garlic cubes, thyme and rosemary and sweat briefly. Add the peppers. Deglaze with the white wine and let the liquid boil briefly, then let the pulpo briefly soak over low heat. Season with lemon juice, salt and pepper. Remove the herbs again.

Arrange the pulpo in a bowl, garnish with basil leaves and serve drizzled with a little olive oil. Go with tomato rice.

COPYCAT RECIPE BIFTEKI

Ingredients for 5 Serving

- 2nd Onions
- 1-2 Garlic cloves
- 1 bunch mixed herbs (flat-leaf parsley, dill, basil, cress)
- 1 kg Ground beef
- 200 g Feta (Greek brine cheese)
- egg
- 1 tsp Sweet paprika powder
- 1 tsp salt
- 1 tbsp olive oil

Preparation time: 30 minutes

Cooking time: 15 minutes

Total: 45 minutes

Peel the onions and garlic and cut them into fine cubes. Wash the herbs and shake them dry. Pluck leaves and stems from the stems and chop finely. Pat the feta cheese dry with kitchen paper and crumble it.

Carefully knead the minced meat in a bowl with onions, garlic, feta and egg. Season with paprika powder, salt and pepper. Form oval meatballs from the mixture with lightly moistened hands.

Heat the olive oil in a pan and fry the bifteki brown on both sides over medium to high heat. Reduce the temperature and finish frying the meat on low to medium heat for about 5–8 minutes.

Spread the bifteki on plates and serve. Zaziki and tomato rice go well with this.

HOMEMADE MEATBALLS COPYCAT RECIPE

Ingredients for 4 Serving

- 2nd   Bread from the previous day
- 200 ml   warm whole milk
- 2nd   Pinch of salt
- small glass of capers (in lake)
- onion
- Clove of garlic
- 2nd   Spring onions
- 1 tbsp   butter
- 100 ml   White wine
- 650 g   mixed minced meat
- 4th   Eggs
- 2 tsp   medium hot mustard
- 1 tbsp   butter
- 2 tbsp   finely chopped flat-leaf parsley
- 1 tbsp   finely chopped rosemary
- Pinch of paprika powder
- Pinch pepper from the mill
- 3 tbsp   olive oil

Preparation time: 30 minutes

Cooking time: 10 minutes

Total: 40 minutes

Season the warm milk with a pinch of salt and soak the rolls in it. In the meantime, drain the capers while catching the brine. Chop the capers finely. Peel the onion and garlic and cut into fine cubes. Clean and wash the spring onions and cut the white to light green part into small rolls.

Heat 2 tablespoons of olive oil in a pan and sauté the onion and garlic cubes until translucent. Deglaze with the white wine and let the liquid boil. Pull the pan off the heat and let the onions cool slightly.

Squeeze out the rolls well and in a bowl with minced meat, onion-garlic mixture capers, spring onions, eggs, season to taste with caper, paprika, salt and pepper.

Form meatballs from the minced meat mixture. Heat the olive oil in a pan and fry the meatballs in it over medium heat for 8-10 minutes, depending on the size, turning occasionally. Remove and drain on kitchen paper.

SPICY MANGO AND PEAR CHUTNEY COPYCAT RECIPE

Ingredients for 4 Serving

- ripe mango
- pear
- ½ Organic cucumber
- ½ red bell pepper
- 2nd tomatoes
- 3rd Spring onions
- ½ red chili pepper
- ½ Bunch of flat-leaf parsley
- Red onion
- Clove of garlic
- 3 tbsp   Brown sugar
- 4 tbsp   sieved tomatos
- pinch of salt
- Pinch pepper from the mill
- Sprinkle of lemon juice
- 2nd Cloves
- Star anise
- 1 tsp Curry powder
- ½ Organic lime zest
- Shot of vegetable broth
- Dash of white wine

Preparation time: 40 minutes

Total: 40 minutes

Peel the mango, cut the meat to the left and right of the stone and dice. Wash and dry the pear, cucumber and paprika, then core each and cut into small cubes.

Slice the tomatoes crosswise on the underside and scald with boiling water. Quench in ice water, then peel, halve, core and cut into cubes without sticking.

Clean, wash and cut the spring onions into rings without root. Wash the chili pepper, remove the stones and also cut into rings.

Wash the parsley, shake dry, pluck the leaves and chop finely. Peel the onion and garlic and cut into fine cubes.

Sprinkle the bottom of a coated pan with the brown sugar and heat the pan. Important: do not stir the sugar, otherwise lumps will form!

As soon as the sugar crystals have completely dissolved, add onion and garlic cubes and briefly sauté in the sugar over medium heat. Gradually add paprika, cucumber, pear and mango.

Add the diced tomatoes with the strained tomatoes. Salt everything well, pepper and drizzle with lemon juice.

Now add the cloves, star anise and curry powder to the pan. Sprinkle with the lime zest. Swirl everything vigorously once, deglaze with the vegetable broth and bring to a boil slightly. Fold in the spring onions and chilli rings, then deglaze with the white wine.

Pull the pan off the stove and stir the chutney thoroughly again, then fold in the parsley. The chutney goes well with fried meat, such as beef sirloin, as well as with fish dishes.

WARM ROMAINE SALAD COPYCAT RECIPE

Ingredients for 2 Serving

- ✓ Romana salad heart

- ✓ Handful of rocket to garnish
- ✓ Handful of basil leaves
- ✓ 150 g   Cherryl tomatoes
- ✓ ½ onion
- ✓ Clove of garlic
- ✓ 2 tbsp   olive oil
- ✓ Dash of white wine
- ✓ 2 tbsp   Balsamic vinegar
- ✓ pinch of salt
- ✓ Pinch pepper from the mill
- ✓ 50 g freshly shaved parmesan shavings

Preparation time: 15 minutes

Total: 15 minutes

Remove the outer, withered leaves from the lettuce. Cut the head into strips, wash the strips and spin dry. Read, wash and dry the rocket. Wash the basil leaves and shake dry. Wash, dry and halve the tomatoes. Peel the onion and garlic and cut into fine cubes.

Heat the olive oil in a pan. Fry the tomatoes, onion and garlic cubes in it over medium to high heat. Deglaze with the white wine. Add Romaine lettuce and basil and stir well. Drizzle with the balsamic vinegar, season with salt and pepper. Swirl the salad well **again**.

Arrange the warm Romaine lettuce on flat plates, sprinkle with the Parmesan and garnish with the arugula. Serve with toasted white bread.

BEEF CARPACCIO WITH A LIGHT TOMATO AND ROCKET TOPPING COPYCAT RECIPE

Ingredients for 2 Serving

- 200 g   Beef fillet
- 5½ tbsp olive oil
- ½ Bunch of arugula
- 100 g   Cherry tomatoes
- Sprig of rosemary
- 2nd Shallots
- Clove of garlic
- 2 tbsp   Pine nuts
- 2nd Pinch of salt
- 1 tbsp   Balsamic vinegar
- Sprinkle of lemon juice
- Pinch pepper from the mill
- Dash of white wine
- Handful of freshly grated parmesan

Preparation time: 20 minutes

Total: 20 minutes

Remove fat and sinews from the fillet of beef, then cut into cubes as thick as a thumb. Cover the cubes between two layers of cling film with a thin layer using the flat side of the meat tenderizer. Lightly brush a large plate with a teaspoon of olive oil and lay the slices next to each other. Cover with cling film and set aside.

Read the arugula, wash and spin dry. Wash, dry and halve the tomatoes. Wash the rosemary, shake dry and pluck the needles. Peel the shallots and garlic and cut into fine cubes.

Roast the pine nuts in a non-fat coated pan over medium heat until golden brown, then lightly salt. Whisk three tablespoons of olive oil, balsamic vinegar and lemon juice. Season with salt and pepper. Marinate the arugula in a bowl with the dressing. Put aside.

Heat the rest of the oil in a pan, sweat the tomato halves, diced shallots and garlic in it over medium heat. Deglaze with the white wine and sprinkle in the rosemary needles. Season with salt and pepper and bring the liquid to a jam over medium heat.

Lightly season the carpaccio with salt and pepper. Spread the arugula on the carpaccio, pour the warm tomatoes on top and garnish with the pine nuts and sprinkle with the parmesan.

TOMAHAWK STEAK WITH MALLORCAN MASHED POTATOES AND TWO TYPES OF VEGETABLES

Ingredients for 3 Serving

- Tomahawk steak (approx. 1 kg)
- 3 tbsp olive oil
- pinch of salt
- Pinch pepper from the mill
- Red onion
- 2nd Garlic cloves
- 2nd Sprigs of rosemary
- 2nd Sprigs of thyme
- 150 ml White wine
- 2 tbsp butter
- 600 g predominantly hard-boiled potatoes
- 1 tsp salt
- 2 tbsp olive oil
- 2nd Shallots
- Clove of garlic
- Shot of vegetable broth
- 1 pinch freshly grated nutmeg
- Sprinkle of lemon juice
- ½ Bunch of arugula

- ✓ 2nd Handful of baby spinach
- ✓ 150 g   brown mushrooms
- ✓ red bell pepper
- ✓ 3rd tomatoes
- ✓ Bunch of spring onions
- ✓ 2nd Shallots
- ✓ Clove of garlic
- ✓ 4 tbsp   olive oil
- ✓ 100 ml   Vegetable broth
- ✓ 1 tbsp   butter
- ✓ pinch of sugar
- ✓ 100 ml   White wine
- ✓ pinch of salt
- ✓ Pinch pepper from the mill

Preparation time: 90 minutes

Total: 90 minutes

Remove the tomahawk steak from the refrigerator 30 minutes before preparation. Preheat the oven to 90 ° C.

Put two tablespoons of olive oil in a large pan or on a grill plate and let it get really hot. Place the steak in the hot oil and sauté briefly, lightly salting the top. Turn the meat over and continue to roast, salting and peppering the other side.

Remove the meat from the pan and place it on the grill of the hot oven. Peel the onion and garlic and roughly dice. Heat the remaining oil in a pan and sweat the onion and garlic cubes in it over medium heat. Wash the rosemary and thyme, shake dry, pluck the rosemary needles, add with the sprigs of thyme and fry briefly. Deglaze with the white wine and season with salt and pepper. Put the meat in the pan, add the butter and froth. Moisten the meat with the steak vinaigrette, put it back in the oven and cook to a core temperature of 54–56 ° C.

In the meantime, peel the potatoes for the mash, cover them with cold water in a saucepan, salt and bring to the boil. Heat the oil in a pan. Peel the shallots and garlic, dice finely and fry over medium to high heat until the shallots lightly brown. Read the arugula, wash, dry and cut roughly.

Read the spinach for the vegetables, wash and drain. Clean the mushrooms, rub dry with kitchen paper if necessary and cut into large pieces. Wash the peppers, dry them, halve them lengthways and cut them into coarse cubes without using the stem. Wash the tomatoes, dry them and cut them roughly without stalks. Clean, wash and cut the spring onions into fine rings without rooting.

Peel the shallots and garlic and dice finely. Heat two tablespoons of olive oil in a pan, fry the mushrooms, peppers and spring onions in it. Deglaze with the vegetable stock and bring the liquid to a minimum. Salt and pepper.

Heat the rest of the oil in a second pan, sauté the shallot and garlic cubes. Add the butter and froth. Sprinkle in a pinch of sugar and briefly swirl the tomato pieces in the pan. Deglaze with the white wine. Season with salt and pepper, then fold in the spinach leaves.

Drain the soft potatoes and let them evaporate, then crush them. Gradually stir in the vegetable broth to the desired consistency, then fold in the shallots and garlic. Season with lemon juice, nutmeg, salt and pepper. Slightly fold in the arugula.

Take the steak out of the oven and let It rest brIefly. Put the mashed potatoes and both vegetables in bowls and serve with the tomahawk steak on a large plate. This goes with a dark jus.

HOMEMADE GNOCCHI IN A TOMATO AND SALMON SAUCE COPYCAT RECIPE

Ingredients for 4 Serving

- 1 kg floury potatoes
- 2 tbsp Salt + 1 pinch to taste
- 2nd Eggs
- 300 g Flour + more for the work surface
- 1 pinch freshly grated nutmeg
- 400 g Salmon fillet (without skin)
- 150 g Boletus or mushrooms
- 200 g Cocktail tomatoes
- Bunch of basil
- Shallot
- Clove of garlic
- 2 tbsp olive oil
- 100 ml dry white wine
- 4 tbsp sieved tomatos
- 100 g cream
- Pinch pepper from the mill
- pinch of salt
- 100 g finely grated parmesan

Preparation time: 60 minutes

Cooking time: 30 minutes

Total: 90 minutes

For the gnocchi, wash the potatoes, bring to the boil in a saucepan with sufficient water and a tablespoon of salt and cook gently for about 20 minutes. Drain the potatoes, let them evaporate, peel while hot and crush them with a fork or press them through the press (see tip). Add the eggs and gradually add enough flour until the dough no longer sticks and is nice to the touch, but still soft. Season with nutmeg and salt.

Lightly dust the work surface with flour and then roll out the dough with your hands into rolls of two cm in diameter. Cut the rolls into finger-thick pieces, shape them into balls with your floured hands and press in the typical grooves with the prongs of a fork so that the sauce can be better absorbed later. Boil plenty of water with a tablespoon of salt in a large saucepan. Let the gnocchi slide in and cook for about four minutes until they rise to the surface. Lift out with a slotted spoon and drain.

Wash the salmon and pat dry with kitchen paper. Check the fillet for bones and pull the existing one. Cut the fish into bite-size cubes. Clean the mushrooms, rub dry with kitchen paper if necessary and cut into pieces depending on the size. Wash, dry and cut the cocktail tomatoes in half. Wash the basil and shake dry. Pluck the leaves and cut them roughly or finely as desired. Peel the shallot and garlic and cut into fine cubes.

Heat two tablespoons of olive oil in a pan and stir in the tomatoes over medium heat until they collapse slightly. Add garlic and half of the basil and stir-fry briefly. Heat the remaining olive oil in a separate hot pan and fry the mushrooms in it.

Add salmon and shallot cubes and fry briefly. Season with salt and pepper. Deglaze with the white wine. Allow the liquid to boil down gently, then pour on the tomatoes and cream and bring to the boil again. Add the gnocchi and swirl in the sauce.

Arrange the gnocchi with the melted tomatoes on plates, sprinkle with grated parmesan and serve garnished with the rest of the basil.

PUFF PASTRY PARCELS WITH SEMOLINA FILLING AND CARAMELIZED FIGS

Ingredients for 2 Serving

- ✓ 500 ml   milk
- ✓ 250 g   honey
- ✓ 6 Figs
- ✓ 350 ml   White wine
- ✓ Dash of white port wine (at will)
- ✓ Cinnamon stick
- ✓ Vanilla bean
- ✓ pinch of salt
- ✓ 300 g   semolina
- ✓ 100 g   Walnut kernels
- ✓ 100 g   Pistachio nuts
- ✓ 5 tbsp   powdered sugar
- ✓ Roll of puff pastry (from the cooling shelf)
- ✓ egg yolk
- ✓ lemon
- ✓ 2nd large tablespoon of Greek yogurt (10% fat)
- ✓ 2nd Sprigs of mint

Preparation time: 35 minutes

Cooking time: 25 minutes

Total: 60 minutes

Preheat the oven to 160 ° C.

Heat the milk in a small saucepan, adding half of the honey. Heat the rest of the honey in a coated, fireproof pan to remove moisture from the mass. Cut the figs crosswise on the underside and place them upright in the pan. When the caramelized honey, deglaze with white wine and white port as you like. Put the cinnamon stick in the pan. Put the pan in the hot oven and let the figs simmer.

During this time, carve the vanilla pod lengthways and scrape out the pulp. Put the vanilla pulp and pod with a pinch of salt in the milk pan. As soon as the milk boils, stir in the semolina with a whisk. Keep stirring, the mass begins to thicken. Transfer to a bowl, removing the vanilla pod.

Chop the walnut kernels. Remove the pan with the figs from the oven and raise the oven temperature to 190 ° C. Roast chopped walnuts and pistachios in a second coated pan, sprinkling with two to three tablespoons of powdered sugar. When the caramelized sugar, spread the nuts on a strip of baking paper and let them cool.

Roll out the puff pastry on the work surface and cut out four circles with a diameter of about 12 cm, for example with a small bowl or a large glass. Place about two tablespoons of semolina on each dough circle and sprinkle with a few caramel nuts. Brush the edge of the dough circles with whisked egg yolk, place a second dough circle and press the edges well. Cut the edges rectangular and press them again with the prongs of a fork.

Spread the puff pastry parcels on a sheet of baking paper and bake in a hot oven for about 15 minutes until golden brown. Wash the lemon hot, rub vigorously dry and rub half of the peel into the fig sauce. Grate the remaining lemon peel in a small bowl. Take the puff pastry pockets out of the oven and sprinkle with the remaining icing sugar.

Spread the puff pastries on plates, and then sprinkle with grated lemon peel and the remaining caramel nuts. Arrange three figs next to each with a nock of Greek yogurt, drizzle with the honey broth from the pan and serve the garnished with mint leaves.

COPYCAT RECIPE MOUSSAKA
Ingredients for 4 Serving

- 500 g predominantly hard-boiled potatoes
- 2nd Pinch of salt
- 2nd Eggplants
- 250 ml   olive oil
- 4th tomatoes
- 2nd red peppers
- yellow bell pepper
- ½ mild green chili pepper
- Red onion
- asian bulb of garlic
- ½ Bunch of flat-leaf parsley
- 2nd Sprigs of rosemary
- 500 g mixed minced meat (beef and pork)
- 2nd Bay leaves
- Pinch of paprika powder
- Pinch of cayenne pepper
- Pinch of pepper
- 3 tbsp   Tomato paste
- Dash of white wine
- ½ Canned tomato sauce (200 g)
- 250 ml   vegetable stock
- ½ Glass of capers (in brine; drained)
- 250 g   Greek hard cheese, grated
- Shallot
- 50 g   butter
- 3 tbsp   Flour
- 500 ml   milk
- Pinch freshly grated nutmeg
- pinch of salt
- Pinch freshly ground pepper

Preparation time: 60 minutes

Cooking time: 30 minutes

Total: 90 minutes

For the moussaka, wash the potatoes thoroughly and cook gently in plenty of salted water for about 20 minutes. In the meantime, wash the eggplants and slice lengthwise without the stalks. Cover the bottom of a pan with oil, heat the oil and sauté the aubergine slices on both sides. Remove and drain on kitchen paper.

Wash the tomatoes and chop them without the stems. Wash the peppers and chilli peppers, halve lengthways, remove the seeds and cut into fine cubes without using the stem. Peel onion and garlic and chop finely. Wash the parsley and rosemary and shake dry. Pluck the parsley leaves and chop them finely. Drain the soft potatoes, let them evaporate and peel while still hot.

Heat 3 tablespoons of oil in a second pan and sauté the onion and garlic cubes until translucent. Add the minced meat and fry. Add the bay leaves, season with paprika, cayenne, salt and pepper. Add tomatoes, peppers, chilli cubes, parsley and sprigs of rosemary. Let the whole thing sweat on low heat. Preheat the oven to 180 ° C.

In the meantime, peel the shallot for the béchmelsauce and cut it into fine cubes. Heat the butter in a pan and sauté the shallot cubes until translucent. Stir in the flour with a whisk and sweat briefly. Gradually add the milk, stirring constantly. Bring everything to a boil and simmer on low heat for about 10 minutes. Season with nutmeg, salt and pepper.

Stir the tomato paste into the minced meat and vegetable mixture and sweat briefly. Deglaze with the white wine and let the liquid almost boil. Fold in the tomatoes, pour in the vegetable broth. Taste again. Cut the potatoes into slices.

Spread the béchamel sauce on the bottom of a baking dish and spread the potato slices on top. Arrange the minced meat mixture on top, place the eggplants and spread another layer of Béchamel sauce on top. Sprinkle the grated cheese on the moussaka and bake in a hot oven on a medium rack for about 30 minutes until golden brown.

SPETSOFAI WITH HERB ZAZIKI COPYCAT RECIPE
Ingredients for 5 Serving

- 9 rough Greek farmer sausages (caraway herb garlic sausage)
- 4th red pointed peppers
- green bell pepper
- 3rd orange carrots
- yellow and purple carrot
- 3rd tomatoes
- Chili pepper
- 2nd Onions
- 2nd Garlic cloves
- 5 tbsp   olive oil
- Bay leaf
- Pinch of paprika powder
- pinch of salt
- Pinch pepper from the mill
- Dash of red wine
- 2 tbsp   Tomato paste
- Dash of white wine
- 400 ml   Vegetable or meat broth
- 2 tsp food starch
- Loaf of flatbread
- Bunch of arugula
- Bunch of flat-leaf parsley
- Bunch of basil
- 2nd yellow chili peppers
- Clove of garlic
- 500 g Greek yogurt (10% fat)
- 3 tbsp   Sour cream
- 4 tbsp   olive oil

- ✓ Dash of milk (at will)
- ✓ ½ Lemon juice
- ✓ Pinch of paprika powder
- ✓ pinch of salt
- ✓ Pinch pepper from the mill

Preparation time: 35 minutes

Cooking time: 30 minutes

Total: 65 minutes

Cut the sausages into bite-size pieces for the Spetsofai. Wash pointed peppers and green peppers, dry, halve lengthways, core and cut into cubes without using a stem. Carefully clean and wash and dry the carrots. Cut the orange carrots into slices, the rest into fine cubes. Wash the tomatoes and chop them without the stems. Wash the chilli, halve lengthways, core and cut into cubes. Peel the onions and garlic. Roughly dice the onions, finely chop the garlic.

Heat three tablespoons of olive oil in a large frying pan and sauté the onions until translucent. Add the carrots with the bay leaf and steam them. In the meantime, heat a further two tablespoons of oil in a second pan and fry or skip the sausage pieces all around. Preheat the oven to 180 ° C.

Add the peppers and diced tomatoes to the carrots in the pan. Season the vegetables with paprika, salt and pepper. Deglaze the fried sausage with the red wine and boil down the liquid. In the meantime stir the tomato paste into the vegetables and briefly sweat. Deglaze with the white wine and boil down the liquid as well. Pour on the broth, add the sausage and cook for another 10 minutes.

Meanwhile, read out the arugula for the zaziki, wash, spin dry and finely chop. Wash parsley and basil, shake dry, pluck the leaves and chop. Wash the chili peppers, dry them, remove the seeds and cut into rings. Peel the garlic and cut it into fine cubes. Mix yogurt, sour cream and olive oil with rocket, herbs, chilli and garlic in a bowl. Add as much milk as you like to make the mixture creamy. Season with lemon juice, paprika powder, salt and pepper. The Spetsofai stir the cornstarch smoothly with a little cold water and bind the contents of the pan with it. Bake the flatbread briefly in the hot oven.

Arrange the spetsofai and herb zaziki on plates and serve with the baked flatbread.

POLPETTONE WITH TOMATO SAUCE COPYCAT RECIPE

Ingredients for 4 Serving

- onion
- 2nd Garlic cloves
- 2 tbsp   olive oil
- 2nd Canned peeled tomatoes (400 g each)
- Bunch of flat-leaf parsley
- 100 g Parmesan
- 300 g   mixed minced meat (beef and pork)
- 500 g   Penne rigate
- egg
- 150 g   White bread or rolls from the previous day
- 3 tbsp   milk
- Scoop of mozzarella
- 2 tbsp Salt + a little more to taste
- 2nd Pinch pepper from the mill

Preparation time: 40 minutes

Cooking time: 30 minutes

Total: 70 minutes

Peel onions and garlic and cut into fine cubes. Heat the olive oil in a large saucepan and sweat the onion with half of the garlic in it until translucent. Pass the peeled tomatoes into the pot through a brisk lot and let the whole thing simmer. In the meantime, wash the parsley for the mince and shake it dry. Pluck the leaves and cut them finely. Grate the parmesan finely. Knead the minced meat in a bowl with two thirds of the parmesan, the remaining garlic, three quarters of the parsley, egg and a good pinch of salt and pepper.

Soak the white bread or bread roll in a little milk and crush it, then add to the mince and knead. Season again with salt and pepper. Pat the mozzarella dry with kitchen paper and cut into cubes. Form a little more than golf ball-sized balls out of the minced meat mass and press a small piece of mozzarella into the middle and close the dumplings again. Spread the dumplings in the tomato sauce and simmer for about 20 minutes. In the meantime, boil plenty of water in a large saucepan with a tablespoon of salt and cook the pasta bite-proof according to the package instructions. Pour the finished pasta into a sieve and let it drain briefly, then add to the sauce in the pan and swirl everything through again. If necessary, season with salt and pepper.

Spread the pasta with the meatballs and sauce on deep plates and serve sprinkled with the remaining parsle.

Roman pot gyros special à la Duchemin COPYCAT RECIPE

Ingredients for 4 Serving

- ✓ 1½ kg   Pork neck with bones, in one piece
- ✓ 5 tbsp   Lemon juice, freshly squeezed
- ✓ 2 toes   Garlic, thinly sliced
- ✓ 5 tbsp   Oregano, dried
- ✓ 2nd Onion (s), cut into rings
- ✓ Something salt and pepper

Working time about 30 minutes

Cooking / baking time approx. 2 hours 15 minutes

Total time about 14 hours 45 minutes

Thoroughly water a Roman pot (approx. 2 hours). Cut the pork neck horizontally with a sharp meat knife at a distance of approx. 1.5 - 2 cm to the bone.

Unfold the individual layers and season well with pepper, salt and oregano. Drizzle a little of the lemon juice on the cut surfaces, cover with a few garlic slices and close again. Then tie the roast well with kitchen twine and then rub vigorously on the outside with pepper, salt and oregano.

Place 1/3 of the onion rings on the bottom of the Roman pot, pour in the remaining lemon juice and put the roast on top. Close the pan and put the roast in the oven at 160 ° C (top / bottom heat) for 2 hours. Then switch off the oven and let the roast cool in it overnight.

The next day, take the roast out of the Roman pot, dispose of the resulting broth and the onion rings from the pot. Remove the kitchen twine from the roast and cut vertically into fine gyro strips.

Then roast them in a hot pan in a little sunflower oil, if necessary add a little salt and / or pepper. Garnish with the remaining raw onion rings. Serve with coleslaw and tzatziki.

COPYCAT RECIPE Suflaki marinade

Ingredients for 4 Serving

- ✓ 4th Turkey escalope or pork escalope
- ✓ ½ cup olive oil
- ✓ 2 tbsp Lemon juice, to taste
- ✓ 2 tbsp Vinegar, to taste
- ✓ 1 teaspoon oregano
- ✓ 2nd Bay leaves
- ✓ salt and pepper

Preparation

Working time about 15 minutes

Total time about 12 hours 15 minutes

Mix all the ingredients together into a marinade and place the schnitzel in it overnight. Either fry in the pan or put on the grill.

French fries, coleslaw and of course tzatziki also taste great.

Beef with Kritharaki from the oven COPYCAT RECIPE

Ingredients for 4 Serving

- ✓ 1 kg Leg of beef boneless
- ✓ 5 Tomato (s) or
- ✓ 1 can   Tomato (peel tomatoes)
- ✓ Salt and pepper, black
- ✓ 3 tbsp   butter
- ✓ 1 tbsp   Tomato paste
- ✓ 200 ml   water
- ✓ 400 g   Kritharaki (rice-shaped pasta)
- ✓ 800 ml   Water, boiling
- ✓ 100 g   Parmesan cheese, freshly grated

Preparation

Working time about 40 minutes

Total time about 40 minutes

Cut the beef into large pieces, removing skins, tendons and fat. Scald, peel, quarter and core the tomatoes (not required for canned tomatoes), stir in the tomato paste with the water. Preheat the oven to 200 ° C.

Heat 2/3 of the butter on a stove in a heavy ovenproof pot (e.g. made of cast iron). Salt and pepper the meat vigorously and sauté all around in the butter. Add the tomato quarters and spread the remaining butter in flakes on top. Pour in the tomato paste water and slide the pot on the middle rail into the oven. Leave to cook for 1 hour.

Lift out the meat and set aside on a plate. Pour the boiling water over the boiling water, add salt if necessary. Put the pasta in the saucepan and stir. Put the pot back in the oven and cook for 25 minutes, then put the meat on the pasta and push in for another 15 minutes, if necessary pour some water, the pasta should have used up almost all the liquid at the end.

Pour the grated cheese over the dish to serve. Serve with a mixed salad.

Sicilian caponata COPYCAT RECIPE

Ingredients for 6 Serving

For the sauce:

- 1 kg Tomatoes)
- 1 bunch basil
- 50 ml olive oil
- 100 ml Boiling water
- Salt and pepper, white
- For the vegetables:
- 1 kg Eggplant
- salt
- Onion (onion)
- 200 g Olives, black without stones
- 300 g Celery
- 1 tbsp Capers
- 50 g Pine nuts
- 100 ml White wine vinegar
- 20 g sugar
- 25 g Almond pencils
- olive oil

Preparation

Working time about 30 minutes

Total time about 12 hours 30 minutes

Quarter the tomatoes for the sauce (with skin) and pour into 0.1 liters of boiling water with olive oil. Reduce the heat to medium and let it simmer for about half an hour. Then pour the tomatoes into a sieve and pass through the sieve (take a wooden spoon and push the tomatoes through the sieve in a circular motion). Chop the basil, add and season with white pepper and a little salt.

Cut the eggplants into cubes of the same size (approx. 2-3 cm). Then salt a little, put in a sieve and cover with a plate. Place a container under the strainer or place the strainer directly in the sink. You should weigh the plate down a bit. The salting must be done absolutely, because the bitter substances pull out of the eggplant. After about half an hour you can pat the eggplant pieces dry on kitchen paper.

Heat a pan on a high heat and fry the eggplant pieces in a little olive oil. Then cut the celery into pieces of approximately the same size as the eggplant and simmer in boiling salted water for 5 min. let it boil. Drain the celery and dab it with kitchen paper.

Cut the onion into slices and sauté in a little olive oil in a saucepan (preferably in a saucepan) until it is slightly glazed. Now add the sauce and the celery and simmer for about half an hour on a medium heat.

Then the pine nuts, capers and halved olives can be added. (You can also add raisins, but that's not really my thing.) Tip: If the pine nuts roast a little in a small pan beforehand, then it tastes better.

Mix the sugar with the wine vinegar and add. The whole thing with slow stirring for about 5 min. let it boil down. Then remove from the stove and let cool. When the mixture is only lukewarm, add the eggplants.

Roast the almond sticks and spread over the dish. Now the whole thing has to go through, preferably overnight in a cool place.

COPYCAT RECIPE Pork fillet in metaxa sauce

Ingredients for 4 Serving

- 1 kg Pork fillet (s)
- 500 g   sweet cream
- 100 g   Herb butter
- 2 gr. Tin / n Tomato paste, 140 g each
- salt and pepper
- Metaxa
- Cayenne pepper
- Marjoram, shredded
- Paprika powder, noble sweet
- Paprika powder, spicy
- olive oil

Preparation

Working time about 15 minutes

Cooking / baking time approx. 15 minutes

Total time about 30 minutes

Cut the fillet into pieces and fry in hot olive oil. Deglaze with Metaxa.

Add the cream and simmer for 10 minutes. Add the herb butter and let it simmer for another 5 minutes.

Tie with the tomato paste and season with the spices.

COPYCAT RECIPE Classic iced tea

Ingredients for 1 Serving

- ✓ 5 tea bags of black tea, (Darjeeling)
- ✓ 650 g ice cubes
- ✓ 0.5 tsp baking soda
- ✓ 1 organic lemon
- ✓ brown sugar

Working time: 15 min.

Preparation

Pour 500 ml of boiling water over the tea bags and let them brew according to the package. Remove the tea bags without squeezing them out and immediately pour the hot tea over 250 g of ice cubes. Stir in the baking soda.

Cut the lemon into slices and place in a carafe with the remaining ice cubes. Pour tea over, sweeten with brown sugar as desired and serve.

Rhubarb iced tea COPYCAT RECIPE

Ingredients for 6 Serving

- ✓ 1 kg rhubarb
- ✓ 30 g ginger, fresh
- ✓ 120 g of sugar
- ✓ 3 bags of hibiscus tea
- ✓ Crushed ice

Working time: 30 min.

Preparation

Clean rhubarb and cut into pieces. Peel and slice the ginger.

Bring rhubarb to the boil in a saucepan with ginger, sugar and 1 liter of water. Add teabags and cover everything over a low heat for 8-10 minutes.

Let the rhubarb juice cool and then pour through a fine sieve.

COPYCAT RECIPE Make ginger ale yourself

Ingredients for 6 Serving

For the syrup

- ✓ 100 g ginger, fresh
- ✓ 180 g cane sugar, as a sugar substitute, for example, birch sugar
- ✓ 100 ml mineral water, quiet
- ✓ For the non-alcoholic drink
- ✓ 2 tbsp syrup
- ✓ 1 lemon
- ✓ 1 bottle of mineral water, carbonated
- ✓ Ice cubes, or crushed ice

Working time: 20 min.

Preparation

Peel and finely grate the ginger. Heat the ginger, sugar and still mineral water in a saucepan until the sugar has dissolved. Syrup boiled once. Let cool down. Then sift out the grated ginger.

Put 2-3 tablespoons of syrup in a glass. Add fresh lemon juice and ice cubes and fill up with cold mineral water (carbonated).

Tip: For serving, cut the basil leaves as you like and add them. And add a dash of whiskey for the cocktail variant.

COPYCAT RECIPE Pineapple iced tea

Ingredients for 12 Serving

- ✓ 1 liter of clear apple juice
- ✓ 4 tea bags red bush tea
- ✓ 1 infusion bag of mint tea
- ✓ 1 can of pineapple slices (in pineapple juice, 446 g)

Working time: 15 min.

Preparation

Freeze 500 ml of clear apple juice in ice cube containers the day before. Scald red bush tea and mint tea with 1 liter of boiling water, leave for 8 minutes. In the meantime, drain the pineapple slices, collecting the juice.

Remove the teabag, add pineapple juice and 500 ml of cold, clear apple juice. It is best to let the tea mixture cool overnight.

Cut the pineapple into small pieces and add to the tea. Wrap filled ice cube trays with 2 frozen ice packs thick in newspaper. Only add ice cubes to the tea.

CONCLUSION

The normal grown-up person is assessed to buy a meal or nibble from an eatery or cheap food around 6 times each week. An expected 30% of youngsters are scheduled to eat inexpensive food on some random day of the week as per the Healthful Food Council. That is a disturbing measure of food expended away from home while the United States faces a weight pandemic. Eating out all the time has its results in more significant segments, higher measures of fat and sodium, and frequently less dietary fiber and vegetables.

Fortunately, eating at home can end up being similarly delicious, time-touchy, and more under a solid way of life most families are taking a stab at. Assume responsibility for the cooking strategies and fixings with regards to your food. Carrying on with a sound way of life can, in any case, incorporate having a cheeseburger or enchiladas; the first caution is to utilize empowering fixings like lean meats and entire grains and stay away from profound browning nourishments. Did you realize that salt included at the table records for about 11% of our day by day consumption for sodium? The rest originates from shrouded guilty parties like handled nourishments and eating out.

COPYCAT RECIPES

MAKING THE MOST DELICIOUS RESTAURANTS DESSERTS RECIPES AT HOME

EASY TO FOLLOW PASTRY RECIPES FOR BEGINNERS

COPYCAT COOKBOOK FOR SWEET AND SAVORY TREATS

BY

Ashley Gosling

SPECIAL DISCLAIMER

All the information's included in this book are given for instructive, informational and entertainment purposes, the author can claim to share very good quality recipes but is not headed for the perfect data and uses of the mentioned recipes, in fact the information's are not intent to provide dietary advice without a medical consultancy. The author does not hold any responsibility for errors, omissions or contrary interpretation of the content in this book.

It is recommended to consult a medical practitioner before to approach any kind of diet, especially if you have a particular health situation, the author isn't headed for the responsibility of these situations and everything is under the responsibility of the reader, the author strongly recommend to preserve the health taking all precautions to ensure ingredients are fully cooked.

All the trademarks and brands used in this book are only mentioned to clarify the sources of the information's and to describe better a topic and all the trademarks and brands mentioned own their copyrights and they are not related in any way to this document and to the author.

This document is written to clarify all the information's of publishing purposes and cover any possible issue.

This document is under copyright and it is not possible to reproduce any part of this content in every kind of digital or printable document. All rights reserved.

© Copyright 2020 Ashley Gosling. All rights reserved

INTRODUCTION

DESSERTS

A dessert is traditionally served as a dessert after a multi-course menu. Alternatively, the dessert can also be enjoyed as a snack in between. Desserts are generally sweet and can, for example, be served layered in a glass or in bowls. Desserts do not necessarily have to be prepared by yourself, but are also often commercially available as ready-to-mix or ready-to-serve portions. Dessert is the culmination of every meal. Indulge yourself in the dessert heaven with a quick apple tiramisu, a tipsy red wine cake, loose curd cheese dumplings, fluffy plum junk or a seductive raspberry parfait ... After the sumptuous meal there is still room.

The dessert is the lasting impression of a menu that you take home with you. Therefore, the dessert should also harmonize with the rest of the menu. Desserts do not always have to be complex. There are many variations that are easy to make or easy to prepare. Whether uncomplicated or sophisticated - you are guaranteed to find the right recipe here!

REASONS WHY COPYCAT RECIPES ARE BETTER THAN EATING AT RESTAURANTS

You realize I love cooking yet imagine a scenario where you required some inspiration to utilize your kitchen for handcrafted suppers.

Here are the leading advantages that ought to urge you to show enthusiasm for cooking!

IT IS A DECENT PRESSURE RELIEVER

Cooking is verifiably the activity that will help you with discarding the weight or the weight created. Right when you cook, you need to get your hands soiled, you achieve something progressively physical, which without a doubt makes you separate the day by day timetable of your day and kick your mental weakness.

This is undoubtedly an action that will require your entire consideration. At the point when you gauge the spread or sugar, or when you whisk the eggs, you get quieter. I would even say cooking can have that reflective or alleviating quality since you get the opportunity to back off and centre.

I can assure you that toward the end, when you get your finished result (for me it was for the most part bread, cakes and so on.) you feel considerably more tranquil and looser. What's more, interestingly, you would then be able to appreciate the food you arranged with your family or companions.

IT CAN MAKE YOU A MORE JOYFUL INDIVIDUAL

It goes past your pressure issue. Studies have demonstrated that cooking can genuinely be a remedial action. Indeed, even merely preparing cupcakes or something straightforward has appeared to improve a person's outlook.

The vibe of the new flour you purchased at the market, the smell of those fresh strawberries, the sound of the whisk beating, every one of those things can invigorate your faculties, which adds to get more endorphins, those important vibe hormones that put a grin all over.

The other explanation is that when you centre around the current second, on your fixings, you can't ruminate over your issues; you need to leave them aside (regardless of whether for a couple of moments).

It indeed encourages you to be all the more genuinely more grounded and thus, more joyful when all are in done.

IT CAN LIFT YOUR CERTAINTY

Moreover, on the off chance that you consider it, you go through hours heating a cake, getting the estimations of every fixing spot on, and setting up your icing to design it. When it's prepared and chilled off, you begin icing your cake and finish it precisely as you need to.

At long last, you feel a solid feeling of achievement, and when you at previous slice into the cake to impart it to your family, you can be pleased that you were the person who made it.

That is somewhat similar to when you get that flood of certainty every time you finish a venture, and you demonstrate the outcomes to other people. This accomplishment can help you to build confidence and develop your assurance to attempt new things in life mainly on the off chance that you were not a decent cook, to begin with, because you realize that with a little exertion, you can do things you were terrible at in any case.

IT CAN HELP WITH MELANCHOLY AND OTHER MENTAL ISSUES

On a progressively certain level, the past advantages of cooking are ground-breaking to such an extent that food is likewise utilized, in numerous psychological wellness facilities, as a significant aspect of the treatment for a lot of states of mind, for example, nervousness, sadness and dependence.

When cooking, patients can genuinely concentrate their brain on something increasingly positive. This entire procedure assists with checking contrary reasoning and lifts their certainty.

IT CAN SUPPORT YOUR COUPLE

Cooking at home is unquestionably an action that could likewise profit your couple, particularly on the off chance that you cook together.

It can be sure to form a more grounded association between both of you.

You get the opportunity to get to know each other, and this additionally empowers correspondence and participation.

Cooking is as I would like to think, some portion of the formula for a stable relationship.

IT UNITES YOUR FAMILY

Notwithstanding how close your family is, cooking is an excellent method to get the entire family in one spot and getting a charge out of a heavenly supper. This is the encapsulation of uniting a family.

A portion of the advantages of cooking for your family are:

- Great food is an excellent method to spur individuals to get together and mingle.
- At the point when you make a social dish, you can find various flavours and allow your family to encounter different sorts of food that they, in any case, would have never tasted.

- The more that you cook supper for your family, the more regularly they get together, and the closer that they become.
- With everything taken into account, cooking can unite your family while simultaneously, ensuring that everybody gets took care of a sound and nutritious supper.

IT'S ENJOYABLE TO MEDDLE WITH VARIOUS FIXINGS

Envision: you're strolling around another store and go over specific fixings that you've never known about. Without intuition, get them.

This may seem like an odd activity; however, if you buy fixings that you're inexperienced with, you can concoct a dish that you've never made and have a great time in doing as such.

The thing about figuring out how to cook is that you need to figure out how to cook conventional dishes that we've all come to know and love. Indeed, doing this is an ensured swarm pleaser, yet there's no innovation here. Cooking ought to be viewed as craftsmanship and as it were, whatever you're cooking is the perfect work of art that wills "stunning" your family.

With new fixings, you can investigate new territories of cooking and can astonish your family with a dinner that they will have never observed coming.

IT MAKES YOU PROGRESSIVELY INNOVATIVE

Cooking doesn't need to be a "follow bit by bit" movement. You don't need to cook something straight out of a formula book (or from a formula site).

The thing is, after you've been preparing adequate nourishment for a couple of months, you'll start to get its hang, and you'll have taken in a scope of various cooking techniques. It's now that you can begin to investigate cooking all alone and concoct your plans and dishes and let your inventiveness juice going.

In the long run, you'll be making dishes that have specific tastes that your family anticipates eating, and that lone you can make. This will point of fact, hold your family returning for additional.

COOKING AS A GATHERING ACTION

In the wake of figuring out how to cook yourself, why not get a portion of your loved ones included?

Cooking is a fabulous route for you to go through the evening with your children while showing them an actual existence exercise or two simultaneously. Teaching your children, the essentials of cooking is significant because recollect that, they'll, in the long run, move out of your home and need to prepare their supper (regardless of whether that is forever and a day early!).

The following are a portion of the reasons that show your children how to cook can be helpful to their lives.

- ❖ It can bring you and your youngsters closer together.
- ❖ As we referenced over, it's a fundamental ability that they'll use later on.
- ❖ Figuring out how to cook urges your youngsters to taste new (and ideally solid) nourishments.
- ❖ Studies have demonstrated that by instructing them to cook, they are bound to eat more advantageous.
- ❖ Cooking is an excellent method to show your youngsters to learn estimations and essential math.
- ❖ Maybe your children are remaining at a companion's home that night. Welcome your very own portion companions over and cook dinner together.

IT CAN GET YOU OUT AND MINGLE

Clearly, on the off chance that you need to cook, you need fixings.

You can purchase online your staple goods however with regards to cooking, nothing beats going yourself to the neighbourhood market and pick the best tomatoes, or choose that particular meat or new fish that you will prepare for today around evening time's supper.

The best thing is to go to a rancher's market to load up on newly gathered vegetables and natural products. I love to proceed to purchase straightforwardly from neighbourhood ranchers and makers.

I love going there to pick my fixings since you genuinely get the items at the pinnacle of newness with the most excellent supplements. Plus, you can converse with others who want to cook to, and makers and ranchers are frequently glad to impart to you tips or new plans that you have never thought of.

LESS EXPENSIVE THAN EATING AT RESTAURANT

Without a doubt, eating well seems like a repetitive and exhausting activity. Yet, a solid eating routine assumes an essential job in keeping up your body weight, dealing with yourself, and keeping up a healthy way of life when all is said in done.

On the off chance that you request food now and again or are living off of prepared suppers, you're going the other way. Try not to stress, however – it's not very late to change things!

Prepared suppers can be delicious, modest, and stylishly satisfying, yet don't let those couple of positive perspectives suck you into getting them.

Before you purchase a prepared feast, take a gander at the dietary data that is composed on the bundling.

You'll rapidly understand that they're fantastically unfortunate and to add to this, you need to cook them in the microwave (besides the not many that are stove cooked). Rapidly dispense with these from your eating routine.

So also, requesting inexpensive food can be a decent treat now and then; however, they should remain as merely that – a treat. In the event that you eat cheap food consistently, you're setting yourself an awful eating routine and to exacerbate the situation and you'll no longer consider it a treat. Except

if you have a different reliable dinner conveyance administration in your town, you should just eat inexpensive food once in a while. By preparing your meal, you know exactly what's going into your cooking and can be guaranteed that you're eating steadily.

MONEY SAVER

Eating out is a decent treat now and again, yet it's a costly treatment. Indeed, there are less expensive spots to eat out (like McDonald's or Subway).

Yet, on the off chance that you are eating from modest foundations consistently, at that point you are carrying on with an unfortunate way of life, and it's an ideal opportunity to roll out an improvement to your life.

Studies have indicated that since 2015, the cost of food supplies has dropped by around 0.5% which in all honesty, is unfathomably bizarre because of the way that staple costs, for the most part, ascend by 2.5% yearly.

On the other hand, a similar report indicated that eatery costs had risen an astounding 2.7% since 2015. Plainly on the off chance that you need to set aside yourself cash, eating at home is the best approach.

It very well may be enticing to eat out (mainly thinking about that you don't need to prepare the dinner), yet when you eat out, you're paying for something other than the food.

Eateries are made to make a benefit, so when they value their food, they consider their staff costs, fixings, cooking, and general eatery costs.

Then again, when you're at home cooking, you should simply consider the cost of your fixings and with the cash that you spare; you can bear to prepare a gourmet feast occasionally, for example, with caviar or lobster.

MAKE YOURSELF SOME SNAPPY MONEY

On the off chance that you genuinely get into cooking and appreciate doing it in your extra time, you could transform it into a side-employment and bring in some cash from what you think about a diversion.

After only half a month of learning some fundamental cooking abilities, you'll become better than the vast majorities ever are.

If you decide to sell a portion of your cooking, here are a few thoughts for you to launch this side-venture. Set up a Basic Website.

With an original site on your side, you can take photos of your cooking and show them off to the world. Not exclusively is a site useful for this. However, it can help you to remember how far you've accompanied your cooking aptitudes and how you've bettered your range of abilities. Utilize Social Media.

Like having a site, utilize your online life profiles to show the photos of your loved ones of the food that you've cooked. On the off chance that you need to make things a stride further, keep in touch with them a rundown of fixings so they can make your suppers themselves. Make YouTube Videos. Making YouTube recordings is an excellent method to flaunt your cooking aptitudes (or any range of abilities so far as that is concerned) and will likewise show potential clients that you realize what you're doing.

When you've begun selling your cooking, who knows, maybe you'll choose to step into the culinary business and become an expert gourmet expert.

RESTAURANTS DESSERTS RECIPES

LAYERED BERRY DISH
Ingredients for serving 4 people

(Preparation time: 60-90 minutes)

Difficulty: Light 420 kcal

- ✓ 500 g mixed berries (e.g. strawberries, raspberries, blueberries, currants; fresh or frozen)
- ✓ 100 g sugar
- ✓ 3 tbsp freshly squeezed lemon juice
- ✓ 3 tsp vegetable binder (e.g. locust bean gum, approx. 10 g)
- ✓ 8-10 mint leaves
- ✓ 500 g Cream curd
- ✓ grated zest of 1 organic lemon
- ✓ 2 packets vanilla sugar
- ✓ 200 g cream
- ✓ 100 g Cantuccini (Italian almond biscuits)

Preparation

- Carefully wash and select the berries, clean the strawberries and quarter them. Let the frozen berries thaw. Puree half of the berries with 75 g sugar and lemon juice.
- Stir in the binding agent with the whisk and continue stirring for 1 min. Rub the mint leaves, cut them into fine strips and set aside 2 tbsp. Place the rest with the remaining berries under the puree.
- Mix the curd with the lemon zest, vanilla sugar and other sugar. Whip the cream until stiff and fold in.

- Roughly crush the cantuccini in a freezer bag with a rolling pin. Alternate the curd cream, cookies and berries in 4-6 glasses. Finish with curd and sprinkle with the other berries. Chill the cream for 1 hour.

BANANA TRIFLE IN THE GLASS
Ingredients for serving 4 people

(Preparation time: 60-90 minutes)

Difficulty: Light 505 kcal

- ✓ 1 small ripe banana
- ✓ 3 tbsps. Limoncello (lemon liqueur)
- ✓ 50 g low-fat quark
- ✓ 1 tbsp. Crème fraiche Cheese
- ✓ 1 teaspoon sugar
- ✓ 50 g Chocolate biscuits (finished product)
- ✓ 1 tbsp dried banana chips (optionally 1/4 tsp unsweetened cocoa powder)

Preparation

- Peel the banana, cut into slices and drizzles with 1 tbsp limoncello.
- Mix the curd with the crème fraîche and the sugar.
- Crumble half of the chocolate biscuits into a glass of 0.3 l and drizzle with 1 tbsp limoncello.
- Put half of the banana slices and the quark cream on each. Crumble the remaining biscuits on top and drizzle with the remaining limoncello. Layer the remaining banana slices and cream. Cover and chill for 1 hour.
- To serve, either crumbles the banana chips over the dessert (the rest tastes like a sweet snack or in breakfast cereal) or dust the cocoa powder through a small sieve.

BANANA LAYER CREAM IN A GLASS
Ingredients for serving 4 people

(Preparation time: 30 minutes)

Difficulty: Light 470 kcal

- ✓ 1 ripe banana
- ✓ 2 tbsp Lemon juice
- ✓ 100 g cream
- ✓ 1 teaspoon vanilla sugar
- ✓ 100 g Chocolate biscuits (finished product)
- ✓ 8 tbsp Marsala (Italian dessert wine; or pineapple juice)
- ✓ 4 tsp Chocolate chips

Preparation

- Crush the banana finely with a fork, mix immediately with lemon juice. Whip the cream with vanilla sugar until stiff and pull it into the sauce.
- Pick up half of the biscuits, place in two glasses and drizzle with 2 tablespoons of Marsala. Add a quarter of the banana cream and sprinkle 1 tsp of chocolate shavings on top.
- Crumble the remaining biscuits on top, soak with Marsala and spread the rest of the cream on top. Sprinkle with the remaining chocolate chips and chill until ready to serve

YOGURT MOUSSE WITH POPPY SEEDS
Ingredients for serving 4 people

(Preparation time: 30 minutes)

Difficulty: Light 420 kcal

- ✓ 1 Vanilla bean
- ✓ 2 tbsp Poppy seeds
- ✓ 2 tbsp sugar
- ✓ 100 g cream
- ✓ 400 g Plain yogurt (3.5% fat)
- ✓ 250 g Seasonal fruits (e.g. strawberries, currants, peaches)
- ✓ 1 Stalks of lemon balm
- ✓ Kitchen strainer plus collecting bowl
- ✓ Kitchen towel made of fabric

Preparation

- Cut the vanilla pod lengthways the evening before and scrape out the pulp. Finely grind the vanilla pulp with poppy seeds and sugar in a blitz chopper. Whip the cream until creamy (not stiff).
- Mix the yoghurt in a bowl with the poppy seed mixture and fold in the creamy cream. Line the sieve with the kitchen towel, pour in the yoghurt-cream mixture and cover with the corners of the kitchen towel. Hang the strainer in a bowl and place in the fridge overnight so that the whey can drain off and an airy cream is created.
- To serve, wash the fruits, peel if necessary, cut them into bite-size pieces and spread them on two plates. Form the yoghurt mousse with two tablespoons and arrange on the fruit. Pluck melissa leaves, rub and garnish the mousse with them.

FROZEN YOGURT WITH RASPBERRY PUREE
Ingredients for serving 4 people

(Preparation time: 60-90 minutes)

Difficulty: Light 180 kcal

- ✓ 600 g Plain yogurt (3.5% fat)
- ✓ ¼ tsp ground vanilla
- ✓ 30 g powdered sugar
- ✓ 1 Organic lime
- ✓ 2nd Protein (size M)
- ✓ salt
- ✓ 1 small bunch of lemon balm
- ✓ 300 g Raspberries
- ✓ 2-3 tbsp apple syrup

Preparation

- Place the yoghurt in a strainer covered with gauze and let it drain in the refrigerator for 4-6 hours. This gives about 300 g of yoghurt mass, with a consistency similar to cream cheese.
- Mix the yoghurt mixture with ground vanilla and powdered sugar. Wash the lime hot and dry. Rub the bowl finely and mix in. Beat the egg whites with a pinch of salt to a firm snow and fold into the mixture.
- Pour into a metal bowl and cover with cling film and place in the freezer. Stir every 30 minutes so that no larger crystals form. After about 3 hours you have a creamy mass of ice cream.
- For the raspberry puree, rinse the lemon balm and pat it dry, put a few leaves aside, finely chop the rest. Read the raspberries, wash and puree with the blender. Swipe through a sieve and mix with apple juice and chopped lemon balm.
- Spread the raspberry puree on plates and garnish with the lemon balm leaves. Cut the frozen yoghurt with a spoon and arrange on the raspberry puree.

GREEK YOGURT WITH HONEY AND PISTACHIOS
Ingredients for serving 1 person

(Preparation time: 30 minutes)

Difficulty: Light 385 kcal

- ✓ 150 g Greek yogurt (10% fat, alternatively cream yogurt)
- ✓ 2 tbsp liquid orange honey (alternatively other honey)
- ✓ 1 tbsp unsalted pistachio nuts
- ✓ some seasonal fruit (e.g. 1 small blue fig, 2 strawberries or a few tangerines)

Preparation

- Whisk the yogurt and 1 tablespoon of honey with a whisk until creamy and pour into a small bowl.
- Roughly chop the pistachio nuts. Drizzle the remaining honey onto the yoghurt. Sprinkle pistachios over it.
- Garnish with a quartered fig, halved strawberries or the tangerine wedges.

CLASSIC RED GROATS

Ingredients for serving 4 people

(Preparation time: 30-60 minutes)

Difficulty: Light 130 kcal

- ✓ 600 g mixed berries and red fruits (e.g. sour cherries, strawberries, raspberries, currants)
- ✓ 1/2 Vanilla bean
- ✓ 1/2 Cherry or black currant juice
- ✓ 3 tbsp. food starch
- ✓ 1-2 tbsp. Cassis liqueur (black currant liqueur, as desired) approx.
- ✓ 3-4 tbsp. sugar

Preparation

- Wash the fruits, clean them and let them drain on a kitchen towel. Stone the cherries, halve or quarter large strawberries, pluck currants from the panicles. Halve the vanilla pod lengthways and scrape out the pulp. Boil the marrow and pod with the fruit juice in a saucepan.
- Mix the starch with 3-4 tablespoons of water and pour into the boiling fruit juice while stirring. Let it cook for 2-3 minutes until the starch binds.
- Add the prepared fruits and the liqueur as desired. Let the fruits heat up briefly in the brew, boil for a maximum of 1-2 minutes - they should neither become mushy nor crumble.
- Remove from the heat and sweeten with more or less sugar, depending on your taste. Let the groats cool. Remove the vanilla pod before serving and serve the groats with only lightly whipped cream or the vanilla sauce.

PANNA COTTA WITH RASPBERRY SAUCE

Ingredients for serving 4 people

(Preparation time: 90 minutes)

Difficulty: Light 540 kcal

- ✓ 2nd Vanilla pods
- ✓ 400 ml milk
- ✓ 600 g cream
- ✓ 50 g sugar
- ✓ 7 sheets white gelatin
- ✓ 500 g fresh raspberries (alternatively thawed frozen raspberries)
- ✓ 150 g powdered sugar
- ✓ 200 g yogurt
- ✓ 6 Small portions or small cups (approx. 180 ml content)

Preparation

- Slice the vanilla pods lengthways, scrape out the pulp. Boil milk, cream, sugar and vanilla pulp briefly in a saucepan, then let simmer over low heat for about 20 minutes.
- Soak the gelatin in cold water for approx. 5 minutes, then squeeze it out and dissolve in the hot cream milk (caution: do not let it boil!) While stirring. Fill the cream milk into small portions or small cups. Cover and refrigerate in the refrigerator for approx. 6 hours until the mixture has set.
- Wash the raspberries, set aside about 3 berries per serving for garnish. Puree the remaining berries with powdered sugar and yoghurt. Pour the panna cotta onto a plate (this works best if you briefly dip the molds in hot water to the edge) and pour the sauce over them. Garnish with raspberries.

FAST CHOCOLATE PUDDING

Ingredients for serving 4 people

(Preparation time: 30 minutes)

Difficulty: medium 490 kcal

- ✓ 150 g Block or dark chocolate
- ✓ 2nd fresh eggs
- ✓ 75 g sugar
- ✓ 1 parcel vanilla sugar
- ✓ 500 ml milk
- ✓ 50 g food starch
- ✓ 30 g Dark chocolate coating

Preparation

- Break the chocolate into pieces. Separate the eggs, set the egg whites aside, whip the egg yolks with 50 g of sugar and the vanilla sugar until creamy with the whisk of the hand mixer.
- Mix 100 ml milk with the cornstarch until smooth. Heat the rest of the milk and let the chocolate melt in it. Stir in the mixed cornstarch and continue stirring until the mixture thickens. Remove the pudding from the heat and stir in the egg yolk cream.
- Do not beat the egg whites with the rest of the sugar too stiff and stir gently under the pudding.
- Place the chocolate pudding in a bowl or four dessert glasses. Cut the chocolate into chips with a sharp knife and sprinkle on the chocolate pudding.

CREPES SUZETTE WITH ORANGE SYRUP

Ingredients for serving 4 people

(Preparation time: 60-90 minutes)

Difficulty: medium 365 kcal

For the crepes:

- 30 g butter
- 80 g Flour
- salt
- 1 teaspoon vanilla sugar
- 200 ml milk
- 2nd Eggs
- 2nd egg yolk
- 1 teaspoon grated organic orange peel
- 2 tbsp Butter for baking

For the syrup:

- 2nd Organic oranges
- 10 pieces Sugar cubes
- 30 g butter
- 2 tbsp Orange liqueur (e.g. Grand Marnier or Cointreau)

Preparation

- Melt the butter for the crepes. Mix the flour with a pinch of salt, vanilla sugar and milk. Stir in the eggs, egg yolks, liquid

- butter and orange peel. Cover the dough and let it rest in the fridge for approx. 2 hours.
- For the syrup, wash the oranges hot and dry them. Grate the sugar cubes on the orange peel until the sugar pieces have a yellow color and are infused with the aromatic oil of the fruit. Halve oranges and squeeze out the juice. Put the butter with the sugar pieces in a pan (picture 1), heat and let them caramelize. Stir in the orange juice and orange liqueur and simmer for approx. 2 minutes.
- Stir the dough. Heat a little butter in the crepe pan, pour in some dough with a small ladle, immediately spread very thinly in the pan with the wooden pusher (picture 2). Bake the crêpe until golden brown on a high heat, turn with a wooden spatula (image 3) and bake the second side. Bake 8 crepes in this way.
- Fold the crêpes into quarters and place them in two large pans. Pour the orange syrup over it and heat it over medium heat. Serve the crêpes Suzette very hot.

CREPES WITH SALTED CARAMEL APPLES

Ingredients for serving 4 people

(Preparation time: 60-90 minutes)

Difficulty: medium

FOR THE CRÊPES:

- ✓ approx. 3 tbsp. butter
- ✓ 1/2 Vanilla bean
- ✓ 200 g Whole milk
- ✓ 125 g Wheat flour (Type 405)
- ✓ 1 Egg (size M)
- ✓ 1 tbsp. sugar
- ✓ sea-salt

FOR THE APPLE:

- ✓ 4th sour apples
- ✓ 50 g butter
- ✓ 2 tbsp strong honey (e.g. garrigue or heather honey)
- ✓ sea-salt
- ✓ 2 tbsp Calvados (apple brandy) or apple juice

TO DISH:

- ✓ 125 g Crème double or 4 scoops of vanilla ice cream

Preparation

- Melt 1 tbsp. butter for the crêpe batter. Slice the vanilla pod lengthways and scrape out the pulp. Whisk the liquid butter, the vanilla pulp (do not throw away the pod, but keep it for the apples), the milk, 75 ml of water, the flour, the egg, the sugar and a pinch of sea salt. Let the dough soak covered for 1 hour.
- In the meantime, peel the apples for the caramel apples, quarter them, cut out the core and cut the quarters into columns. Fry the butter in a pan. Add the honey, the vanilla pod and 1 pinch of sea salt, then add the apple wedges. Approx. Braise for 5 minutes until the apple wedges are soft but not yet crumbling. Pour in the calvados or apple juice and bring to a boil briefly. Cover the apples warm or let them cool down as desired.
- Heat about 1 teaspoon of butter in a pan. Let a quarter of the dough flow in with a small ladle and bake a thin crepe on both sides in medium heat for 2-3 minutes.
  - Take out the crepe and keep warm covered. Do the same with the rest of the dough and bake three more crepes in 1 teaspoon of butter. Arrange the crêpes with the apples and, if desired, with 1 clack of creamy double cream or 1 scoop of vanilla ice cream.

CREPES WITH SOUR CHERRY RAGOUT
Ingredients for serving 4 people

(Preparation time: 60-90 minutes)

Difficulty: medium 530 kcal

- ✓ 30 g butter
- ✓ 150 g Flour
- ✓ salt
- ✓ 150 ml milk
- ✓ 100 ml carbonated mineral water
- ✓ 4th Eggs
- ✓ 400 g Sour cherries

- ✓ 400 ml Cherry juice or currant juice (alternatively 1 glass of sour cherries; 720 g drained weight)
- ✓ 1 tbsp powdered sugar
- ✓ 30 g food starch
- ✓ 50 g Cane sugar
- ✓ 1 parcel vanilla sugar
- ✓ 2 tbsp Cassis syrup (as desired)
- ✓ Fat for baking

Preparation

- Melt the butter. Mix the flour with 1 strong pinch of salt and stir until smooth with the milk and mineral water. Mix in the eggs and the melted butter. Leave the dough covered for about 30 minutes.
- In the meantime, wash, halve and stone the cherries. (Drain the cherries from the glass in a sieve and collect the juice (400 ml).) Mix the cherries and powdered sugar. Stir 100 ml of juice with corn-starch until smooth. Bring the remaining juice with sugar and vanilla sugar to the boil in a saucepan. Stir in the corn-starch and bring to the boil again while stirring. Mix in the cherries and stir in the cassis syrup. Let the cherry ragout cool down at room temperature.
- Stir the dough. Heat some fat in a coated pan. Add a small ladle of dough and bake 8 thin crepes one after the other over high heat. Keep finished crepes warm in the oven at 80 °. Warm the cherry ragout and spread on the crepes, serve immediately.

CREPES WITH ORANGE SAUCE
Ingredients for serving 6 people

(Preparation time: 30-60 minutes)

Difficulty: medium 245 kcal

- ✓ 40 g butter
- ✓ 150 ml milk
- ✓ 50 g cream
- ✓ 25 g Corn flour
- ✓ 50 g gluten-free corn-starch
- ✓ salt
- ✓ 2nd Eggs
- ✓ 3rd Organic oranges
- ✓ 10 g butter
- ✓ 50 g sugar
- ✓ 1 tbsp Lemon juice
- ✓ 2 cl Orange liqueurs (at will)

Preparation

- Melt the butter for the crepes. Put the milk and cream in a bowl. Sift the flour and starch over it, add a pinch of salt and whisk through well with a whisk until a smooth dough is formed, then stir in the eggs. Add 2 tablespoons of the melted butter dropwise and stir until it is completely mixed with the dough.
- Heat a coated pan (16 cm Ø) and brush with a little melted butter. Pour ½ ladle of dough into the pan and spread it over the pan base by swivelling it. Place the lid on the pan and bake the crêpe on the underside over medium heat until it is lightly browned at the bottom and almost stocked at the top, then turn and bake open on the second side. Bake further crêpes from the remaining dough in the same way and keep them warm.
- For the sauce, use a sharp knife to cut the peel off the oranges and the white skin into the flesh and remove the fruit fillets between the white cuticles, collecting the juice in a plate.

- Put the butter in the pan, melt on a medium heat and melt the sugar while stirring. Deglaze with the orange and lemon juice. Add the orange fillets, refine the sauce as you like with the liqueur and let it sit briefly on the switched off hob. Fold the crêpes twice and arrange them on four preheated plates with the sauce

WARM RICE CASSEROLE WITH RASPBERRIES AND PEACHES
Ingredients for serving 4 people

(Preparation time: 60-90 minutes)

Difficulty: medium

- ✓ 300 ml milk
- ✓ Mark of 1 vanilla bean
- ✓ 80 g rice pudding
- ✓ 4th ripe peaches
- ✓ 100 g sugar
- ✓ 50 g butter
- ✓ 150 ml Peach juice
- ✓ 400 g fresh raspberries
- ✓ 2nd Eggs (size M)
- ✓ 1 pinch salt
- ✓ Butter for the mold
- ✓ Powdered sugar for dusting

Preparation

- Boil milk, add vanilla pulp and rice. Let the rice swell in medium heat in about 20 minutes. Stir more often. Remove the pan from the heat and let the rice cool.
- In the meantime, wash the peaches, pat dry, halve and stone. Sprinkle the cut surfaces with a little sugar and place with this side in a large pan with melted butter. Fry and turn for about 4 minutes. Pour in the peach juice and let it boil down like a syrup.

- Place the peach halves side by side in a buttered gratin dish with the cavity facing upwards and drizzle with syrup. Spread raspberries on top.
- Preheat the oven to 225 ° C. Separate the eggs. Whisk egg yolks with 3 tablespoons sugar. Stir in the cooled milk rice. Beat the egg whites with the salt very stiffly. Gradually pour in the remaining sugar. Lift the egg whites under the rice mass.
- Spread rice mass over the peaches. Bake the peaches in the oven until golden brown in about 15 minutes. Dust fresh from the oven with powdered sugar and serve.

WARM CHOCOLATE CAKES
Ingredients for serving 4 people

(Preparation time: 30minutes)

Difficulty: Light 450 kcal

- ✓ 100 g Dark chocolate (at least 70% cocoa content)
- ✓ 75 g soft butter
- ✓ 50 g + 1 tsp. icing sugar
- ✓ salt
- ✓ 2nd Eggs (size M)
- ✓ 2 tbsp. Flour
- ✓ 1 ripe mango
- ✓ 125 g Raspberries
- ✓ 4th ovenproof dishes (approx. 100 ml content)
- ✓ Butter and flour for the molds
- ✓ Powdered sugar for dusting

Preparation

- Preheat the oven to 160 ° (fan oven 140 °). Spread the molds with a little butter and dust thinly with flour. Break the chocolate into pieces and melt in a hot water bath.

- Put the soft butter, 50 g powdered sugar and 1 small pinch of salt in a mixing bowl and stir until foamy with the hand mixer for 2-3 minutes. Add the eggs one after the other and fold in. Stir in the melted chocolate. Sieve the flour on top and fold in with a spatula. Spread the dough on the ramekins and bake the cakes in the oven (center) for about 12 minutes.
- In the meantime, peel the mango, cut the flesh from the stone and puree in a tall mixing bowl with a hand blender. Wash the raspberries and drain on kitchen paper. Puree with 1 tsp icing sugar and strain through a fine sieve to remove the seeds.
- Take the chocolate cakes out of the oven, throw them out of the molds and arrange them on dessert plates with mango and raspberry sauce. Serve immediately with powdered sugar so that the core of the cake is still hot.

BAKED BANANA WITH HONEY
Ingredients for serving 2 people

(Preparation time: 30 minutes)

Difficulty: Light 415 kcal

- ✓ 2nd not too ripe bananas
- ✓ 1 tbsp butter
- ✓ 2 tbsp Liquid honey
- ✓ Cinnamon powder
- ✓ 1 tbsp Coconut flakes
- ✓ 2 balls vanilla ice-cream

Preparation

- Peel and halve the bananas lengthways. Heat the butter in a pan and sauté the bananas for 2-3 minutes on both sides until lightly browned. Then drizzle with 1 tablespoon of honey, sprinkle with 1 pinch of cinnamon.

- Place bananas on two plates, drizzle with the remaining honey and sprinkle with the coconut flakes. Arrange the vanilla ice cream next to it.

TYPICAL GERMAN MARBLE CAKE

Ingredients for serving 12 pieces

(Preparation time: 60-90 minutes)

Difficulty: Light 425 kcal

- ✓ 250 g soft butter
- ✓ 225 g sugar
- ✓ 1 parcel vanilla sugar
- ✓ 4th Eggs (size M)
- ✓ 500 g Flour
- ✓ 1 parcel baking powder
- ✓ 170 ml milk
- ✓ 3 tbsp unsweetened cocoa powder
- ✓ Fat and bread crumbs for the shape
- ✓ Powdered sugar for dusting
- ✓ Spring form pan with cupcake insert

Preparation

- Mix the butter with 200 g of sugar and vanilla sugar until the sugar has dissolved. Gradually mix in the eggs. Mix the flour with the baking powder and sieve over it, add 125 ml milk and mix everything to smooth dough. Preheat the oven to 175 °. Grease the mold, sprinkle with breadcrumbs. Pour in two thirds of the dough.

- Mix the rest of the dough with the cocoa powder, 25 g of sugar and the rest of the milk. Blot over the light dough and circle with a fork.
- Smooth the surface, bake the cake in a hot oven (center, fan oven 160 °) for a good 1 hour. Insert a wooden stick as a test: If it can be pulled out cleanly, the cake is ready.
- Remove from the oven and let cool briefly. Loosen the spring form pan and let the cake cool on a wire rack. Dust with icing sugar to serve.

VANILLA PUDDING

Ingredients for serving 4 people

(Preparation time: 60-90 minutes)

Difficulty: Light 370 kcal

- ✓ 500 ml milk
- ✓ 40 g food starch
- ✓ 1 Vanilla bean
- ✓ 40 g sugar
- ✓ salt
- ✓ 100 g Dark chocolate
- ✓ 100 g cream
- ✓ 1 tbsp. honey

Preparation

- Take 6 tbsp. of the milk and stir in the cornstarch. Slice the vanilla pod lengthways, scrape the pulp into the remaining milk, and add the pod, the sugar and a pinch of salt.

- Bring the milk to the boil, stir in the mixed cornstarch and let everything rise once until the mixture is thick. Remove the pan from the heat and remove the vanilla pod.
- Pour the pudding into a glass bowl and let it cool lukewarm, stirring occasionally.
- Crumble the chocolate and melt with the cream and honey over the hot water bath while stirring. Let it cool down again and pour it into the pudding.
- Mix in lightly with a wooden spoon handle as desired, so that a stripe pattern is created. Let cool completely and serve in the glass bowl.

CHOCOLATE PUDDING WITH SPONGE CAKE

Ingredients for serving 4 people

(Preparation time: 60-90 minutes)

Difficulty: Light 430 kcal

- ✓ 80 g Ladyfingers
- ✓ 50 g Dark chocolate (at least 70% cocoa)
- ✓ 60 g soft butter
- ✓ 4th Eggs
- ✓ 50 g sugar
- ✓ 100 ml milk
- ✓ Butter and breadcrumbs for the mold

Preparation

- Grease a pudding mold with its lid thoroughly and sprinkle with breadcrumbs. Half fill a high saucepan with space for the pudding mold

- with the lid on and boil the water. Put the ladyfingers in a freezer bag and finely crumble with the rolling pin.
- Grate the chocolate finely. Mix the soft butter with the whisk of the hand mixer until it is foamy. Separate the eggs. Add egg yolks and sugar to the butter and stir everything thoroughly for 2 minutes. Mix the biscuit crumbs with the milk and stir in the chocolate with the egg yolk cream. Beat the egg whites to stiff egg whites and fold in gently.
- Pour the mixture into the pudding mold and close the lid. Place the pan in the saucepan with boiling water. The water should reach half the shape. Let the pudding cook on low heat for 1 hour. The water has to bubble gently at all times.
- After 1 hour remove the lid of the pudding mold and check with a wooden stick whether the pudding is cooked. If there is dough left on the chopstick, continue cooking the pudding for 10-15 minutes.
  - Remove the form from the water bath and let it stand for 5 minutes. Use a small knife to loosen the pudding from the edge of the form and drop it on a plate. Serve immediately.

WARM SEMOLINA PUDDING

Ingredients for serving 4 people

(Preparation time: 30-60 minutes)

Difficulty: Light 185 kcal

- ✓ 200 ml milk
- ✓ 50 g Durum wheat semolina
- ✓ 1/2 Organic lemon
- ✓ 3rd Eggs (M)
- ✓ 3 tbsp sugar
- ✓ Butter for greasing
- ✓ 4th Soufflé cases or flat, wide preserving jars (100–125 ml each)

Preparation

Weigh the ingredients and prepare them.

- Bring the milk to a boil in a small saucepan and pull the saucepan off the heat. Add the semolina to the milk and stir in, put the pot back on the stove and let the semolina cook for about 4 minutes, stirring over low heat. Take off the heat, let the semolina cool down.
- Preheat the oven to 140 °, immediately pushing a deep baking sheet into the oven (center). Boil a good 1½ liters of water and pour onto the baking sheet.
- Wash the lemon hot and dry it, grate the peel finely and squeeze out 1 teaspoon of juice. Stir both under the semolina porridge. Separate eggs, stir egg yolks under the semolina porridge. Beat the egg whites with sugar until stiff. First stir a third of the egg snow under the porridge, then stir in the rest with a whisk.
- Grease the tins or jars with butter and pour in the semolina. Carefully place the jars in the hot water bath in the oven and let the pudding freeze

in approx. 25 minutes. Take the semolina pudding out of the oven, let it cool briefly and serve warm.

VEGAN COCONUT SEMOLINA PUDDING WITH MANGO

Ingredients for serving 4 people

(Preparation time: 90 minutes)

Difficulty: Light 350 kcal

- ✓ 1 Organic lemon
- ✓ 400 g Coconut milk
- ✓ 100 g sugar
- ✓ 1/2 tsp Agar-agar powder (from the health food store)
- ✓ Cinnamon powder
- ✓ salt
- ✓ 60 g Durum wheat semolina
- ✓ 1 ripe mango
- ✓ 3rd Mint leaves
- ✓ 4th Portion cups (approx. 8 cm ∅, alternatively lintel glasses)

Preparation

- For the semolina pudding, wash the lemon hot and dry. Then rub the peel and squeeze out the juice. Bring the coconut milk to the boil in a saucepan with 200 ml of water, 60 g of sugar, agar and 1 pinch of cinnamon powder and salt. Sprinkle in the semolina and cook over medium heat while stirring in about 5 minutes to a thick mass.
- Remove the mixture from the heat, stir in the lemon zest and season with 1-2 teaspoons of lemon juice. Rinse the molds cold, pour in the semolina and let them cool lukewarm. Then cover and cool for approx. 2 hours.

- Peel the mango, cut the flesh flat from the stone and dice. Caramelize 20 g of sugar in a saucepan in a light brown. Add the mango cubes and 2 tablespoons of lemon juice and simmer for 3 minutes, and then remove from the heat. Wash the mint leaves and pat dry. Grate finely with 20 g sugar in a mortar until the sugar turns green.
- Pour the semolina pudding onto four dessert plates and arrange the mango compote all around. Sprinkle with a little mint sugar and serve.

RICE PUDDING WITH MOCHA SHOT

Ingredients for serving 4 people

(Preparation time: 90 minutes)

Difficulty: Light 360 kcal

For the rice pudding:

- ✓ 1 Cardamom capsule
- ✓ 80 g Rice flour
- ✓ 1 Msp. Cinnamon powder
- ✓ 20 g peeled almonds
- ✓ 750 ml milk
- ✓ 50 g sugar
- ✓ 1 pinch ground bourbon vanilla

For the mocha shot:

- ✓ 1 tbsp ground mocha
- ✓ 3 tbsp sugar
- ✓ 25 g Perlsago

Furthermore:

✓ 4 tsp ground pistachios (as desired)

Preparation

- Open the cardamom capsule, crush the seeds in a mortar and put them in a saucepan with rice flour, cinnamon powder and almonds. Stir in the milk, bring to the boil with constant stirring and simmer for about 5 minutes on low heat.
- Put the sugar and vanilla in the saucepan and let everything steep for 2 minutes over low heat. Spread the milk cream over four moistened dessert glasses and let them set in the fridge for at least 2 hours.
- In the meantime, bring 200 ml of water with the mocha powder and the sugar to a boil in a cezve (an Arabic mocha pot) over low heat for the mocha shot. If you don't have a cezve at home, just take a small saucepan. Stir gently in between. Bring the mocha to the boil briefly, then filter through a fine tea strainer.
- Pour the mocha into a saucepan, add Perl sago, bring to the boil briefly, then cover and simmer for 25-30 minutes over low heat. Stir again and again. Then let it cool a little and spread it on the rice pudding. Chill the dessert for at least 30 minutes, sprinkle the pistachios as you like, then eat them.

BAKED RICE PUDDING

Ingredients for serving 6 people

(Preparation time: 30-60 minutes)

Difficulty: Light 295 kcal

- ✓ 100 g rice pudding
- ✓ 1 l milk
- ✓ 150 g sugar
- ✓ 1 pinch salt
- ✓ 1 tbsp Rice starch
- ✓ 2nd Egg yolks
- ✓ 1 Vanilla bean
- ✓ 6 ovenproof cases

Preparation

- Rinse the rice under running cold water and drain. Bring to the boil well covered with water. Simmer on low heat for 10 minutes. Drain the rest of the water, then stir in the milk, sugar and salt.
- Bring the rice to the boil again and continue to cook for about 15 minutes until it is soft. Mix the rice starch with 1 tablespoon of water, mix into the rice. Cook for 2-3 minutes, stirring, until the food becomes slightly thick. But it should remain juicy.
- Fill the rice in six ovenproof portions and let it cool down a bit. Mix the egg yolks with 1 tablespoon of water. Scrape out the vanilla pulp and stir in. Carefully spread the mixture on the rice surface.

- Place the ramekins on the roasting tray, pour in some water. Slide the tray into the top of the oven. Bake under the grill or on top heat until a medium brown crust has formed. Let the rice cool and serve in the tins.

PINEAPPLE AND GINGER RICE PUDDING

Ingredients for serving 4 people

(Preparation time: 60-90 minutes)

Difficulty: Light 890 kcal

- ✓ 50 g glazed ginger
- ✓ 50 g dried pineapple
- ✓ 300 g Long grain rice (not parboiled)
- ✓ salt
- ✓ 75 g White chocolate
- ✓ 3rd Eggs (size M)
- ✓ 4 tbsp sugar
- ✓ 125 g Creme fraiche Cheese
- ✓ 150 g Dark chocolate coating
- ✓ 200 ml milk
- ✓ Butter and breadcrumbs for the mold

Preparation

- Dice the ginger, put it in a saucepan with pineapple and ½ l water and bring to the boil. Sprinkle in the rice, add a pinch of salt and cover and cook the rice over a low heat until bite-proof in 15 minutes. Preheat the oven to 200 °.

- Chop the chocolate finely. Separate the eggs, whisk egg yolks, beat the egg whites with 2 tablespoons of sugar until stiff. Grease a small tin (25 cm) and sprinkle with crumbs. Stir the crème fraiche under the cooked rice, let it cool a little, then add the chocolate, the egg yolks and the egg whites.
- Pour the rice mixture into the mold, smooth the surface and bake the pudding in the oven (centre, fan oven 180 °) for 20 minutes. Then cover the pudding with aluminium foil and cook the pudding in the oven for another 25 minutes.
- Chop the couverture for the sauce. Heat the milk with the remaining 2 tablespoons of sugar and let the chocolate melt in it. Stir vigorously with the whisk. Turn the pudding over, portion it and serve with the chocolate sauce.

VEGAN VANILLA TART WITH QUINCE

Ingredients for serving 12 pieces

(Preparation time: 90 minutes)

Difficulty: Light 290 kcal

- ✓ 170 g Flour (type 550)
- ✓ 75 g powdered sugar
- ✓ 100 g cold vegan margarine
- ✓ 1 pinch salt
- ✓ vegan margarine for the mold
- ✓ Flour for work and for the form
- ✓ 250 g dried legumes
- ✓ 200 ml Soy cream for cooking
- ✓ 150 ml Vegetable milk
- ✓ 3 tbsp Agave syrup
- ✓ 1 pack Custard powder
- ✓ 700 g Quinces

- ✓ 1 Organic lemon
- ✓ 1 stick cinnamon
- ✓ 1 teaspoon Bourbon vanilla powder
- ✓ 6 Cardamom capsules
- ✓ 100 g sugar
- ✓ 50 g Pistachios

Preparation

- Grease the mold and sprinkle with flour. Quickly knead the flour, icing sugar, margarine, salt and 1-2 tablespoons of cold water into a dough with your hands. Roll out the dough slightly larger than the form, place in the form and cut off any excess edges. Approx. Chill for 30 minutes. Preheat the oven to 200 °.
- Prick the dough several times with a fork, cover with baking paper and add legumes. Pre-bake in the middle of the oven for about 10 minutes. Then remove the baking paper and legumes and bake the base in about 20 minutes.
- Mix the soy cream, milk and agave syrup. Mix 5 tablespoons of it with pudding powder until smooth. Bring the rest to the boil, stir in the mixed pudding powder, bring to the boil and simmer for 1-2 minutes while stirring. Allow to cool, stirring frequently.
- Rub the quinces, quarter them, remove the seeds and cut the quarters into slices approx. 3 mm thick. Wash and dry the lemon hot, grate the peel and squeeze out the juice. Bring both to the boil with 600 ml of water, quince, cinnamon and vanilla powder and cook for about 2 minutes. Cover the quinces and let them steep for about 15 minutes over low heat. Open cardamom capsules, remove the seeds. Take out the quinces, bring the broth to a boil over medium heat to approx. 200 ml.
- Melt the sugar in a saucepan, do not stir. Deglaze with quince sauce and spices, add cardamom seeds. Allow everything to simmer in a syrup-like manner over medium heat in about 15 minutes.

- Spread the pudding on the tart base, spread the quinces on it and pour the syrup on. Chop pistachios. Sprinkle the tart with it and chill for approx. 1 hour.

FLORENTINE APPLE PIE
Ingredients for serving 12 pieces

(Preparation time: 90 minutes)

Difficulty: Light 415 kcal

For the short crust pastry:

- 100 g soft butter
- 50 g sugar
- salt
- 1 Egg yolk (size M)
- 150 g Flour (Type 405)
- 1/2 tsp Baking powder (3 g)
- 1/2 tsp grated organic lemon peel
- FOR THE APPLE Topping:
- 5 sour apples (e.g. Boskop or Braeburn)
- 3 tbsp sugar

FOR THE VANILLA CREAM:

- 800 ml milk
- 85 g sugar
- 2nd Egg yolk (size M)
- 65 g Custard powder

FOR THE FLORENTINE DIMENSION:

- 75 g butter
- 90 g Raw cane sugar

- ✓ 90 g honey
- ✓ 100 g Flaked almonds

ALSO:

- ✓ Flour to work with
- ✓ 2 tbsp apricot jam
- ✓ approx. 50 g Biscuit crumbs (alternatively bread crumbs)

Preparation

- Prepare a dough for the shortcrust pastry from the specified ingredients and let it rest in the refrigerator wrapped in cling film for at least 2 hours.
- Quarter the apples for the apple topping, peel and remove the core. Cut the quarters lengthways into approx. 1 cm thick columns. Bring ½ l water with 3 tablespoons of sugar to a boil and blanch the slits in it for approx. 5 min., Pour into a sieve and drain.
- Preheat the oven to 190 °. Roll out the dough on the flour-dusted work surface into a circle with a diameter of approx. 38 cm, line the shape with it and form a 5 cm high edge. Spread the apricot jam on the shortcrust pastry and spread the biscuit crumbs on top. Place the apples in a circle and overlap slightly.
- Boil 650 ml milk with the sugar for the vanilla cream. Mix the egg yolks with the remaining milk and the pudding powder. Pour the mixture into the milk and bring to the boil a few times with stirring. Pour the vanilla cream immediately onto the apples and bake the cake in the oven (center) for approx. 30 minutes.
- Shortly before the end of the baking time for the Florentine mass, simmer butter, sugar and honey in a saucepan for about 4 minutes, then mix in the almond leaves. Take the cake out of the oven and spread the almond paste on top. Bake the cake until golden in another 30 minutes. Let the Florentine apple cake cool in the mold.

- You can also do without blanching the apples - the cake tastes even more aromatic with fresh apples. However, it doesn't look quite as pretty because it collapses slightly when baking.

ALMOND PANNA COTTA WITH MATCHA POWDER

Ingredients for serving 6-8 people

(Preparation time: 90 minutes)

Difficulty: Light 230 kcal

- ✓ 100 g peeled almonds
- ✓ 50 g Cocoa butter (health food store)
- ✓ 4 tbsp Coconut sugar
- ✓ 1 tbsp Soy cream
- ✓ 200 ml Almond milk
- ✓ 1 Organic lime
- ✓ 1 teaspoon Matcha powder (5 g)
- ✓ 1 large, ripe pear
- ✓ 100 ml Aronia juice
- ✓ 2 tbsp Lemon juice
- ✓ 1 pack Gelling sugar without cooking for 250 g of fruit

Preparation

- Soak the almonds in cold water for at least 2 hours (preferably 12 hours overnight). Pour the almonds into a sieve, rinse them cold and let them drain.
- Melt the cocoa butter and puree it with almonds, coconut blossom sugar, soy cream and almond milk. Wash the lime hot and dry, rub the peel

finely and squeeze out the juice. Mix both with the matcha powder under the almond cream.
- Distribute the cream in 6 - 8 glasses and let it set in the freezer in about 1 hour. Then take out and put in the fridge for about 30 minutes.
- In the meantime, peel, quarter, core and purée the pear finely in the blender. Mix 135 g of pear puree with aronia juice and lemon juice and mix in the gelling sugar.
- Take the almond cream out of the fridge about 30 minutes before serving. Spread the aronia and pear sauce over the cream and serve.

COCONUT PANNA COTTA WITH STRAWBERRY SAUCE

Ingredients for serving 2 people

(Preparation time: 90 minutes)

Difficulty: Light 330 kcal

- ½ Vanilla bean
- ½ Organic lime
- 250 g Coconut milk
- 2 tbsp sugar
- ½ tsp Agar Agar
- 200 g Strawberries
- 2 tbsp powdered sugar
- 1 stem mint

Preparation

- Scrape the pulp out of the half of the vanilla pod. Wash the lime halves hot and dry. Grate ½ teaspoon of peel finely. Squeeze out the juice.

- Place the coconut milk with the vanilla pulp and the scraped out pod in a saucepan. Stir in the sugar and the lime peel, bring to the boil once, stir until smooth and then simmer for about 10 minutes on a lower heat.
- Mix the agar agar with 2 tablespoons of water and stir with the whisk under the coconut mixture and let everything simmer for approx. 2 minutes. Then remove from the heat and let cool slightly.
- Remove the vanilla pod. Pour the cream into two bowls or glasses, filling only half of the glasses so that the strawberry sauce fits in later. Cool the panna cotta a little and then let it set in the fridge in about 2 hours.
- Wash the strawberries and remove the calyx. Roughly chop the berries, put them in a tall beaker with just 2 tablespoons of powdered sugar and mash them finely with the blender. Then stir in 1 - 2 tsp lime juice. Season the strawberry sauce again.
- Wash the mint and shake well dry, pluck the leaves. Spread the strawberry sauce over the coconut panna cotta and garnish the dessert with mint leaves. Serve immediately

MASCARPONE CHOCOLATE CREAM

Ingredients for serving 4 people

(Preparation time: 30 minutes)

Difficulty: Light 445 kcal

- ✓ 100 g Dark chocolate
- ✓ 1 Organic orange
- ✓ 1 tbsp Liquid honey
- ✓ 250 g Mascarpone

Preparation

- Break the chocolate into pieces and melt in a cup in a hot water bath. Wash the orange hot and dry, cut thinly half of the peel and chop finely. Squeeze out the juice.
- Stir the lukewarm chocolate with the orange peel and juice and the honey thoroughly under the mascarpone using the hand mixer. Spread in dessert bowls, dust with powdered sugar and serve.

VEGAN PUMPKIN PANNA COTTA WITH WARM CRANBERRY COMPOTE

Ingredients for serving 4 people

(Preparation time: 90 minutes)

Difficulty: medium

FOR THE PANNA COTTA:

- 250 g Butternut squash (alternatively Hokkaido squash)
- 100 g Almonds
- 1 Vanilla pod (alternatively tsp bourbon vanilla powder)
- 2 tbsp Maple syrup
- 1/2 tsp Agar Agar
- 1/3 tsp Locust bean gum (alternatively arrow root starch)
- 1 Organic lemon

FOR THE CRANBERRY COMPOTE:

- 1 Vanilla bean
- 200 g Cranberries (alternatively frozen cranberries)
- 3 tbsp Maple syrup
- 1/2 tsp Locust bean gum
- 1 teaspoon Cinnamon powder

ALSO:

- 4th Glasses (approx. 200 ml each)
- 1 stem Mint (alternatively lemon balm)
- Other panna cotta variants

Preparation

- Wash and peel the pumpkin, remove the seeds and fibers. Cut the pumpkin meat into approx. 2 cm cubes. Puree the almonds with 300 ml water in a blender and strain through a fine sieve or pass cloth. Collect the almond milk.
- Cut the vanilla pod lengthways and scrape out the pulp. Boil the pumpkin, almond milk, vanilla pulp, pod and maple syrup in a saucepan. Cover and cook over low heat in about 15 minutes.
- Remove the vanilla pod 2 minutes before the end of the cooking time, stir in the agar agar and locust bean gum and continue to simmer for approx. 2 minutes. Puree the mass in the blender (if the blender is not strong enough, pass it through a sieve). Wash the lemon hot, pat dry, rub the peel and fold it under the pumpkin mass.
- Pour the mixture into the cold rinsed glasses. Allow the panna cotta to cool in the glasses and then put in the fridge for 2-3 hours.
- For the compote, cut the vanilla pod lengthways before serving and scrape out the pulp. Place in a saucepan with the other ingredients for the cranberries and 50 ml of water, stir well, bring to the boil and simmer for 2 minutes. Then remove from the stove.
- Pour the panna cotta onto four dessert plates and add the warm cranberry compote. Wash the mint and shake it dry, pluck the leaves and garnish the panna cotta with it.

CHIA PUDDING WITH APPLE PULP AND CINNAMON

Ingredients for serving 2 people

(Preparation time: 60-90 minutes)

Difficulty: Light 455 kcal

- ✓ 4 tbsp Chia seeds
- ✓ 400 ml Milk (cow's milk or vegetable milk at will)
- ✓ 500 g Apple pulp (unsweetened applesauce)
- ✓ 2 Tea spoons ground cinnamon
- ✓ 1 teaspoon ground vanilla
- ✓ 2 tbsp Maple syrup
- ✓ 2 tbsp sliced almonds

Preparation

- Soak the chia seeds in the milk for about 12 hours (or overnight), preferably in the refrigerator. (The mixture is initially very fluid; it becomes firmer overnight). Stir the chia seed mix from time to time so that no lumps form.
- The next morning, stir the apple pulp with cinnamon powder, ground vanilla and maple syrup into the chia pudding with a spoon.
- Spread the pudding over two glasses, sprinkle with the sliced almonds and enjoy immediately.

MESQUITE PUDDING

Ingredients for serving 4 people

(Preparation time: 90 minutes)

Difficulty: Light 255 kcal

- ✓ 4 tbsp Sunflower seeds
- ✓ 4 tbsp white chia seeds
- ✓ 60 g dried apricots
- ✓ 2 tbsp Mesquite powder
- ✓ 400 ml Almond milk
- ✓ 100 g Physalis
- ✓ 1 tbsp dried goji berries
- ✓ 2 tbsp Almond flour

Preparation

- Soak the sunflower seeds in cold water for at least 2 hours. Allow chia seeds, dried apricots, mesquite powder and almond milk to swell in a blender for approx. 30 minutes.
- In the meantime, remove the physalis from the shells, wash and halve. Grind goji berries and almond flour in a lightning chopper. Drain the sunflower seeds into a sieve, rinse them cold and let them drain and add them to the chia seed mixture. Puree the mixture in a blender and pour into four glasses or bowls.
- Put the physalis on top and sprinkle with the goji berry crumbs. Either serve the cream immediately or chill in the fridge for about 30 minutes so that the cream becomes a little firmer.

POPPY SEED AMARANTH PUDDING WITH A COMPOTE OF PHYSALIS
Ingredients for serving 4 people

(Preparation time: 90 minutes)

Difficulty: medium 550 kcal

For the pudding

- ✓ 300 ml milk
- ✓ 100 g Amaranth
- ✓ 30 g dried apricots
- ✓ ½ Organic orange
- ✓ 60 g butter
- ✓ 100 g Whole grain bread crumbs
- ✓ 1 pack Whole cane sugar
- ✓ 70 g Whole cane sugar
- ✓ 1 Msp. Ground carnations
- ✓ 3rd Eggs (M)
- ✓ 50 g ground poppy seeds
- ✓ 30 g chopped almonds
- ✓ salt

For the compote

- ✓ 300 g Physalis (cape gooseberries)
- ✓ 1 Organic lime
- ✓ 200 ml freshly squeezed blood orange or orange juice
- ✓ 40 g Whole cane sugar
- ✓ ½ Cinnamon stick
- ✓ 2 heaped teaspoons vegetable binder (e.g. locust bean gum)
- ✓ 150 g cream

Preparation

- Bring the milk to the boil, sprinkle the amaranth on top and swell for 45 minutes over low heat, stirring occasionally, then let it cool. Meanwhile, finely dice the apricots.
- Wash the orange halves hot, dry them, finely grate 1 teaspoon peel and set aside, squeeze 2 tablespoons of juice. Drizzle apricots with it. Grease a pudding mold (approx. 1.5 l) including the lid well with approx. 10 g butter and sprinkle with approx. 20 g bread crumbs, shake out any excess crumbs.
- Mix the remaining butter, the vanilla sugar and 50 g of whole cane sugar very creamy with the whisk of the hand mixer in about 5 minutes. Then add the orange peel and the clove powder and stir in briefly.
- Separate the eggs and stir the egg yolks individually into the butter mixture. Add the amaranth porridge and stir in. Then stir in the remaining breadcrumbs, poppy seeds, almonds and drained apricots.
- Beat the egg whites with a pinch of salt until stiff, while pouring in the remaining sugar. Stir a third of the egg snow into the pudding mixture, fold in the rest. Fill the mass into the prepared mold and close it tightly. Place the mold in a saucepan and pour enough water so that half of it is in the water. Put the lid on the pot. Cover and cover the poppy seed amaranth pudding over low heat for approx. 1 hour.
- Remove the bracts from the physalis for the compote. Wash the lime hot, dry, rub the peel finely and squeeze out the juice. Bring the lime peel and juice, orange juice, 5 tablespoons of water, sugar and cinnamon stick to the boil in a small saucepan. Add the physalis and stew for about 2 minutes. Whisk the binder with 3 tablespoons of water and stir in. Bring the compote to a boil, then let it cool.
- Remove the finished pudding from the saucepan and let it stand for approx. 10 minutes, then open it. Detach the pudding from the edge, drop it on a plate and cut into portions. Whip the cream semi-stiff and serve with the physalis compote to the pudding.

HORSERADISH CREME BRULEE

Ingredients for serving 4 people

(Preparation time: 60-90 minutes)

Difficulty: Light 310 kcal

- ✓ 200 g cream cheese
- ✓ 100 g sour cream
- ✓ 60 g horseradish
- ✓ 1 tbsp. Aceto balsamic bianco
- ✓ 1 Clove of garlic
- ✓ salt
- ✓ pepper
- ✓ 4th egg yolk
- ✓ 3rd radish
- ✓ 2 tbsp Trout caviar or salmon caviar
- ✓ 2 tbsp Garden cress
- ✓ Lime juice
- ✓ 2 tbsp Raw cane sugar
- ✓ 8 - 12 slices Bread (quite small, e.g. Pumper nicktaler, thin baguette slices and pretzel slices)

Preparation

- Preheat the oven to 120 °. For the cream, mix the cream cheese and sour cream with the horseradish and vinegar. Peel and press the garlic. Season the cream with salt and pepper, then stir in the egg yolks.
- Divide the cream into four ovenproof flat serving tins (125 ml each), place the tins on a deep tray or in a baking dish. Pour hot water into the baking tin or baking dish up to

about 1 cm below the rim of the tins. Allow the cream to bake in the middle of the oven for 45 minutes.
- Remove the stocked cream from the oven and let cool. As soon as the cream has reached room temperature, cover the moulds and chill for 1 hour.
- For the topping, clean the radishes and cut them into thin slices, then into fine strips. Mix with caviar and cress, season with a little lime juice and set aside.
- Sprinkle the chilled creams evenly with sugar. Caramelize with a Bunsen burner or under the grill. To do this, swirl the burner flame over the sugar until it has melted and turns brown. Or preheat the grill on the highest setting. Let the moulds caramelize in the oven (top) light brown. Attention: The cream must be evenly covered with sugar; otherwise uncovered areas will quickly turn dark.
- Place the moulds with the finished crème brûlée on a plate and place the topping in the centre. Serve the bread with it.

COTTAGE CHEESE PUDDING WITH CHERRY RAGOUT

Ingredients for serving 6 people

(Preparation time: 60-90 minutes)

Difficulty: medium 450 kcal

- ✓ 350 g Sweet cherries
- ✓ 1 tbsp butter
- ✓ 1 teaspoon sugar
- ✓ 3 tbsp port wine
- ✓ 2 branches thyme
- ✓ 60 g skinned almonds
- ✓ 2 tbsp sugar
- ✓ 120 g Butter + some butter for the mold
- ✓ 1/2 Vanilla bean
- ✓ 90 g Powdered sugar + some powdered sugar for dusting
- ✓ 5 Eggs (M)
- ✓ 100 g Quark
- ✓ 30 g Flour

Preparation

- For the cherry ragout, wash the cherries and pluck the stems, cut the fruit in half and remove the seeds. Melt the butter in a pan. Add the cherries and sugar and braise for 2 minutes. Deglaze with the port wine and let the liquid boil down. Rinse off the thyme and shake it dry, remove the leaves and stir into the cherries. Place the cherry ragout in a bowl and let cool.
- Roughly chop the almonds for the curd pudding. Put the sugar in a small pan with 2 tablespoons of water and let it

caramelize until golden brown. Add the almonds to the caramel with 1 tsp butter and mix in. Spread the almond paste flat on baking paper and let cool. Then break into pieces and roughly chop in the Blitzhacker.

- Preheat the oven to 190 ° (better: 170 ° convection) with a deep baking sheet. Halve the vanilla pod lengthways and scrape out the pulp. Place the vanilla pulp with the remaining butter and powdered sugar in a mixing bowl and whip until creamy with the electric hand mixer in about 5 minutes. Separate the eggs and gradually stir the yolks into the butter and sugar mixture. Then mix in the curd. Mix the crushed almonds with the flour and stir into the egg mixture.
- Do not whisk the egg whites with the electric hand mixer and fold them under the almond paste. Lightly grease 6 ovenproof jars (each about 150 ml) with butter. Put a strip of baking paper in each jar, which is slightly higher than the jars and protrudes all around the edge.
- Spread the curd cheese mixture on the glasses and place the glasses on the baking sheet in the oven. Pour boiling water so that the molds are about 2 cm high in the water. Allow the puddles to freeze for 35-40 minutes, after 10 minutes reduce the oven temperature to 170 ° (better: 150 ° convection). Take the quark puddings out of the oven, dust with powdered sugar and serve hot or lukewarm with the cherry ragout.

CREME BRULEE WITH VANILLA AND SAFFRON

Ingredients for serving 2 people

(Preparation time: 60-90 minutes)

Difficulty: medium

- ✓ 200 g cream
- ✓ 50 ml milk
- ✓ 2 Msp. Saffron powder
- ✓ 1/2 Bourbon vanilla bean
- ✓ salt
- ✓ 4 tbsp light cane sugar or brown sugar
- ✓ 2nd Eggs (size S or M)
- ✓ 2nd ovenproof flat molds (approx. 150 ml each)
- ✓ ovenproof flat form or roasting pan
- ✓ Kitchen gas burner (at will)

Preparation

- Mix the cream and milk with the saffron powder in a small saucepan. Preheat the oven to 140 ° (convection not suitable). Place the molds in the larger ovenproof form. Fill this with boiling water to just under 1 cm below the rim of the molds. Remove the molds and place the water bath in the heating oven.
- Slit the vanilla pod lengthways and scrape out the pulp with a knife. Put the pod and the pulp together with 1 pinch of salt and 2 tablespoons of sugar in the saffron cream. Bring them to a boil while stirring. After boiling, pull the mixture off the stove and let it cool for a good 5 minutes.
- In the meantime, stir the eggs well in a bowl, but do not stir until frothy. Stir the cream mixture without the vanilla pod slowly under the eggs and pour everything into the molds immediately. Place them in the water bath in the hot oven and let the cream freeze in 25-30 minutes; the

surface should become a little bit firm and give in slightly to pressure with the fingertip.
- Remove the tins from the oven, let them cool slightly and put them in the fridge for at least 4 hours. To serve, sprinkle the remaining sugar evenly on the well-chilled cream and caramelize with a gas burner. Serve the crème brûlée immediately.

ITALIAN TIRAMISU

Ingredients for serving 12-16 portions

(Preparation time: 60-90 minutes)

Difficulty: Light 295 kcal

- ✓ 4th Egg yolk (M)
- ✓ 1 Egg (M)
- ✓ 80 g sugar
- ✓ 800 g Mascarpone
- ✓ 150 ml cold espresso (not too strong)
- ✓ 6 cl Orange or coffee liqueur
- ✓ 250 g Ladyfingers
- ✓ 2-3 tbsp Cocoa powder

Preparation

- Weigh the ingredients and prepare them.
- Fill a small saucepan 3 cm high with water, bring to the boil and keep hot. Prepare a metal bowl that can later be placed on the water pot without the bottom of the bowl touching the water.

- Put the egg yolks, egg and sugar in the bowl and whisk until light creamy with the whisk of the hand mixer.
- Place the bowl on the water pot and continue to whisk the mixture vigorously and without a break until it is thick and foamy - this takes 7-8 minutes. Whisk as much as possible in the shape of an eight - this way, the mixture is shaken particularly evenly and thoroughly.
- Remove the bowl from the water bath and allow the foam to cool to room temperature, whisking well with a whisk every now and then.
- In between, whisk the mascarpone with the whisk of the hand mixer until it looks a little different than whipped cream. The mascarpone edges are sharper, the tips thinner. Stiffly beaten mascarpone resembles creamy beaten butter.
- Add the mascarpone to the foam and fold in evenly with the whisk.
- Mix the espresso and the liqueur in a deep plate. Gradually dip half of the ladyfingers into portions in the coffee mixture and lay them on the bottom of a tall dish (approx. 20 x 30 cm).
- Spread half of the mascarpone cream on the ladyfingers in the tin. Dip the remaining biscuits in the coffee mixture, distribute in the mold and cover with the rest of the cream, smooth out. Let the tiramisu soak in the refrigerator for at least 4 hours.
- Then pour the cocoa powder into a small fine sieve and evenly dust the tiramisu with it.
- Cut rectangular pieces from the tiramisu, lift them out of the mold and arrange on plates. Serve.

LEMON TIRAMISU

Ingredients for serving 8 pieces

(Preparation time: 60-90 minutes)

Difficulty: Light 395 kcal

- ✓ 3rd Organic lemons
- ✓ 4th Eggs
- ✓ 1 pinch salt
- ✓ 100 g powdered sugar
- ✓ 100 g Flour
- ✓ 1 Str. EL cornstarch
- ✓ 15 tbsp Limoncello (Italian lemon liqueur)
- ✓ 4th Egg yolks
- ✓ 5 tbsp sugar
- ✓ 1 parcel vanilla sugar
- ✓ 200 g Mascarpone
- ✓ 3 tbsp chopped pistachios (as desired)
- ✓ Butter and flour for the mold

Preparation

- Preheat the oven to 180 °. Wash 1 lemon hot, grate zest. Separate eggs. Beat the egg whites with salt until stiff, gradually add the powdered sugar. Add 4 egg yolks one after the other. Mix the flour, starch and lemon zest, fold in.
- Grease the mold, dust with flour. Spread the dough smooth in it and bake in the oven (center, circulating air 160 °) in 35-40 minutes until golden yellow. Let cool down.
- Cut the cake across, soak the cut surfaces with 10 tbsp limoncello. Wash the remaining lemons hot, grate the peel, squeeze out the juice.

- Mix the egg yolks, sugar, vanilla sugar and citrus peel with the whisk of the mixer until creamy white. Stir in mascarpone in tablespoons, adding spoonfuls of lemon juice and other limoncello.
- Spread a third of the cream on the bottom, put the top on and brush with the rest of the cream. Chill for 3 hours. Sprinkle with pistachios as you like before serving.

STRAWBERRY TIRAMISU

Ingredients for serving 4 people

(Preparation time: 60-90 minutes)

Difficulty: Light 635 kcal

- ✓ 1 parcel gluten-free custard powder
- ✓ 250 ml Milk (1.5% fat)
- ✓ 120 g sugar
- ✓ 1 kg Strawberries
- ✓ 100 g cream
- ✓ 200 g low-fat quark
- ✓ 3 tbsp. Almond liqueur (at will)
- ✓ 24th gluten-free ladyfingers
- ✓ 250 ml orange juice
- ✓ 4 tbsp. chopped pistachio nuts

Preparation

- Prepare the custard according to the package, but only with 250 ml milk and 40 g sugar. Place the pudding in a bowl and place cling film directly on the pudding surface so that no skin forms. Chill the pudding until it cools completely.

- In the meantime, wash, clean and quarter the strawberries or cut them into slices.
- Whip the cream until stiff. Add lean quark, remaining sugar and the liqueur as desired in a bowl and whip until creamy with the whisk of the hand mixer, stirring in the spoonful of the cold pudding. Finally, fold in the whipped cream under the cream.
- Place half of the ladyfingers in a rectangular baking dish (approx. 28 × 22 cm) and drizzle with half of the orange juice. Cover the biscuits with half the strawberries and half the cream. Then put the remaining ladyfingers on top, drizzle with orange juice, layer strawberries and cream on top and finally sprinkle with the chopped pistachios. Chill Tiramisu covered for at least 4 hours before serving.

GINGER BREAD TIRAMISU

Ingredients for serving 8 people

(Preparation time: 90 minutes)

Difficulty: Light

- 125 g chopped almonds
- 250 g sugar
- 1 teaspoon Cinnamon powder
- 1 teaspoon ginger bread spice
- Clove powder
- 2 tbsp Rum (at will)
- 250 g Liquid honey
- 125 g soft butter
- 450-480 g gluten-free flour, light
- 1 parcel baking powder
- 300 ml red wine
- 1 teaspoon Cinnamon powder
- 1 parcel Mulled wine spice
- 1 parcel Cream pudding powder
- 100 g sugar
- 500 ml Milk, 1.5% fat
- 200 ml cream
- 400 g Mascarpone (Italian cream cheese)
- Mark of 1 vanilla bean
- Baking dish (approx. 20 x 30 cm); 2-3 tbsp cocoa powder for dusting
- 3rd Eggs (size M)

Preparation

- Preheat the oven to 200 ° (fan oven 180 °). For the gingerbread chopped almonds and 50 g sugar caramelize in a pan over medium heat and let cool slightly.
- Mix the remaining sugar and eggs with the whisk of the hand mixer until frothy. Stir the cinnamon and gingerbread spice, 1 pinch of cloves, possibly rum, honey and the butter in flakes under the egg cream. Add caramelized almonds.
- Mix the flour with baking powder, sieve on the dough and work in with the kneading hooks of the hand mixer. The result is a very compact, firm dough.
- Spread the gingerbread dough on a baking sheet covered with baking paper, bake in the preheated oven (center) for approx. 30 minutes. Let cool down.
- For the mulled wine, put red wine with cinnamon and mulled wine seasoning in a saucepan, bring to the boil and let cool.
- For the cream, mix the pudding powder with 50 g sugar and 6 tablespoons milk. Bring the rest of the milk to the boil, stir in the pudding powder, bring to the boil and allow to thicken. Chill the pudding, then mix with the hand blender.
- Whip the cream until stiff and chill. Mix the mascarpone with the remaining sugar until creamy. Stir in the vanilla pulp and the cold pudding. Finally fold in the whipped cream.
- Cut the gingerbread plate into pieces. Place half of the gingerbread in the mold and soak in half of the mulled wine. Spread half of the mascarpone cream on top, repeat this layering. Chill the tiramisu for about 2 hours. Dust with cocoa powder before serving.

WHITE MOUSSE CAKE

Ingredients for serving 12 pieces

(Preparation time: 90 minutes)

Difficulty: Light

- ✓ 4th Eggs
- ✓ 250 g sugar
- ✓ 200 ml oil
- ✓ 200 ml milk
- ✓ 200 g acc. Almonds
- ✓ 300 g Flour
- ✓ 1 pack baking powder
- ✓ 200 ml milk
- ✓ 400 g White chocolate
- ✓ 2nd Eggs
- ✓ 300 g cream
- ✓ 50 g Flaked almonds

Preparation

- Preheat the oven to 200 ° for the floor. Prepare the mold. Measure out all ingredients and have them ready to hand. Beat the eggs with the sugar thick and creamy in a mixing bowl in 2-3 minutes.
- Add oil and milk while stirring. Mix in the flour, the ground almonds and the baking powder, stir in quickly. Pour the dough into the baking pan and bake in the oven (bottom, fan oven 180 °) for 40-45 minutes. Let cool down.
- Warm the milk for the mousse, chop the chocolate and let it melt. Let it cool a little, then separate the eggs, stir in the yolks.

Beat the egg whites and cream separately and fold in one after the other.

- Divide the floor twice across. Place a cake ring around the base, coat with 1/3 of the mousse, lay on the second base, also cover with 1/3 of the mousse. Put the lid on and spread the remaining mousse on the cake. Toast almond leaves without fat in a pan and sprinkle with the cake. Chill for 3 hours.

MOUSSE-AU-CHOCOLATE SPREAD

Ingredients for serving 1o pieces

(Preparation time: 60minutes)

Difficulty: Light 115 kcal

- ✓ 100 g Dark chocolate
- ✓ 2 tbsp milk
- ✓ 1 pack Bourbon vanilla sugar
- ✓ 1 tbsp sugar
- ✓ 1 tbsp Cocoa powder
- ✓ 3 tbsp ground almonds (best freshly grated in a nut mill)
- ✓ ½ tsp Cinnamon powder
- ✓ 100 g cream

Preparation

- Break the chocolate into pieces and place in a small saucepan with milk, vanilla sugar and sugar. Heat everything over a gentle heat while stirring until the chocolate has melted.

- Add cocoa, almonds and cinnamon to the chocolate mixture and stir until the cream is smooth. Let the mass cool down a bit.
- Whip the cream until stiff and use a spoon to loosely pull it under the chocolate cream. Pour the chocolate mass into a jar with a screw cap, close well and put in the fridge for about 30 minutes before serving. Spread on toast bread, croissants or bread rolls for breakfast and top with a few banana slices as desired.
- Shelf life: chilled 5–6 days.

VEGAN CHOCOLATE NOUGAT MOUSSE WITH MANGO FOAM

Ingredients for serving 4 people

(Preparation time: 60 minutes)

Difficulty: medium 995 kcal

- ✓ 600 ml whipped cream
- ✓ 3 pack Cream fixers (if necessary, observe package instructions for cream)
- ✓ 100 g vegan nougat chocolate (health food store)
- ✓ 200 g Dark chocolate (at least 70% cocoa)
- ✓ 1 Msp. Bourbon vanilla powder
- ✓ Agave syrup
- ✓ 1-2 tsp Agar Agar
- ✓ 1 very ripe mango (alternatively 50 g mango brandy, health food store)
- ✓ Agave syrup (at will)
- ✓ 1 Cream siphon
- ✓ 2nd CO cartridges
- ✓ Decorative fruits (e.g. 4 physalis or 50 g raspberries)
- ✓ 1 Dessert ring (8 cm Ø)

Preparation

- Whisk 400 g of cream for the nougat mousse the day before or in the morning on the day of eating. Chop the chocolate and melt it gently in a water bath. Mix the lukewarm chocolate and vanilla powder under the cream and whip the mixture well again. If the mass is too dry, sweeten with agave syrup.
- Mix the remaining cream with the agar agar in a small saucepan, bring to the boil and simmer for 1 min., Stirring constantly. If the mass thickens too quickly, dilute with a little water. Take off the stove and let it cool lukewarm, stirring constantly. Fold the agar cream under the chocolate cream and whisk everything well again. Chill the mousse for at least 5 hours or overnight.
- Peel the mango, cut the pulp from the core and mash very finely with 100 ml of water. Pass the mixture (or the finished mango pulp) through a fine sieve and, if necessary, season with a little agave syrup.
- Fill the mango mark into the cream siphon and insert 2 CO_2 cartridges. Shake well and chill the siphon for at least 1 hour.
- To serve, wash the fruit if necessary and pat dry. Portion by portion, place the dessert ring on a pre-cooled plate, pour in a quarter of the mousse, press down a little with a spoon and pull off the ring. Spray each of the Mango-Air into a bowl and use a spoon to carefully distribute it around the mousse as a mirror. Garnish with a few fruits and serve immediately.

COTTAGE CHEESE MOUSSE WITH PEACHES

Ingredients for serving 4 people

(Preparation time: 90 minutes)

Difficulty: Light 395 kcal

- ✓ 4 sheets gelatin
- ✓ 400 g lowfat quark
- ✓ 75 g powdered sugar
- ✓ 1 parcel vanilla sugar
- ✓ 3 tbsp Lilac flower syrup (alternatively lime syrup)
- ✓ 2 tbsp freshly squeezed lemon juice
- ✓ 250 g cream
- ✓ 750 g Peaches
- ✓ 1/2 Vanilla bean
- ✓ 2 tbsp sugar
- ✓ 200 ml orange juice
- ✓ Mint leaves for garnish

Preparation

- For the mousse, soak the gelatin in cold water according to the package instructions. Put the curd in a bowl (press the homemade curd into the bowl through the potato press) and stir until smooth with the icing sugar, vanilla sugar and syrup.
- Dissolve the gelatin dripping wet in the lemon juice over low heat. Stir in 2 tablespoons of curd cream and stir this mixture quickly into the rest of the curd cream.
- Whip the cream until stiff and also stir into the quark cream. Place the mousse in a bowl and cover and chill for approx. 3 hours.
- Bring water to a boil in a saucepan for the peaches. Put the peaches briefly in the boiling water, lift out, skin and halve. Remove the seeds and cut the peach halves again. Cut the vanilla pod lengthways, scrape out the

pulp and place in a saucepan with sugar and orange juice. Bring to the boil and simmer for 3 minutes.
- Add the peaches and let them steep for about 5 minutes. Lift them out with a slotted spoon and put them in a bowl. Allow the broth to boil down like syrup, pour over the peaches and let cool. Spread the mousse with the peaches on dessert glasses and garnish with mint leaves.

ALMOND BUTTERMILK MOUSSE WITH APRICOT COMPOTE

Ingredients for serving 4 people

(Preparation time: 90 minutes)

Difficulty: Light 485 kcal

- 1/2 Vanilla bean
- 200 g cream
- 2 tbsp white almond butter (from the health food store)
- 1 1/2 tsp Agar Agar
- 1-2 tbsp Amaretto (alternatively 2-3 drops of bitter almond oil)
- 300 g Buttermilk
- 2nd fresh protein (M)
- salt
- 75 g sugar
- 500 g Apricots
- 1/2 Vanilla bean
- 75 g sugar
- 200 ml fresh pressed orange juice
- 3 tbsp freshly squeezed lemon juice
- 2 Tea spoons food starch
- 3-4 tbsp amaretto (at will)

Preparation

- For the mousse, slit the vanilla pod lengthways and scrape out the pulp. Put the marrow with the pod, cream and almond sauce in a saucepan, stir in the agar and bring to the boil. Add the Amaretto and cook everything for 2 minutes, stirring. Remove from the heat, remove the vanilla pod and stir in the buttermilk. Let the cream cool. Beat the egg whites with a pinch of salt until stiff, gradually pouring in the sugar. Keep beating until a shiny egg snow has formed. As soon as the cream gels slightly, fold in the egg whites. Fill the cream into small portions, cover with cling film and let it set in the fridge in 4 hours.
- For the compote, wash the apricots, halve lengthways and remove the stones, cut the halves into wedges. Slice the vanilla pod lengthways and scrape out the pulp. Caramelize the sugar in a saucepan. Pour in the orange and lemon juice (caution, it can splash!)
- Add the vanilla pulp and cook everything over medium-high heat, stirring, until the caramel has dissolved. Mix the starch with 5 tablespoons of water, add and let simmer for 2 minutes. Add apricots and amaretto as desired and let it heat up. Take it from the stove and let it cool off. Pour the mousse onto a plate and arrange with the compote.

ORANGE CURD MOUSSE WITH MIXED BERRY COMPOTE

Ingredients for serving 4 people

(Preparation time: 60 minutes)

Difficulty: Light 465 kcal

- ✓ 1 Organic lime
- ✓ 3rd Oranges
- ✓ 3 tbsp Cherry water (at will)
- ✓ 1 teaspoon Agar Agar
- ✓ 2nd fresh egg yolk (M)
- ✓ 75 g powdered sugar
- ✓ 1 parcel vanilla sugar
- ✓ 400 g lowfat quark
- ✓ 200 g cream
- ✓ 400 g mixed berries (e.g. blueberries, raspberries, strawberries or frozen berries)
- ✓ 2 1/2 tbsp sugar
- ✓ 1/2 tsp food starch

Preparation

- Wash the lime hot and dry, rub off the peel and squeeze out the juice. Squeeze oranges. Measure out 150 ml of juice, mix with the lime juice and, if you like, put it in a saucepan with kirsch. Stir in the agar, bring to a boil and simmer for 2 minutes.
- Whisk egg yolks, powdered sugar and vanilla sugar in a mixing bowl with the whisk of the hand mixer until creamy. Stir the orange mixture quickly into the egg mixture, then stir in the quark and lime zest immediately. Whip the cream until stiff and fold in as well. Cover and leave to solidify in the fridge in at least 5 hours.
    - In the meantime, wash the berries for the compote, clean them and let them drain. Caramelize sugar in a saucepan. Deglaze with

the remaining orange juice and cook over high heat, stirring, until the caramel has completely dissolved. Mix the starch with 5 tablespoons of water, add to the juice and cook for 2-3 minutes until the orange juice binds slightly. Add the berries, bring to the boil, remove from the heat and let cool. Cut the mousse from the mousse and serve with the compote.

MARZIPAN MOUSSE WITH AMARETTO

Ingredients for serving 4 people

(Preparation time: 90 minutes)

Difficulty: Light 360 kcal

- 5 sheets white gelatin
- 150 g Raw marzipan
- 2nd Eggs (M)
- 2nd Egg yolk (M)
- 5 tbsp Amaretto (alternatively water plus 3 drops of bitter almond oil
- 1 1/2 tbsp sugar
- 250 g cream

Preparation

- Soak the gelatin in cold water according to the package. Finely grate the marzipan on a raw vegetable grater and add the eggs, egg yolks, the amaretto and the sugar to a bowl.
- Hang the bowl in a saucepan of boiling water so that the bottom of the bowl does not touch the water. Whisk everything thickly with the whisk of the hand mixer in 5

- minutes. Squeeze out the gelatin and quickly dissolve in the warm cream, remove the bowl from the water bath.
- Let the cream cool in the refrigerator for 10-15 minutes until it starts to gel. Whip the cream until stiff and carefully but carefully fold under the gelling cream. Cover the bowl with cling film and let the cream solidify in the refrigerator in at least 4 hours.
- To serve, cut off the marzipan mousse with a large spoon.

COTTAGE CHEESE AND POPPY SEED MOUSSE WITH CHERRY WATER

Ingredients for serving 6 people

(Preparation time: 90 minutes)

Difficulty: Light 280 kcal

- ✓ 50 g ground poppy seeds
- ✓ 6 tbsp Cherry water (at will)
- ✓ 5 sheets white gelatin
- ✓ 1 pack vanilla sugar
- ✓ 150 g sugar
- ✓ freshly squeezed juice of 1 lemon
- ✓ 250 g cream
- ✓ 500 g low fat quark

Preparation

- Roast the poppy seeds in a non-fat pan over medium-high heat, stirring, until they smell. Deglaze with 60 ml water and possibly 3 tbsp cherry water, let the liquid boil down completely. Let the poppy seeds cool.

- In the meantime, soak the gelatin in water according to the package. Mix the vanilla sugar, sugar, lemon juice, any remaining cherry water and 50 g of cream until the sugar has dissolved. Add the curd and poppy seeds and stir until smooth. Whip the rest of the cream until stiff.
- Squeeze out the gelatin and dissolve in a small saucepan over low heat. Add 1 tablespoon of curd cream, stir well, add a spoon and stir well again, then stir the gelatin quickly with a whisk under the remaining curd, fold in the cream. Cover the mousse and let it set in the fridge in about 5 hours.
- Cut off the mousse with a tablespoon of cams and serve - for example with spiced cherries or cassis pears.

GOOD MOOD FRUIT SALAD

Ingredients for serving 4 people

(Preparation time: 30 minutes)

Difficulty: Light 145 kcal

- 1 Apple
- 150 g grapes
- 1 kiwi
- 1 banana
- 1 orange
- 2 tbsp dried cranberries (dried fruit shelf)
- 2 tbsp Agave syrup

Preparation

- Wash the apple and grapes. Peel the kiwi, banana and orange. Cut everything into small pieces. (Bananas stay firmer if you quarter them lengthways and then cut them into thumb-thick slices - that makes cubes.)
- Mix the fruit and cranberries with the agave syrup.

FRUIT SALAD WITH LEMON FOAM

Ingredients for serving 4 people

(Preparation time: 30 minutes)

Difficulty: Light 225 kcal

- ✓ 4th ripe nectarines
- ✓ 200 g Raspberries
- ✓ 1 tbsp Pistachio nuts
- ✓ 4th very fresh egg yolk (size M)
- ✓ 4 tbsp sugar
- ✓ Juice of 1 lemon
- ✓ 1/8 l prosecco (or non-alcoholic sparkling wine)

Preparation

- Peel the nectarines with a small sharp knife and cut the pulp into slices from the stone. Read out the raspberries, wash them carefully and drain them on kitchen paper. Spread the fruit mixed in four glasses or on dessert plates. Roughly chop the pistachios.
- Prepare a saucepan with a suitable metal mixing bowl for a hot water bath, pour approx. 5 cm of water into the saucepan and heat. Mix the egg yolks in the bowl with the

sugar and whisk for 3-4 minutes with the whisk of the hand mixer.
- Place the bowl over the hot water bath and pour the lemon juice and prosecco into the egg yolk cream while stirring continuously until an airy foam forms. Remove the bowl from the water bath and continue to beat the foam for 1-2 minutes until it is only lukewarm.
- Pour the lemon foam over the fruit salads and sprinkle the pistachios. Serve the dessert immediately.

VEGAN AMARANTH PUDDING WITH FRUIT SALAD

Ingredients for serving 4 people

(Preparation time: 60 minutes)

Difficulty: Light

- ✓ 200 g Amaranth grains
- ✓ 1 l soy milk
- ✓ 6 Apricots
- ✓ 2 tbsp Walnut kernels
- ✓ 4 tbsp Pomegranate seeds
- ✓ 60 g sugar
- ✓ Cinnamon powder
- ✓ 3 tbsp food starch
- ✓ 2 pack Bourbon vanilla sugar
- ✓ 1 pinch salt
- ✓ 300 g cold whippable soy cream
- ✓ 1 pack Cream fixer

Preparation

- For the pudding on the evening before, cover the amaranth with sufficient water and let it swell for 12 hours. Pour into a colander the next day and drain. Boil the amaranth and soy milk in a saucepan, then cover and simmer over low heat for 25 minutes.
- In the meantime, wash, halve, stone and cut the apricots for the fruit salad and cut them into wedges. Roughly chop the walnut kernels. Mix the apricot slices, nuts, pomegranate seeds and 1 tablespoon of sugar, season with a pinch of cinnamon.
- Mix the starch, vanilla sugar, remaining sugar, salt and ½ tsp cinnamon. Stir the mix into the amaranth and let simmer for about 2 minutes. Let the pudding mixture cool lukewarm in the pot.
- Whisk the soy cream with the hand mixer until foamy. Sprinkle in the cream fixer and continue beating until the cream is firm and foamy. Fold the whipped cream under the pudding mixture. Fill the pudding in four glasses and arrange the fruit salad on it.

QUICK FRUIT SALAD WITH SABAYON

Ingredients for serving 4 people

(Preparation time: 30 minutes)

Difficulty: medium 135 kcal

- ✓ 2nd fully ripe figs
- ✓ 1 kiwi
- ✓ 100 g each seedless blue and green grapes
- ✓ 100 g Strawberries
- ✓ 1 pear
- ✓ 6 tbsp freshly squeezed lime juice
- ✓ 2nd Egg yolks
- ✓ 1 tbsp sugar
- ✓ grated peel of 1 organic lime
- ✓ 1 tbsp chopped almonds

Preparation

- Wash the figs and quarter them lengthways. Peel the kiwi, quarter lengthways and slice transversely. Wash the grapes, pluck from the stems and cut in half.
- Briefly rinse, clean and halve the strawberries. Quarter the pear, core, peel and cut into fine slices. Arrange the fruit decoratively on four plates, drizzle with 2 tablespoons of lime juice.
- Mix the egg yolks with the sugar, 2 tablespoons of warm water and the remaining lime juice and the grated lime peel in the kettle and beat in a hot, non-boiling water bath until the mixture is thick and creamy.
- Remove from the water bath, continue to beat for 1-2 minutes next to the stove and spread lukewarm over the fruit. Sprinkle with the almonds.

TROPICAL FRUIT SALAD WITH COCONUT CREAM

Ingredients for serving 4 people

(Preparation time: 60minutes)

Difficulty: Light 295 kcal

- 150 g small strawberries
- 100 g Raspberries
- 1 pear
- 1 Apple
- 1 banana
- 2nd Kiwi fruit
- 1 1/2 tbsp lemon juice
- 2 tbsp sugar
- 4 tbsp Grated coconut
- 150 g cream

Preparation

- Wash the strawberries carefully and cut out the sepals. Pick raspberries. Peel the pear, apple, banana and kiwi fruit. Quarter the pear and apple, core and cut into wedges. Slice the banana. Quarter the kiwis lengthways, separate the stalk from the center and cut the kiwis into thin slices.
- Mix the lemon juice with 1 tablespoon of sugar, mix in the fruit and let marinate for 15-30 minutes.
- Mix the grated coconut with 1 teaspoon of sugar in a pan and roast without fat while stirring over medium heat until golden yellow. Be careful not to burn them! Put on a plate.
- Do not whip the cream until stiff, pour in the remaining sugar and mix in the coconut flakes. Spread the fruit salad on plates and garnish with the coconut cream.

EXOTIC FRUIT SALAD WITH COCONUT-LIME YOGHURT

Ingredients for serving 4 people

(Preparation time: 30 minutes)

Difficulty: Light 175 kcal

- ✓ 3rd Tangerines
- ✓ 1 papaya
- ✓ 300 g Pineapple pulp
- ✓ 50 ml orange juice
- ✓ 5 tbsp Lime juice
- ✓ honey
- ✓ 300 g Greek or Turkish yogurt (10% fat)
- ✓ 50 g coconut cream

Preparation

- Peel the tangerines, divide them into individual segments and divide them crosswise. Peel and halve the papaya, remove the seeds and dice the pulp. Dice the pineapple pulp as well.
- Mix all the prepared fruits, add the orange juice and 1 tablespoon of lime juice and season with a little honey.
- Place the yoghurt with coconut cream and 4 tablespoons of lime juice in a blender jar and puree until smooth. Season the cream with honey to taste. Divide the coconut-lime yogurt into four deep plates and arrange the fruit on it.

GINGER FRUIT SALAD WITH VANILLA SAUCE

Ingredients for serving 6 people

(Preparation time: 60-90 minutes)

Difficulty: Light 280 kcal

- ✓ 1 Vanilla bean
- ✓ 1/4 l milk
- ✓ 250 g cream
- ✓ 1 tbsp food starch
- ✓ 2nd fresh egg yolk
- ✓ 60 g sugar
- ✓ 1 ripe mango
- ✓ 3rd ripe peaches

- ✓ 1 small ripe honeydew melon
- ✓ 250 g Strawberries
- ✓ 1 piece fresh ginger (approx. 4 cm)
- ✓ 4th Stems of mint
- ✓ 1 Organic lime
- ✓ 70 g powdered sugar

Preparation

- Slice the vanilla pod for the sauce, scrape out the pulp. Put both in a saucepan with 200 ml milk and the cream and simmer for 5 minutes, stirring occasionally, over low heat.
- In the meantime, mix the starch well with the egg yolks, remaining milk and sugar. Pour into the pot while stirring and bring to the boil once, stirring constantly. Take it from the stove and let it cool off. (Fish out the pod before serving!)
- For the salad, peel the mango thinly, cut diagonally from the core and dice finely. Wash, halve, core and dice peaches. Cut the melon into wedges, remove the seeds with a spoon, cut the pulp from the skin and dice. Wash and clean the strawberries and quarter or halve them depending on their size.
- Peel and finely chop the ginger. Wash the mint, pluck the leaves and cut them into strips.
- Wash the lime hot. Rub the peel finely, squeeze out the juice and mix both with sugar, ginger and mint. Mix gently under the fruit and cover and let the salad cover in the refrigerator for 25-30 minutes.

FRUIT SALAD WITH VANILLA SAUCE

Ingredients for serving 10 people

(Preparation time: 30 minutes)

Difficulty: Light 135 kcal

- ✓ 400 g Cream pudding with vanilla flavor
- ✓ 400 ml milk
- ✓ 1 kg fresh fruit (e.g. orange, banana, apple, berries, kiwi, grapes)

Preparation

- For the sauce, simply stir the cream pudding into the cold milk.
- Wash and clean the fresh fruit. Halve or quarter larger fruits. Mix the fruit and eat with the sauce.

FRUIT SALAD WITH YOGHURT CREAM

Ingredients for serving 4 people

(Preparation time: 30 minutes)

Difficulty: Light 405 kcal

- ✓ 1 Charentais melon
- ✓ 500 g soft seasonal fruit
- ✓ 50 g Pine nuts
- ✓ 2 tbsp Coconut flakes
- ✓ 1 cup Cream (200 ml)
- ✓ 1 parcel vanilla sugar
- ✓ 1 cup Vanilla Yogurt (150 g)

Preparation

- Divide the melon once, remove the seeds and scrape out the pulp with an ice cream spoon so that the peel is not destroyed. Cut the pulp into 1 cm cubes.
- Wash the rest of the fruit well and cut it into small pieces. Mix all the fruit well in a large bowl and arrange in the melon bowls. What no longer fits in comes in small bowls.
- Roast the pine nuts briefly in a non-fat pan, add coconut flakes for a few seconds. Spread both evenly over the fruit salad.
- For the yoghurt cream, whip the cream stiffly together with the vanilla sugar using the hand mixer. Stir in the vanilla yogurt and let it flow in slowly just before the cream becomes really stiff. Serve with fruit salad.

Pancakes with apple sauce

Ingredients for serving 4 people

(Preparation time: 60-90 minutes)

Difficulty: Light 630 kcal

For the dough

- ✓ 250 g Flour (Type 405)
- ✓ 500 ml milk
- ✓ 4th Eggs
- ✓ 2 tbsp sugar
- ✓ salt

For the apple sauce

- ✓ 1 kg sour apples (e.g. Boskop or Cox Orange)
- ✓ 3 tbsp sugar

- ✓ 2 tbsp Lemon juice
- ✓ Butter for frying

Preparation

- Mix the flour and milk well with a whisk for the dough. Mix in the eggs, sugar and 1/2 tsp salt. Allow to swell for 30 minutes.
- In the meantime, wash the apples for the applesauce and remove the stems. Cut the apples into rough pieces and put them in a saucepan. Pour in 200 ml of water and bring to the boil. Cook the apples in a closed pot for about 20 minutes over medium heat, stirring occasionally so that nothing burns.
- Rotate the soft apple pieces through the Lotte fleet (pass mill). Sweeten to taste with 2-3 tablespoons of sugar and 1-2 tablespoons of lemon juice. If you do not have a fleet of Lotte, stroke the apple pieces through a coarse mesh sieve. Another option: peel, quarter, core and cook the apples as described. Then puree with the blender, so the applesauce is particularly fine. Let cool down.
- Heat 1-2 teaspoons of butter in a pan, pour a ladle of dough into it and spread it over the bottom of the pan by tilting the pan. First bake the pancake on one side, then turn and bake light brown on the second side. Make eight pancakes this way.

Back to childhood pancakes

Ingredients for serving 2 people

(Preparation time: 60-90 minutes)

Difficulty: Light

- ✓ 3rd Eggs (size M)
- ✓ 1 pinch salt

- ✓ 150 ml milk
- ✓ 150 ml Sparkling water
- ✓ 200 g Flour
- ✓ Butter for baking

Preparation

- Whisk the eggs with salt, milk and mineral water in a bowl. Gradually add the flour and stir in until a smooth dough has formed. Let the dough soak for approx. 30 minutes.
- Heat some butter in a coated pan. Add a ladle of pancake batter and spread well by swirling.
- Bake the pancake until medium brown on both sides in 2-3 minutes until golden brown. Gradually process the rest of the dough as well. Fill the finished pancakes at will, e.g. B. with applesauce.

Buckwheat pancakes with applesauce

Ingredients for serving 4 people

(Preparation time: 60-90 minutes)

Difficulty: Light 815 kcal

- ✓ 350 ml milk
- ✓ 250 g Buckwheat flour
- ✓ salt
- ✓ pepper
- ✓ 800 g Apples (Elstar)
- ✓ 2 tbsp Raisins

- ✓ 2 tbsp Lemon juice
- ✓ 50 g sugar
- ✓ 2nd Eggs
- ✓ 6 tbsp oil
- ✓ 125 g Bacon
- ✓ 4 tbsp Cranberries (glass)

Preparation

- Warm milk, Mix the flour with the milk, lightly salt and pepper. Allow to swell for 30 minutes.
- Peel, quarter, clean, dice and slowly heat with raisins, lemon juice and sugar and cover and simmer for 15 minutes until the apple pieces disintegrate. Let cool down.
- Heat the oven to 75 °. Stir the eggs into the batter.
- Heat some oil in a pan. Briefly fry 2 slices of bacon, pour a little batter over them and roast over medium heat for about 4 minutes, turn and fry on the other side for 3-4 minutes. Keep the pancakes warm in the oven, process the remaining dough as well. Serve pancakes with apple sauce and cranberries.

Crepes with caramelized pineapple

Ingredients for serving 2 people

(Preparation time: 30 minutes)

Difficulty: Light 290 kcal

- ✓ 100 g Flour
- ✓ 1 egg
- ✓ 200 ml milk
- ✓ 50 ml strong espresso
- ✓ 1/2 fresh pineapple
- ✓ 3 tbsp butter
- ✓ 1 tbsp sugar
- ✓ 2 tbsp Maple syrup or honey
- ✓ 40 g dried cranberries

Preparation

- Mix the flour, egg, milk and espresso and let it soak for 10 minutes. Peel the pineapple, cut in half and remove the stalk. Slice.
- Foam 2 tablespoons of butter in a wide pan. Stir in sugar and syrup or honey. Caramelize the pineapple in golden yellow. Mix in the cranberries.
- Gradually bake six to eight thin crepes from the dough in a little butter. Serve with the pineapple.

Currant tonka terrine in a crepe coat vegan

Ingredients for serving 4 people

(Preparation time: 90 minutes)

Difficulty: Light 395 kcal

FOR THE CRÉPETEIG:

- ✓ 1 teaspoon vegan margarine
- ✓ 100 ml soy milk
- ✓ 1 little orange
- ✓ 50 g Wheat flour (Type 405)
- ✓ 1 tbsp sugar
- ✓ 1 teaspoon Egg substitute powder (substitute soy flour)
- ✓ 1 pinch salt

FOR THE FILLING:

- ✓ 100 g Red currants
- ✓ 300 ml whipped cream
- ✓ 1 1/2 pck. Cream fixer (if necessary; observe packing instructions for the cream)
- ✓ about 1/4 Tonka bean (delicatessen)
- ✓ 2 crossed TL Agar Agar
- ✓ Sugar (at will)
- ✓ 1 teaspoon vegan margarine for roasting
- ✓ Terrine shape (900 ml content)

Preparation

- For the crepes, melt the margarine in the soy milk in a saucepan over low heat and let cool. Squeeze the orange.

Mix all the dry ingredients for the crepe dough and stir until smooth with the cooled milk mixture and the orange juice. Chill the dough until ready to use.

- Pluck, wash and drain the currants from the stem for the filling. Whip up the plant cream according to the package instructions, grate the tonka bean. Mix the 80 ml water with the agar agar in a small saucepan, bring to the boil and cook for 1 min. Allow the mixture to cool with stirring for 2-3 minutes and fold into the cream. Beat the clay cheese cream well again and chill.
- For the crepes, melt 1/2 tsp margarine in a coated pan (approx. 26 cm Ø), add half of the crepe dough and spread well by swirling. Bake the crepe in approx. 1 min. Light brown, turn, bake for another 10 seconds from the other side and let cool on a plate. Bake a second crepe from the rest of the dough.
- Line the terrine shape with the crepes. Pour in the cream, press on a little and spread the currants on top. Fold the crepe edges over and tap the bottom of the form a few times on the work surface. Let the terrine soak in the fridge for at least 4 hours, preferably overnight. Before serving, tumble out of the mold and cut into slices.

Lemon crepes with berries

Ingredients for serving 6 people

(Preparation time: 90 minutes)

Difficulty: Light 280 kcal

For the dough:

- 40 g Flour
- salt
- 200 ml milk
- 30 g Cane sugar
- 2nd Eggs

For the lemon cream:

- 4 sheets gelatin
- 2nd egg yolk
- 50 g sugar
- 100 ml White wine
- 100 ml Lemon juice
- 1 teaspoon grated zest of 1 organic lemon
- 4 tbsp milk
- 200 g cream
- Butter for baking
- 150 g Berries (e.g. raspberries or blackberries)
- Powdered sugar for dusting

Preparation

- For the dough, stir in the flour with a pinch of salt, milk and cane sugar. Stir in the eggs one at a time. Leave the dough covered for about 30 minutes.
- In the meantime, soak the gelatine in a little water for the lemon cream. Mix egg yolks with sugar over the hot water bath until creamy. Mix in the white wine, lemon juice and zest. Warm the milk, drain the gelatine and dissolve in it. Stir in the cream. Cover and cover the cream in the fridge for approx. 45 min. Whip the cream until stiff and fold it under the cream towards the end of the gel time.
- Stir the dough. Heat a little butter in the crepe pan, add a little batter with a small ladle and immediately spread very thinly in the pan with the wooden pusher. Bake the crêpe until golden brown, turn and bake the second side. Bake 6 thin golden-brown crepes in this way. Let cool down covered.
- Spread the lemon cream over the crepes, roll up the crepes and cover and chill. Read the berries, wash them and pat them dry. Cut the crêpes diagonally into 3 pieces. Arrange with the berries and dust with icing sugar.

Crespelle with raspberries

Ingredients for serving 4 people

(Preparation time: 90 minutes)

Difficulty: medium 680 kcal

- 150 g Flour
- salt
- baking powder
- 200 ml milk
- 100 ml Mineral water
- 3rd Eggs
- 1 tbsp Clarified butter
- 400 g Raspberries
- 50 g powdered sugar
- 2 tbsp Raspberry spirit
- ½ Organic lemon
- 1 branch mint
- 250 g ricotta
- 50 g sugar
- 1 egg yolk
- 2 tbsp butter
- Butter for the mold

Preparation

- Mix the flour with 1 pinch of salt and baking powder. Mix in milk, mineral water and 2 eggs thoroughly with a whisk. Let the fairly liquid dough soak for about 30 minutes.
- Melt 1 teaspoon of clarified butter in a pan. Pour dough into the pan with a ladle and spread evenly in it by swiveling the

pan. Bake on medium heat for about 1 minute, turn and bake for another 1 minute. Bake about 8 pancakes in this way.
- Preheat the oven to 200 °. Spread a flat ovenproof dish with butter. Read the raspberries, but do not wash them. Mix the berries with powdered sugar and raspberry spirit as desired. Wash the lemon half hot and dry, rub the peel finely. Wash the mint and shake it dry, pluck the leaves and chop them finely.
- Mix the ricotta with the sugar, the remaining egg and the egg yolk. Mix in the lemon zest and mint, carefully fold in the raspberries.
- Spread the mixture on the pancakes, roll up the pancakes and place them side by side in the mold. Cut the butter into flakes and spread on top. Bake the crespelle in the oven (center) for about 30 minutes until they are nicely browned.

Gâteau des crepes with rose cream

Ingredients serving size for a baking ring

(Preparation time: 90 minutes)

Difficulty: medium

Serving size

FOR THE CREAM:

- 200 g Cème double (or 100 g mascarpone and cream each)
- 100 g cream
- 40 g powdered sugar
- scraped out marrow of 1/2 vanilla bean
- 4 tbsp Rose water

FOR THE DOUGH:

- 300 g Flour
- 8th Eggs
- 120 g sugar
- salt
- 600 ml Milk (3.8% fat)
- 100 g melted butter
- 1/2 tsp ground anise
- grated zest of 1/2 organic lemon

FOR THE DECORATION:

- 100 g Rose jam
- 2 tbsp Rose water
- sweetened rose petals
- candied lemon julienne

Preparation

- For the cream, whip the crème double with cream, powdered sugar, vanilla pulp and rose water for 3-4 minutes, then refrigerate. Mix the flour, eggs, sugar and 1 pinch of salt for the dough and slowly pour in the milk. Mix in the butter, then stir in anise and lemon zest. Heat the pan without fat and add 3 - 4 tablespoons of batter. Bake the crepe wafer-thin on each side in 3 - 4 minutes until golden yellow. Bake a total of 14 crepes from the dough as described.
- Place the baking ring on the baking sheet and line it with cling film over the edge. Set aside 4 crepes and line the back ring with 3 crepes, leaving the ends of the crepes hanging over the edge.
- Spray the cream with the piping bag thinly onto the crêpes base. Cover with 1 crepe, again spray a thin layer of cream. Continue like this until all crepes are used up. Finally, spray a layer of cream and fold the overhanging crepe edges inwards. Cover with film and cool for at least 3 hours.
- For decoration, heat the jam in the pot until it is liquid. Stir in the rose water and pour everything through the sieve, allow to cool briefly. Detach the Gâteau from the back ring and remove the foil. Spread half of the jam on the Gâteau, soak the other 4 crêpes with the other half and drape them on the Gâteau. Decorate with sweetened rose petals and leaves and lemon julienne.

Filled espresso crepes

Ingredients for serving 2 people

(Preparation time: 20 minutes)

Difficulty: Light 310 kcal

- ✓ 100 g Flour
- ✓ 1 egg
- ✓ 200 ml milk
- ✓ 50 ml strong espresso
- ✓ 150 g Quark (20% fat9
- ✓ 150 g Natural yoghurt
- ✓ 2 tbsp. sugar
- ✓ 150 g Sour cherries
- ✓ approx. 2 tbsp. butter
- ✓ Powdered sugar for dusting

Preparation

- Mix the flour with the egg, milk and espresso. Let the dough soak for approx. 5 minutes. In the meantime, mix the curd with the yoghurt and sugar thoroughly. Wash the cherries, remove the stones and stir into the quark and yoghurt mixture.
- Gradually bake thin crêpes from the dough in a little butter in a coated pan. Brush with the curd yoghurt cream and roll up. Dust with icing sugar to serve.

Cappuccino and chocolate crepes

Ingredients for serving 4 people

(Preparation time: 30-60 minutes)

Difficulty: Light 505 kcal

- ✓ 80 g Flour
- ✓ salt
- ✓ 2 Tea spoons Instant espresso powder
- ✓ 30 g sugar
- ✓ 150 ml milk
- ✓ 2nd Eggs
- ✓ 2 tbsp melted butter
- ✓ 100 g White chocolate
- ✓ 50 g Creme fraiche Cheese
- ✓ 100 g cream
- ✓ Butter for baking
- ✓ 2nd candied orange slices
- ✓ Powdered sugar for dusting

Preparation

- Mix the flour, a pinch of salt, espresso powder and sugar and stir until smooth with the milk. Mix in the eggs and butter. Let the dough rest for approx. 30 minutes. Break the chocolate into pieces.
- Warm crème fraîche, melt chocolate in it and let cool. Whip the cream until stiff, stir in the chocolate cream. Cover and refrigerate.
- Stir in the dough. Heat a coated pan and spread thinly with butter. Add some dough. Bake 8 thin crepes, keep warm. Arrange crêpes with chocolate cream and orange slices, dust with icing sugar.

Iced almond crepes with raspberry sauce

Ingredients for serving 4 people

(Preparation time: 90 minutes)

Difficulty: Light 440 kcal

- ✓ 60 g Flour
- ✓ salt
- ✓ 1 teaspoon sugar
- ✓ 150 ml milk
- ✓ 2nd Eggs
- ✓ 1 tbsp melted butter
- ✓ 40 g Flaked almonds
- ✓ 2 tbsp powdered sugar
- ✓ 300 g Frozen raspberries
- ✓ 150 g cream
- ✓ 50 g Mascarpone
- ✓ Butter for baking
- ✓ Mint leaves for garnish
- ✓ Powdered sugar for dusting (at will)

Preparation

- Mix the flour with a pinch of salt, sugar and milk until smooth. Add the eggs one by one and stir in, stir in the melted butter. Leave the dough covered for about 30 minutes. In the meantime, mix the flaked almonds with 1 tsp icing sugar. Bring the raspberries and the remaining powdered sugar to a boil in a saucepan, let them cool a little and then pass through a sieve.
- Heat a coated pan and spread with butter. Add a small ladle of dough, sprinkle a quarter of the sugared almond flakes on it and bake 4 thin crepes one after the other. Let cool down.

- Whip the cream until stiff, carefully stir in the mascarpone and two thirds of the raspberry sauce. Spread the cream on the crêpes and smooth out, roll up the crêpes loosely and place them in a freezer-proof form. Cover the mold and freeze the crêpes for at least 3 hours.
- Remove the crepes from the freezer approx. 15 minutes before serving and place them in the refrigerator. Cut into slices 2-3 cm thick to serve. Arrange on plates with the remaining raspberry sauce and mint leaves. Dust with icing sugar as desired.

Rice pudding with cranberries

Ingredients for serving 4 people

(Preparation time: 30-60 minutes)

Difficulty: Light 585 kcal

- ✓ 1/2 l milk
- ✓ salt
- ✓ 250 g rice pudding
- ✓ 3 tbsp sugar
- ✓ 340 g Cranberries
- ✓ 200 g sugar
- ✓ 1 piece Zest of an untreated lemon (approx. 5 cm)

Preparation

- For the milk rice, boil the milk with 1/2 liter of water and a pinch of salt, add the rice. Cook the rice softly over a low heat in approx. 20 minutes, stirring often. Finally stir in the sugar.
- In the meantime, wash and drain the cranberries. Boil 1/4 l of water with sugar and lemon zest, add the cranberries and

let them boil for about 5 minutes until they burst open. Serve the milk rice with the cranberries.

Cranberry-coconut parfait with chocolate-ginger sauce

Ingredients for serving 4 people

(Preparation time: 30-60 minutes)

Difficulty: medium 655 kcal

- ✓ 4th egg yolk
- ✓ 90 g sugar
- ✓ 200 ml Coconut milk
- ✓ 200 g cream
- ✓ 70 g dried cranberries
- ✓ 140 g cream
- ✓ 30 g sugar
- ✓ 100 g Dark chocolate
- ✓ 1 teaspoon Ginger powder
- ✓ rectangular form
- ✓ 1 tbsp oil

Preparation

- For the parfait, heat a little water to a low boil in a saucepan. Whisk the egg yolks in a metal bowl with a whisk until foamy. Let the sugar pour in and continue beating until the mixture is light creamy. Place the bowl on the hot water bath and continue beating until the egg yolk mixture is lukewarm.
- Gradually fold in the coconut milk. Remove the bowl from the saucepan, place in a large bowl with ice-cold water and beat cold with a whisk.
- Whip the cream until stiff and fold it under the coconut cream. Finely chop 50 g cranberries. Brush the mold with oil and line with cling film.

- Pour in the parfait mass and smooth it out. Sprinkle with the chopped cranberries, cover with the excess film and freeze for at least 4 hours or overnight.
- For the sauce, heat the cream and sugar in a saucepan and remove from the heat. Roughly chop the chocolate and let it melt in the cream while stirring. Stir in the ginger powder and let the sauce briefly so that the aroma can develop.
- Take the parfait out of the freezer and carefully drop it. Peel off the foil and cut the parfait into slices. Arrange with the chocolate and ginger sauce on four plates, garnish with the remaining cranberries.

Sweet onion cake with cranberries

Ingredients for 1 baking sheet

(Preparation time: 90 minutes)

Difficulty: Light 190 kcal

- ¼ milk
- 4 tbsp tasteless oil
- 400 g Spelled flour (Type 630)
- 1 pinch salt
- 50 g Beet syrup
- 1 cube Yeast (42 g)
- Flour to work with
- 400 g Red onions
- 500 g fresh or frozen cranberries
- 1 Vanilla bean
- 200 g Brown sugar
- 100 g Raisins
- 400 ml Currant nectar
- 1 tbsp vegetable binding agent (e.g. Biobin)
- 4 sts Proteins

- ✓ 2 Tea spoons Lemon juice
- ✓ 100 g Brown sugar
- ✓ 75 g Flaked almonds
- ✓ Piping bag with perforated nozzle

Preparation

- Heat the milk lukewarm for the dough. Put the oil, flour, salt and syrup in a bowl and crumble the yeast. Use the kneading hooks on the hand mixer until the dough comes off the edge of the bowl. Then knead with your hands on the floured work surface in 5 minutes to an elastic dough. Cover and let rise in a warm place for 45 minutes.
- For the compote, peel the onions and dice them small. Rinse and read fresh cranberries, thaw the frozen cranberries. Slice the vanilla pod lengthways and scrape out the pulp. Melt the sugar in a saucepan over medium heat. Turn onions and cranberries in, add vanilla pulp and raisins. Pour in currant nectar, bring to the boil and let everything boil down thickly in about 10 minutes.
- Preheat the oven to 200 ° (fan oven 180 °). Line a baking sheet with parchment paper. Stir the binder under the compote and let it cook on low heat for 2 minutes until it is lightly bound. Take off the stove.
- Knead the dough again, roll out to the size of the sheet and line the sheet with it, forming an edge. Spread the compote on the dough. Bake in the middle of the oven for about 15 minutes. In the meantime, whisk the egg whites for the meringue, adding lemon juice. Let the sugar pour in and continue beating until a firm meringue is formed. Crumble the almond leaves and fold in.
- Take the sheet out of the oven. Pour the meringue into the piping bag and sprinkle on the cake as a grid or like a graffiti. Bake in the oven at 180 ° (bottom, fan oven 160 °) for another 12-15 minutes until the meringue is golden brown.

Apple cranberry crumble

Ingredients for serving 4 people

(Preparation time: 60-90 minutes)

Difficulty: Light 815 kcal

- ✓ 50 g Walnut kernels
- ✓ 70 g Flaked almonds
- ✓ 750 g Apples
- ✓ 2 tbsp freshly squeezed lemon juice
- ✓ 180 g fresh or frozen cranberries
- ✓ 150 g sugar
- ✓ 1 1/2 tsp Cinnamon powder
- ✓ 4 tbsp Rum (at will)
- ✓ 100 g cold butter
- ✓ 200 g Flour
- ✓ Butter for the mold

Preparation

- Preheat the oven to 180 °, grease a round baking dish (approx. 20 cm Ø) thoroughly with butter. Roughly chop the walnuts and roughly crumble the almond leaves.
- Peel, quarter, core and cut apples into pieces or slices, mix immediately with lemon juice. Roughly chop cranberries (wash fresh fruit beforehand), mix with just under 2 tablespoons of sugar and half of the cinnamon and add to the mold with the apples. Drizzle with rum if desired.
- Cut butter into small pieces, mix with flour, remaining sugar and cinnamon and grate quickly between your hands to form crumbs. Also rub in the walnuts and almonds, spread the crumbs over the apples and press them down lightly.

- Bake the crumble in the oven (center, fan 160 °) for 40 minutes, and then raise the temperature to 200 ° (fan 180 °) and bake for another 10 minutes. Allow the crumble to cool briefly, then serve with vanilla ice cream or with vanilla sauce.

Cranberry baked apple

Ingredients for serving 4 people

(Preparation time: 30-60 minutes)

Difficulty: Light 340 kcal

- ✓ 70 g dried cranberries
- ✓ 100 g Walnut kernels
- ✓ 1 tbsp Maple syrup
- ✓ 1 teaspoon Cinnamon powder
- ✓ 4th medium sized apples
- ✓ Half a lemon juice
- ✓ 600 g Vanilla yogurt
- ✓ Fat for the shape

Preparation

- First, chop the cranberries and walnuts into large pieces with a knife. Then mix both with the maple syrup and cinnamon.
- Then you grease a small baking dish and preheat the oven to 200 ° (convection 180 °). Then you wash the apples, use an apple cutter to prick out the core and some pulp and drizzle the hole with a little lemon juice.
- Pour as much nut and berry mixture into the apple holes as possible. You can spread the rest of the filling on the bottom of the mold. Then put the apples in the mold and let them

bake in the hot oven (center) for about 15 minutes. An apple with 150 g of vanilla yogurt becomes a real meal.

Cranberry-Buchteln

Ingredients for serving 4 people

(Preparation time: 90 minutes)

Difficulty: medium 600 kcal

- ✓ 1 small apple (approx. 130 g)
- ✓ 1 teaspoon freshly squeezed lemon juice
- ✓ 50 g dried cranberries
- ✓ 350 g Flour
- ✓ salt
- ✓ 1 parcel Dry yeast
- ✓ 50 g sugar
- ✓ 1 parcel vanilla sugar
- ✓ 75 g butter
- ✓ ⅛ l milk
- ✓ Butter for the pot

Preparation

- Peel and quarter the apple, remove the core. Cut the pulp into very fine cubes. Drizzle with lemon juice. Chop cranberries.
- Mix the flour, a pinch of salt, yeast, sugar and vanilla sugar in a bowl. Melt 50 g butter in a small pot, pour in the milk and warm it lukewarm. Add the lukewarm milk and butter mixture to the flour mixture and knead quickly. Knead in apple cubes and cranberries. Cover and let the dough rise for 1 hour in a warm place.

- Water the Roman pot. Knead the dough again and shape it into 8 balls of the same size. Grease the Roman pot and put the dough balls in it. Bake covered at 220 ° (fan oven 200 °) for 50 minutes.
- Remove the lid 10 minutes before the end of the cooking time and distribute the remaining butter in pieces on the booklets. Bake open Bayeln. In addition, a vanilla sauce tastes particularly good.

Da Capo smoothie

Ingredients for serving 4 long drink glasses

(Preparation time: 90 minutes)

Difficulty: medium

- ✓ 400 g Cocktail tomatoes
- ✓ 8 tbsp sugar
- ✓ 240 g Strawberries
- ✓ 8 cl Cranberry fruit drink
- ✓ 4 cl Lime juice (best freshly squeezed)
- ✓ 8th Basil leaves
- ✓ 8 cl ice cold soda water

Preparation

- For the tomato sauce, wash the cocktail tomatoes, dry them, halve lengthways and put them in a saucepan. Add 400 ml of water and sugar and bring to the boil once. Simmer open on low heat for 15-20 minutes. Hang a fine sieve in a bowl. Pour the tomatoes into the sieve and let them drain in 2-3 hours.

- Fish the peels out of the cooled tomato paste and throw them away; put the tomato paste in the blender. Measure 4 cl of the drained juice and add.
- Put the undefrosted strawberries with the cranberry fruit drink and the lime juice in the blender as well. Mix everything until a homogeneous liquid is formed. Wash the basil leaves and pat dry. Add with 10 tablespoons of crushed ice and soda water and mix everything again.
- Spread the contents of the mixer over the long drink glasses. Put 1 branch of basil in each of the drinks and serve the smoothies with the drinking straws immediately.

Pear and cranberry sauce

Ingredients for serving 4 people

(Preparation time: 30 minutes)

Difficulty: Light 170 kcal

- ✓ 250 g fresh cranberries
- ✓ 1 pear
- ✓ 120 g sugar
- ✓ Lemon juice

Preparation

- Wash and drain the cranberries. Peel the pear, remove the core and finely dice the pulp.
- Bring the berries to the boil with the pear cubes, 150 ml of water and the sugar and let them boil gently over medium heat until the berries are soft and burst open.
- Puree the sauce and season with sugar and lemon juice.

Yogurt mousse with raspberries and cranberries

Ingredients for serving 4 people

(Preparation time: 60-90 minutes)

Difficulty: Light 160 kcal

- ✓ 200 g fresh cranberries
- ✓ 50 ml Apple juice
- ✓ 100 g Raspberries
- ✓ 3 sheets gelatin
- ✓ 1 tbsp Elderflower syrup
- ✓ 200 g Natural yoghurt
- ✓ 100 g cream

Preparation

- Wash the cranberries, put them in a saucepan with the apple juice and bring to a boil over medium heat until the cranberries start to crumble. Let the mass cool. Pick out raspberries and wash only if necessary. Add raspberries to the cranberries when they are only lukewarm.
- Soak the gelatine in cold water according to the package. Bring the elderflower syrup to the boil. Take the gelatine leaves individually out of the water, squeeze them out, add them to the syrup and dissolve in them while stirring.
- First stir the syrup with 3-4 tablespoons of yoghurt and then mix it with the rest of the yoghurt. Whip the cream until stiff and fold it under the yoghurt. Cool the mousse in the refrigerator for about 1 hour.
- To serve, cut the mousse from the mousse, arrange on four dessert plates and spread some of the berry coulis around it.

White choc cranberry cookies

Ingredients for serving 20 pieces

(Preparation time: 30-60 minutes)

Difficulty: Light 155 kcal

- 80 g Almond pencils
- 120 g butter
- 50 g White chocolate
- 80 g dried cranberries
- 150 g Flour
- ½ tsp baking powder
- ½ tsp salt
- 1 large pinch Cinnamon powder
- 1 Egg (L)
- 150 g Brown sugar
- ½ tsp Vanilla pulp
- 50 g melted white chocolate (at will)

Preparation

- Preheat the oven to 180 °. Line a baking sheet with parchment paper. Lightly roast the almonds in a coated pan without fat, remove and let cool. Froth the butter in a saucepan and simmer gently until golden brown and fragrant. Then fill in a bowl and set aside.
- Roughly chop the chocolate and cranberries. Mix the flour with baking powder, salt and cinnamon. Mix the egg with sugar, liquid butter and vanilla pulp. First stir the flour mixture into the butter mixture. Then carefully mix in the almonds, chocolate and cranberries.
- Remove even portions from the dough with a tablespoon and place them on the tray at a distance of about 8 cm.

Press the piles a little flatter and, if necessary, shape them round with a damp finger.
- Bake the cookies in the oven (center) in approx. 15 minutes light brown. Take out, pull the baking paper on a wire rack and let cool. Decorate with melted white chocolate as desired in strips.

Cranberry almond spiral

Ingredients for serving 4 12 pieces

(Preparation time: 90 minutes)

Difficulty: medium 375 kcal

- ✓ 1 amount of sweet yeast dough
- ✓ 100 g dried cranberries
- ✓ 6 tbsp Amaretto
- ✓ 100 g Raw marzipan
- ✓ 3 tbsp milk
- ✓ 40 g Almonds
- ✓ 1 egg

Preparation

- Prepare the dough according to the basic recipe. Soak the cranberries in 4 tablespoons of Amaretto. Heat the raw marzipan in a saucepan with 2 tablespoons of Amaretto and the milk while stirring over low heat. Chop the almonds and roast them in a pan without fat.
- Knead the dough again briefly and roll it out on a floured work surface to a rectangle (approx. 60 × 40 cm). Spread the marzipan mixture on the dough. Sprinkle cranberries and almonds on top. Roll up the dough from one long side.

- Halve the dough roll lengthways, with the exception of the upper 5 cm, using a sharp knife, so that two coherent strands of dough are formed. Strands, beginning at the connected end, cross each other loosely and lay them into a braid. Then wrap the strand of dough around the top, creating a spiral.
- Place the bread on a baking sheet covered with baking paper and let it rest covered for approx. 30 minutes. Meanwhile preheat the oven to 180 °. Whisk the egg and brush the dough spiral with it. Bake in the hot oven (center) for approx. 35 minutes. Take it out and enjoy it warm.

White chocolate bars with poppy seeds and cranberries

Ingredients for serving 16 pieces

(Preparation time: 60-90 minutes)

Difficulty: Light

- ✓ 200 g sugar
- ✓ 50 g cream
- ✓ 40 g butter
- ✓ 10 g ground poppy seeds
- ✓ 50 g Red wine (alternatively cranberry juice)
- ✓ 200 g fresh cranberries (alternatively frozen cranberries, thawed)
- ✓ 400 g white couverture
- ✓ 30 g Clarified butter
- ✓ fat-soluble red food coloring in powder form
- ✓ high baking frame, set to approx. 14 x 25 cm
- ✓ Oil for the frame
- ✓ Sugar thermometer
- ✓ Bowl of ice water

Preparation

- Place the frame on baking paper and apply a thin layer of oil on the inside. Cook 150 g sugar with cream and butter in a saucepan at 114 °. Quench the pot in ice water, stir in the poppy seeds and whisk the mixture vigorously with a wooden spoon until it becomes thick and crystalline. Fill in the frame and let something solidify.
- Caramelize the rest of the sugar in a saucepan until golden brown, then deglaze with the red wine. Add cranberries and cook gently in about 5 minutes. Puree with a hand blender and push through a fine sieve. Weigh 150 g puree and reheat. Chop 300 g of white couverture, add and melt. Stir until the mixture is smooth. Fill this mass onto the mass in the frame, cover with foil and let it rest overnight.
- Melt the clarified butter in a saucepan and let it cool down a bit. Chop, melt and temper the rest of the white chocolate coating. Mix in the clarified butter. Remove 2 - 3 tbsp and put in a small bowl. Mix with the paint and pour into a piping bag.
- Spread the white chocolate coating on the cranberry mixture. Quickly apply a few thin lines next to each other with the red couverture, run through with a wooden stick at right angles to the lines. Let the couverture set in about 2 hours. Remove the frame, cut the whole into 16 bars of approx. 3.5 × 5 cm. Store cool.

Apple pancakes with honey curd

Ingredients for serving 2 people

(Preparation time: 30 minutes)

Difficulty: Light 550 kcal

For the pancakes:

- ✓ 4th Eggs (M)
- ✓ 2 tbsp milk
- ✓ 1 tbsp honey
- ✓ 50 g Wholemeal flour
- ✓ 2nd Apples
- ✓ 2 tbsp oil

For the honey curd:

- ✓ 100 g Quark (20% fat)
- ✓ 4 tbsp milk
- ✓ 1 tbsp honey

Preparation

- For the pancakes, whisk the eggs with milk and honey in a bowl. Stir in the wholemeal flour and let the dough rest for about 5 minutes.
- In the meantime, mix the curd with milk and honey for the honey curd. Chill until serving.
- Peel the apples and grate roughly on a kitchen grater except for the core. Immediately lift the grated apple under the dough so that it does not change color.
- In a small, coated pan (20 cm Ø), let 1 tablespoon of oil become hot over medium heat. Put half of the dough in the pan and spread evenly in it.

Bake the pancake for about 3 minutes, then turn and bake for about 3 minutes from the second side. Then remove from the pan and keep warm. Heat the remaining oil in the pan and bake a second pancake from the remaining dough.
- Let the finished pancakes slide on two plates. Spread half of the honey quark on top, fold into quarters and serve immediately.

Fast apple roses

Ingredients for 6 pieces

(Preparation time: 30-60 minutes)

Difficulty: Light 200 kcal

- ✓ 2nd Apples
- ✓ 2 tbsp Lemon juice
- ✓ 1 Roll of puff pastry (rectangular; 275 g;
- ✓ 3 tsp Peach jam
- ✓ 6-piece muffin tin

Preparation

- Preheat the oven to 220 °. Halve the apples and remove the core. Cut the apples crosswise into thin slices and cook with lemon juice and 500 ml of cold water in a bowl in the microwave at 650 watts for approx. 3 minutes. Drain and let cool.
- Unroll the puff pastry and roll out to approx. 30 × 45 cm, then cut transversely into 6 strips. Heat the jam with 2 teaspoons of water in the microwave at 650 watts for approx. 30 seconds. Brush the puff pastry strips with it and then cover the apple wedges so that they protrude slightly

over the edge and the lower half of the strips remains free. Then fold the free half of the dough over the apple wedges.
- Roll up the strips. Place apple roses in 1 muffin tin and bake in the hot oven (center) for approx. 20 minutes until they are lightly browned.

Quinoa parfaits with apple pulp and peanut butter

Ingredients for serving 2 people

(Preparation time: 30-60 minutes)

Difficulty: medium 750 kcal

- ✓ 160 g Quinoa
- ✓ 500 ml Milk (cow's milk or vegetable milk at will)
- ✓ 2 Tea spoons ground cinnamon
- ✓ 4 tbsp Peanut butter
- ✓ 120 g greek yogurt
- ✓ 2 tbsp honey
- ✓ 1 Apple
- ✓ 8 tbsp Apple pulp (alternatively: unsweetened applesauce)

Preparation

- Rinse the quinoa cold in a colander. Place in a saucepan with milk and cinnamon powder and bring to the boil. Then cover and simmer over medium-high heat for approx. 15 minutes until all of the liquid has been absorbed.
- In the meantime, mix the peanut butter with the yoghurt and honey in a bowl. Wash, quarter and core the apple. Cut the apple quarters into bite-size pieces.

- Put a quarter of cooked quinoa in two glasses. Then alternately add a quarter of apple pulp, peanut sauce and apple pieces to the quinoa layer. Repeat layering until all ingredients are used up. Finish off the top layer with apple pieces.

Baked apple cupcakes

Ingredients for serving 12 pieces

(Preparation time: 90 minutes)

Difficulty: Light 347 kcal

FOR TOPPING:

- 2nd Apples (approx. 170 g each; e.g. boskop)
- 1 tbsp Raisins
- 2 tbsp Flaked almonds
- 1 teaspoon Cinnamon powder
- 1 tbsp sugar
- 50 g Raw marzipan
- 30 g butter
- 100 g Mascarpone
- 100 g Double cream cheese

FOR THE DOUGH:

- 175 g Flour
- ½ pck. Baking powder (8 g)
- salt
- 100 g butter
- 100 g sugar

- ✓ scraped out marrow of 1 vanilla pod (alternatively 1 tsp vanilla extract)
- ✓ 2nd Eggs
- ✓ 125 ml milk
- ✓ 140 g Biscuits (e.g. speculoos)
- ✓ 12 Paper cases

Preparation

- Preheat the oven to 175 °. For the topping, peel, quarter, core the apples and place them in a flat baking dish. Mix raisins, flaked almonds, cinnamon and sugar. Roughly grate the raw marzipan and stir in. Spread this mixture over the apples and top with the butter in flakes. Add 4 - 5 tablespoons of water.
- Bake the apples in the oven (center) for about 45 minutes until they are soft. Take out of the oven (start the oven), put in a tall mixing beaker and puree. Let the puree cool.
- In the meantime, mix the flour with baking powder and a pinch of salt. Mix the butter and sugar with the whisk of the hand mixer until creamy in about 5 minutes. Stir in the vanilla. Stir in the eggs one at a time. Stir in the flour mixture alternately with the milk at a low setting. Set aside 6 biscuits to decorate, roughly chop the rest and fold under the dough. Place a paper case in each of the recesses in the muffin tray. Fill the batter into the tins. Bake in the middle of the oven for 18-20 minutes. Take out the cupcakes, let them cool briefly, remove them from the tin and let them cool on a wire rack.
- Beat the mascarpone and cream cheese briefly with the whisk of the hand mixer. Briefly add the cooled apple mass. Fill into a piping bag with a large perforated nozzle (14 mm ⌀) and spray as tufts on the cupcakes. Carefully break the biscuits aside in half and decorate the tufts with ½ biscuits each.

Hazelnut brownies

Ingredients for serving 8 pieces

(Preparation time: 30-60 minutes)

Difficulty: Light 210 kcal

- ✓ 50 g Dark chocolate (70% cocoa mass)
- ✓ 50 g butter
- ✓ 1 egg
- ✓ 100 g Brown sugar
- ✓ 50 g Flour
- ✓ 2 tbsp Hazelnut kernels
- ✓ 50 g Nut nougat mass

Preparation

- Line the form with baking paper. Preheat the oven to 175 °. Melt chocolate and butter in a water bath, let cool. Whisk the egg, stir into the cream with sugar and flour. Roughly chop the hazelnut kernels, dice the nut nougat and fold in both.
- Fill the dough into the mold and bake in the oven (center, convection 160 °) for about 20 minutes. Let cool in the mold, then detach and cut into eight pieces.

Brownies with pieces of almond

Ingredients for serving 1 square baking pan

(Preparation time: 30-60 minutes)

Difficulty: Light

- ✓ 250 g Dark chocolate coating (at least 60% cocoa content)
- ✓ 250 g butter
- ✓ 65 g Whole milk couverture
- ✓ 50 g whole unshelled almonds
- ✓ 4th Eggs (M)
- ✓ salt
- ✓ 100 g sugar
- ✓ 150 g ground peeled almonds (almond flour)
- ✓ 1 Msp. Cinnamon powder
- ✓ Cocoa powder or powdered sugar for dusting (at will)

Preparation

- Preheat the oven to 160 ° (fan oven). Line the baking pan with baking paper. Melt the dark chocolate coating and the butter in a metal bowl over the hot water bath. Roughly chop the whole milk couverture and almonds.
- Beat the eggs with 1 pinch of salt and sugar in a metal bowl over the hot water bath with a whisk in 2-3 minutes until thick and creamy. Pour into the food processor and beat cold. Gradually add the dissolved chocolate and butter mixture to the egg mixture and stir well. Finally, fold in the almond flour and cinnamon carefully.
- Pour the dough into the mold and sprinkle with chopped whole milk couverture and chopped almonds. Bake the cake in the oven for 25-30 minutes. Then take out of the oven and let cool in the mold on a wire rack.

- To serve, remove the cake from the mold and cut into rectangular pieces. Dust with cocoa or powdered sugar as desired.
- The chopped almonds for sprinkling the brownies can also be replaced with macadamia nuts, cashew nuts or pecans - roughly chop them for this.

Pumpkin-coconut brownies

Ingredients for serving 20 brownies

(Preparation time: 60-90 minutes)

Difficulty: Light

- ✓ 500 g Nutmeg cubes
- ✓ 280 g sugar
- ✓ 200 g Flour
- ✓ 180 g Grated coconut
- ✓ 2 Tea spoons baking powder
- ✓ 200 g dark block chocolate
- ✓ 150 g butter
- ✓ 5 Eggs
- ✓ salt
- ✓ 150 g white couverture

Preparation

- Drain half of the pumpkin with 30 g of sugar in a sieve. Cook and puree the rest with 50 g sugar for 6 min. Preheat the oven to 180 °. Mix the flour, 100 g grated coconut and baking powder. Melt chocolate with butter.

- Beat the eggs with a pinch of salt until fluffy, add 200 g of sugar. Mix in the chocolate mass, flour and pumpkin. Spread the mixture on a baking sheet covered with baking paper and bake for about 30 minutes (middle; air circulation 160 °).
- Melt couverture in a water bath and spread on the cooled brownies. Sprinkle with grated coconut.

Blondies with raspberries

Ingredients for serving 20 pieces

(Preparation time: 30-60 minutes)

Difficulty: Light 205 kcal

- ✓ 100 g white couverture
- ✓ 225 g soft butter
- ✓ 190 g sugar
- ✓ 1 teaspoon Vanilla sugar or 1/2 tsp vanilla extract
- ✓ 3rd Eggs (M)
- ✓ 225 g Flour
- ✓ 1 teaspoon baking powder
- ✓ 150 g Frozen raspberries
- ✓ Powdered sugar for dusting

Preparation

- Preheat the oven to 180 °. Line a rectangular baking dish (approx. 26 × 20 cm) with baking paper. Crumble the baking paper vigorously once and unfold it again. In this way it adapts well to the baking dish. Finely chop the couverture with a large knife or rub it on the kitchen grater and set aside.

- Mix the butter, sugar and vanilla sugar or vanilla extract in a bowl with the whisk of the hand mixer until creamy for approx. 1 min. Work in the eggs one by one. Mix the flour and baking powder and stir in together with the chocolate coating.
- Quickly fold two thirds of the frozen raspberries into the batter. Pour the mixture into the mold, spread evenly with a spatula and sprinkle with the remaining raspberries.
- Put the mold in the oven (center) and bake the blondies for 35-40 minutes. Take out, lift out of the mold with the baking paper, cut into 20 cubes approx. 6 × 5 cm and let cool. Before serving, sprinkle with powdered sugar.

Nutmeg blondies with Brazil nuts

Ingredients for serving 1 square baking pan

(Preparation time: 60-90 minutes)

Difficulty: medium

- 70 g Brazil nut kernels
- 165 g white couverture
- 125 g butter
- 50 g Whole grain rice flour
- 50 g ground peeled almonds (almond flour)
- 1 heaped teaspoon Locust bean gum (approx. 6 g)
- 3rd Eggs (M)
- 70 g sugar
- grated peel of 1 organic orange
- 3 Msp. freshly grated nutmeg
- 3 Msp. Mace (Macis)
- Butter for the mold
- Whole grain rice flour for the mold
- Powdered sugar for dusting (at will)

Preparation

- Preheat the oven to 185 ° (top and bottom heat). Grease the mold with butter and sprinkle with rice flour. Roast the Brazil nuts lightly in a non-fat pan without stirring, then let them cool and roughly chop.
- Chop 125 g of white couverture and melt with the butter in a metal bowl over the hot water bath. Roughly chop the remaining white chocolate coating and mix with Brazil nuts. Mix rice flour and almond flour with locust bean gum.
- Beat the eggs with sugar, orange peel, nutmeg and mace in a metal bowl over the hot water bath with a whisk in 4 - 6 minutes until thick and creamy. Pour into the food processor and beat cold. Add the chocolate and butter mixture little by little, then stir in the flour mixture. Finally, add the Brazil nut mixture.
- Pour the dough into the mold and prebake in the oven for 10-15 minutes until it starts to brown. Reduce the oven temperature to 170 ° (convection) and bake the cake in about 20 minutes. Take out and let cool in the mold on a wire rack. For serving, dust with icing sugar as desired and cut into pieces.
- Macis, also called mace, is the fine, net-like coat of nutmeg. It is considered an independent spice and has a long tradition in baking. Its flower-like scent further underlines the muscat aroma.

Blondies with white chocolate

Ingredients for serving 16 pieces

(Preparation time: 30-60 minutes)

Difficulty: Light 260 kcal

- ✓ 150 g white couverture
- ✓ 150 g butter
- ✓ 2nd Eggs (M)
- ✓ 150 g sugar
- ✓ 200 g Flour
- ✓ ½ tsp ground vanilla
- ✓ salt
- ✓ 100 g Macadamia nuts (roasted and salted)

Preparation

- Preheat the oven to 180 °. Chop couverture and melt with the butter over the hot water bath. Let lukewarm cool down. Mix the eggs and sugar until foamy with the whisk of the hand mixer for 2 minutes. Stir in the chocolate mixture. Mix in the flour, vanilla and a pinch of salt.
- Cover the bottom of the baking tin with baking paper. Pour the dough into the tin and smooth it out. Roughly chop the macadamia nuts and sprinkle on top.
- Bake in the oven (center) for approx. 20 minutes so that the surface is crispy but the inside is still soft. Take out of the oven and let cool in the mold.

Chocolate cube brownies

Ingredients for serving 4 65 pieces

(Preparation time: 30-60 minutes)

Difficulty: Light 65 kcal

- ✓ 200 g Dark chocolate
- ✓ 150 g Milk chocolate
- ✓ 100 g butter
- ✓ 100 g ground almonds
- ✓ 2 heaped tablespoons Flour
- ✓ 100 g sugar
- ✓ 5 Eggs (M)
- ✓ 1 pinch salt
- ✓ 1 Brownie shape (approx. 24 x 24 cm)

Preparation

- Do not chop the two types of chocolate too finely. Melt 100 g dark chocolate and whole milk chocolate and the butter in a small saucepan while stirring over low heat.
- Preheat the oven to 200 ° (fan oven 180 °), line the brownie mold with baking paper. Mix the almonds with the flour.
- Only stir the sugar, eggs and salt with the whisk of the hand mixer, do not beat until frothy. Then stir in the chocolate and butter mixture, quickly stir in the almond and flour mixture. Spread the dough in the tin and smooth it out. Sprinkle with the rest of the milk chocolate and lightly press into the dough. Bake in the middle of the oven for 15-18 minutes. Allow to cool in the mold.
- Place the remaining dark chocolate in a small bowl and melt over the hot water bath. Brush the cake with the chocolate and let it dry. Then cut the cake into approx. 3 cm brownies.

Cheese cream brownies

Ingredients for serving 8 pieces

(Preparation time: 60-90 minutes)

Difficulty: Light 250 kcal

- 50 g Dark chocolate (70% cocoa mass)
- 50 g butter
- 1 egg
- 100 g sugar
- 50 g Flour
- 25 g soft butter
- 75 g cream cheese
- 40 g sugar
- 1 egg
- 20 g Flour

Preparation

- Line the form with baking paper. Preheat the oven to 175 °. Chop chocolate and melt with butter in a water bath. Let it cool down, whisk the egg, stir in the sugar with the chocolate mass, then stir in the flour.
- Mix the very soft butter and cream cheese with a whisk for the cream cheese cream. Mix in the sugar and egg, finally the flour.
- Spread the chocolate batter into the mold and pour the cream cheese cream on top. Mix the dough with a fork so that it is marbled. Bake in the oven (center, fan oven 160 °) for 30-35 minutes. The dough should still be soft. Allow to cool in the mold, then use the baking paper to remove it from the mold and cut it into eight pieces.

Baileys brownies with nut crust

Ingredients for serving 16 pieces

(Preparation time: 30-60 minutes)

Difficulty: Light

- ✓ 200 g Dark chocolate (50-65% cocoa content)
- ✓ 150 g butter
- ✓ 1/2 tsp soluble cocoa powder
- ✓ 3rd Eggs (M)
- ✓ 150 g light brown raw cane sugar (e.g. Muscovado)
- ✓ 50 g White sugar
- ✓ 1/4 tsp ground cinnamon
- ✓ 1/4 tsp fine sea salt
- ✓ 125 g Flour
- ✓ 25 g weakly deoiled cocoa powder
- ✓ 60 ml Baileys (whiskey cream liqueur)
- ✓ 50 g chopped hazelnuts
- ✓ Brownie shape (20 x 20 cm)

Preparation

- Preheat the oven to 190 ° (fan oven 170 °), line the brownie tin with baking paper. Chop the chocolate finely and melt it together with the butter and coffee powder in a metal bowl over the hot water bath, stirring occasionally.
- Beat the eggs in a bowl with the whisk of the hand mixer or the food processor briefly, add both types of sugar, stir creamy in at least 3 minutes. Stir in the chocolate butter, cinnamon and salt, then sieve the flour and cocoa over it, add the baileys and keep stirring until you have a homogeneous dough.

- Pour the dough into the mold, spread it evenly and sprinkle the nuts evenly over it. Bake in the oven (middle) for 28-30 minutes. Take out, after 10 minutes lift the pastry plate out of the mold using the baking paper and let it cool completely on a wire rack. Then cut into 16 equal pieces.

Apple and cinnamon waffles

Ingredients for serving 10 waffles

(Preparation time: 30-60 minutes)

Difficulty: Light 220 kcal

- 50 g butter
- 300 g Wheat flour
- 1 teaspoon baking powder
- 3 tbsp. Cane sugar
- 2 Tea spoons Cinnamon powder
- 3rd Eggs (M)
- ¼ l milk
- 200 g Natural yoghurt
- 200 g sour apples
- 1 pinch strong salt
- fat for waffle iron

Preparation

- Melt the butter and let it cool lukewarm. Mix the flour, baking powder, sugar and cinnamon together.
- Separate the eggs. Mix egg yolks, milk, yoghurt and liquid butter thoroughly. Then gradually add the flour mixture and stir in.

- Wash, quarter, core and roughly grate the apples. Stir in the dough. Beat the egg whites with salt until stiff and fold in.
- Preheat the waffle maker, thinly grease the baking surfaces. Place about 2 tablespoons of dough in the middle of the lower baking surface and close the waffle iron. Bake the waffle in about 2 minutes until it is crispy and light brown. Take out the waffle, place it on a wire rack and do the same with the rest of the dough.

Basic waffle recipe

Ingredients for serving 2 people

(Preparation time: 30-60 minutes)

Difficulty: Light 1210 kcal

- ✓ 50 g soft butter
- ✓ 1 egg
- ✓ salt
- ✓ 1 teaspoon honey
- ✓ 150 g Whole meal spelled flour (or 100 g +50 g grated nuts)
- ✓ 200 ml Water, juice or milk
- ✓ some oil for the waffle maker
- ✓ 1 Msp. baking powder

Preparation

- Beat the butter until fluffy, then stir in the egg.
- Mix the baking powder, a pinch of salt and the honey with the flour. Gradually stir this flour mixture and the liquid alternately into the butter and egg mixture. Let the dough soak for approx. 10 minutes.

- Preheat the waffle iron, brush the baking surfaces with a little oil. Put 3-4 tablespoons of dough in portions in the middle of the waffle iron, close the lid and bake the waffles in approx. 3-5 minutes until golden yellow. Bake as many waffles until the batter is used.

Chocolate waffles

Ingredients for serving 8 waffles

(Preparation time: 30-60 minutes)

Difficulty: Light 355 kcal

- ✓ 125 g soft butter
- ✓ 75 g sugar
- ✓ 1 parcel Bourbon vanilla sugar
- ✓ 3rd Eggs (M)
- ✓ 250 g Wheat flour (Type 405)
- ✓ ½ tsp baking powder
- ✓ 1 level tablespoon cocoa
- ✓ 150 ml milk
- ✓ 50 g bittersweet chocolate
- ✓ 1 pinch salt
- ✓ Fat for the waffle maker

Preparation

- Beat the butter, sugar and vanilla sugar until fluffy. Separate the eggs. Stir the egg yolks into the butter-sugar mixture. Mix the flour, baking powder and cocoa. Add alternately with the milk. Stir in the grated chocolate. Beat the egg whites with salt until stiff and fold in.

- Preheat the waffle maker, thinly grease the baking surfaces. Place about 3 tablespoons of dough in the middle of the lower baking surface and close the waffle iron.
- Bake the waffle in about 2 minutes until it is crispy and light brown. Take out the waffle, place it on a wire rack and do the same with the rest of the dough.

Rice waffles

Ingredients for serving 8 waffles

(Preparation time: 60-90 minutes)

Difficulty: Light 215 kcal

- ✓ 100 g Risotto rice or milk rice
- ✓ 400 ml Whole milk
- ✓ ½ Vanilla bean
- ✓ 40 g sugar
- ✓ 3rd Eggs
- ✓ 80 g Wheat flour
- ✓ ½ level tsp. baking powder
- ✓ salt
- ✓ 100 ml cream
- ✓ soft butter for waffle iron
- ✓ 2 tbsp. powdered sugar
- ✓ ¼ tsp. Cinnamon powder

Preparation

- Put the rice in a sieve, rinse with cold water and drain. Boil 250 ml of milk in a saucepan, stir in the rice with a wooden spoon. Halve the vanilla pod lengthways with a pointed, sharp knife and scrape out the vanilla pulp

- with the back of the knife. Add the vanilla pulp and pod to the rice. Bring to the boil, then simmer over medium heat for about 20 minutes. Stir frequently so that the rice pudding does not stick to the bottom of the pot.
- Place the rice pudding and sugar in a large mixing bowl and stir with the whisk of the hand mixer. Stir in the eggs one by one. Mix in each egg completely before adding the next one. Then stir the mixture for another 5 minutes.
- Mix the flour with the baking powder, sieve on the rice and egg cream and stir in quickly with the spatula. Mix in a pinch of salt, cream and remaining milk with the spatula so that the dough is smooth. Cover and leave to rest at room temperature for 10 minutes.
- Preheat the waffle iron at medium heat. When the baking temperature is reached, brush the baking surfaces with a little soft butter. Place 3 - 4 tablespoons of dough in the middle of the lower baking surface. Close the waffle maker without pressure. Bake the waffle until golden yellow in about 3 minutes. Place on a wire rack to cool down. Bake more waffles until the batter is used up.
- Mix the powdered sugar with the cinnamon powder in a cup. Dust the still warm waffles with it and serve immediately.

Hearty waffles

Ingredients for serving 2 people

(Preparation time: 30 minutes)

Difficulty: Light 660 kcal

- ✓ 75 g soft butter
- ✓ 2nd Eggs
- ✓ salt
- ✓ 100 g Whole wheat flour
- ✓ 1/2 tsp baking powder
- ✓ 40 g grated mountain cheese (45% fat in dry matter)
- ✓ 2 tbsp chopped parsley
- ✓ 100 g sour cream (10% fat)
- ✓ Nutmeg, freshly grated
- ✓ pepper
- ✓ Oil for the waffle maker

Preparation

- Mix the butter until frothy. Add the eggs and a pinch of salt and beat until creamy. Mix the flour with the baking powder. Mix in the flour, cheese, parsley and 4 tablespoons of sour cream one after the other. Season the dough with some nutmeg and pepper.
- Preheat and grease the waffle iron on a medium setting. Place the dough on the lower baking surface and bake golden yellow waffles one after the other in 2-3 minutes. Mix the remaining sour cream until smooth and serve with the waffles.

CONCLUSION

While eating in restaurant is a reward for some families, it has become a standard comfort for some individuals. You get benefits in the regions of nourishment, wellbeing and financial matters when you limit feasting out and start eating your own one of a kind copycat plans food.

Copycat food permit you to control the fixings in your food, so you can utilize common fixings rather than unfortunate prepared nourishments. Handled nourishments, often served in eateries or accessible in premade suppers from the supermarket, will in general be high in sodium, fat and included sugars. As per the BBC, the World Wellbeing Association suggests enormously diminishing the admission of prepared nourishments. Eating natively constructed nourishments lets you include all the newer products of the soil to your weight control plans with the goal that you can concentrate on every regular fixing.

Sirtfood Diet

Cookbook for Beginners with Easy and Healthy Recipes for a Rapid Weight Loss. Burn your Body Fat and Improve your Metabolism with the Sirt Foods.

ASHLEY GOSLING

Copyright © 2020 Ashley Gosling

All rights reserved.

DEDICATION

This book is dedicated to everyone who wants to live a healthier lifestyle and challenge himself of herself with this noble purpose. Every little success is a great success in reality.

Every little step matters.

DISCLAIMER

All the informations included in this book are given for instructive, informational and entertainment purposes, the author can claim to share very good quality recipes but is not headed for the perfect data and uses of the mentioned recipes, in fact the informations are not intent to provide dietary advice without a medical consultancy.

The author does not hold any responsibility for errors, omissions or contrary interpretation of the content in this book.

It is recommended to consult a medical practitioner before to approach any kind of diet, especially if you have a particular health situation, the author isn't headed for the responsibility of these situations and everything is under the responsibility of the reader, the author strongly recommend to preserve the health taking all precautions to ensure ingredients are fully cooked.

All the trademarks and brands used in this book are only mentioned to clarify the sources of the informations and to describe better a topic. All the trademarks and brands mentioned own their copyrights and they are not related in any way to this document and to the author.

This document is written to clarify all the informations of publishing purposes and cover any possible issue. This document is under copyright and it is not possible to reproduce any part of this content in every kind of digital or printable document. All rights reserved.

Spinach Green Juice

Prep Time   10 min

Servings 1

INGREDIENTS

- 1 bunch spinach
- 1 kiwi fruit
- 1 apple
- large stalks green celery, including leaves
- half a lemon, juiced
- 1 tsp. matcha green tea

DIRECTIONS

1. Extract the juice of spinach, apple and kiwi fruit.
2. Pour a Half juice into a glass, then add the matcha, lemon juice and mix well with fork.
3. Once the matcha is dissolved add the
4. remainder of the juice.
5. Mix well.
6. Pour some water on top.
7. Enjoy!

NUTRITIONAL INFORMATION

Calories Per Servings, 181 kcal, 1.72 g Fat, 39.64 g Total Carbs, 10.41 g

Protein, 12.2 g Fiber

Berries Green Juice

Prep Time 10 min
Servings 1

INGREDIENTS

- 1 bunch mint leaves
- 1 apple
- ¼ cup mix berries
- 1/8 tsp. ginger
- half a lemon, juiced
- 1 tsp. matcha green tea

DIRECTIONS

1. Extract the juice of mint leaves, apple and berries.
2. Pour a Half juice into a glass, then add the matcha, lemon juice and mix well with fork.
3. Once the matcha is dissolved add the
4. remainder of the juice.
5. Mix well.
6. Pour some water on top.
7. Enjoy!

NUTRITIONAL INFORMATION

Calories Per Servings, 121 kcal, 0.49 g Fat, 32.2 g Total Carbs, 0.85 g Protein, 5.3 g Fiber

Broccoli Green Juice

Prep Time   10 min

Servings 1

INGREDIENTS

- 1 bunch spinach
- 1 apple
- 1 cup broccoli
- 1/8 tsp ginger.
- half a lemon, juiced
- 1 tsp. matcha green tea

DIRECTIONS

1. Extract the juice of spinach, apple and broccoli florets.
2. Pour a Half juice into a glass, then add the matcha, lemon juice and mix well with fork.
3. Once the matcha is dissolved add the
4. remainder of the juice.
5. Mix well.
6. Pour some water on top.
7. Enjoy!

NUTRITIONAL INFORMATION

Calories Per Servings, 187 kcal, 1.89 g Fat, 40.33 g Total Carbs, 11.56 g Protein, 13 g Fiber

Mix Green Juice

Prep Time   10 min

Servings 1

INGREDIENTS
- 1 bunch parsley
- 1 apple
- 1 cucumber
- half a lemon, juiced
- 1 tsp. matcha green tea

DIRECTIONS

1. Extract the juice of parsley apple and cucumber.
2. Pour a Half juice into a glass, then add the matcha, lemon juice and mix well with fork.
3. Once the matcha is dissolved add the
4. remainder of the juice.
5. Mix well.
6. Pour some water on top.
7. Enjoy!

NUTRITIONAL INFORMATION

Calories Per Servings, 146 kcal, 1.16 g Fat, 33.93 g Total Carbs, 3.53 g Protein, 7.8 g Fiber

Celery Green Juice

Prep Time   10 min

Servings 1

INGREDIENTS

- 5 -8 stalks celery with leaves
- 1 apple
- half a lemon, juiced
- 1 tsp. matcha green tea

DIRECTIONS

1. Extract the juice of celery and apple.
2. Pour a Half juice into a glass, then add the matcha, lemon juice and mix well with fork.
3. Once the matcha is dissolved add the
4. remainder of the juice.
5. Mix well.
6. Pour some water on top.
7. Enjoy!

NUTRITIONAL INFORMATION

Calories Per Servings, 118 kcal, 0.55 g Fat, 30.07 g Total Carbs, 1.33 g Protein, 6.2 g Fiber

Kale Green Juice

Prep Time   10 min

Servings 1

INGREDIENTS

- 2 bunch kale
- 1 apple
- 2 stalk celery with leaves
- half a lemon, juiced
- 1 tsp. matcha green tea

DIRECTIONS

1. Extract the juice of kale, apple and celery.
2. Pour a Half juice into a glass, then add the matcha, lemon juice and mix well with fork.
3. Once the matcha is dissolved add the
4. remainder of the juice.
5. Mix well.
6. Pour some water on top.

Enjoy!

NUTRITIONAL INFORMATION

Calories Per Servings, 171 kcal, 1.67 g Fat, 39.53 g Total Carbs, 6.54 g Protein, 9.8 g Fiber

Spinach & Apple Juice

Prep Time   10 min

Servings 1

INGREDIENTS

- 1 bunch baby spinach
- 1 apple
- half a lemon, juiced
- 1 tsp. matcha green tea

DIRECTIONS

1. Extract the juice of spinach, and apple.
2. Pour a Half juice into a glass, then add the matcha, lemon juice and mix well with fork.
3. Once the matcha is dissolved add the
4. remainder of the juice.
5. Mix well.
6. Pour some water on top.

Enjoy!

NUTRITIONAL INFORMATION

Calories Per Servings, 178 kcal, 1.69 g Fat, 39.13 g Total Carbs, 10.29 g Protein, 11.9 g Fiber

Cucumber Green Juice

Prep Time   10 min

Servings 1

INGREDIENTS

- 1 cucumber
- 1 green apple
- half a lemon, juiced
- 1 tsp. matcha green tea

DIRECTIONS

1. Extract the juice of cucumber and apple.
2. Pour a Half juice into a glass, then add the matcha, lemon juice and mix well with fork.
3. Once the matcha is dissolved add the
4. remainder of the juice.
5. Mix well.
6. Pour some water on top.

Enjoy!

NUTRITIONAL INFORMATION

Calories Per Servings, 124 kcal, 0.69 g Fat, 31.13 g Total Carbs, 1.75 g Protein, 5.8 g Fiber

Creamy Spinach Juice

Prep Time   10 min

Servings 1

INGREDIENTS

- 1 bunch spinach
- ½ cup soy milk
- half a medium green apple
- half a lemon, juiced
- 1 tsp. matcha green tea

DIRECTIONS

1. Extract the juice of spinach and apple.
2. Pour a Half juice into a glass, then add the matcha, lemon juice and mix well with fork.
3. Once the matcha is dissolved add the remainder of the juice.
4. Mix well.
5. Pour some water on top.
6. Enjoy!

NUTRITIONAL INFORMATION

Calories Per Servings, 185 kcal, 3.35 g Fat, 32.68 g Total Carbs, 13.28 g Protein, 10 g Fiber

Parsley Green Juice

Prep Time   10 min

Servings   1

INGREDIENTS

- 1 bunch parsley
- 1 apple
- large stalks green celery, including leaves
- half a lemon, juiced
- 1 tsp. matcha green tea

DIRECTIONS

Extract the juice of parsley apple and stalk.

1. Pour a Half juice into a glass, then add the matcha, lemon juice and mix well with fork.
2. Once the matcha is dissolved add the
3. remainder of the juice.
4. Mix well.
5. Pour some water on top.
6. Enjoy!

NUTRITIONAL INFORMATION

Calories Per Servings, 124 kcal, 0.87 g Fat, 31.9 g Total Carbs, 2.47 g Protein, 6.7 g Fiber

Apple Porridge

Prep Time   10 Min

Servings   4

INGREDIENTS

- 2 apples, chopped
- 3 cups walnut milk
- 1 tsp. cinnamon
- 2 tsp. dates syrup
- TOPPING
- Blueberries
- dark chocolate
- apple slice
- walnuts

DIRECTIONS

1. Mix all ingredients together in a bowl that fits inside the bowl of your slow cooker.
2. Place the bowl in your slow cooker, and fill your slow cooker with 1 cup of water to surround the bowl.
3. Cook on LOW 6-8 hours, stirring occasionally.
4. Carefully remove the bowl.
5. Top with banana slice and berries.
6. Serve and enjoy!

NUTRITIONAL INFORMATION

Calories Per Servings, 227 kcal, 7.04 g Fat, 36.45 g Total Carbs, 6.95 g Protein, 4.3 g Fiber

Spinach Omelet

Prep Time   20 min

Servings 2

INGREDIENTS

- 2 cups baby spinach, finely chopped
- 1 cup, chopped onion
- 1 cup buckwheat flour
- ¼ cup water
- salt & pepper to taste
- 1 tsp. paprika powder
- 1 tsp. oregano
- olive oil for frying

DIRECTIONS

1. Mix flour, spinach, salt, pepper, oregano and paprika in a bowl and mix well.
2. Add water slowly in the mixture to make a thick batter.
3. Place a frying pan over medium heat and grease with olive oil.
4. Pour ¼ cup mixture in skillet and spread it evenly.
5. Once cooked, flip and cook for another 2-3 minutes.
6. Once the omelet is cooked remove from heat.
7. Serve with spinach leaves, tomato slice, and cucumber slice.
8. Enjoy!

NUTRITIONAL INFORMATION

Calories Per Servings, 283 kcal, 3.02 g Fat, 57.39 g Total Carbs, 14.52 g Protein, 12.5 g Fiber

Tofu & Kale Toast

Prep Time   10 min

Servings 4

INGREDIENTS

- 1 tsp. capers, drained and loosely chopped
- sea salt and black pepper
- 1 tsp. sesame seeds
- 1/4 cup guacamole
- 8 oz. tofu, firm and drained
- 4 slices buckwheat bread
- 4 oz. kale
- 1 tbsp. olive oil

DIRECTIONS

1. Heat olive oil in pan over medium heat and fry tofu until golden brown from all sides.
2. Add capers, salt and pepper to a mixing bowl.
3. Taste and adjust seasonings as needed.
4. Toast bread on heated griddle for 2-3 minutes per side.
5. Spread guacamole on each bread slice and arrange in plate.
6. Arrange tofu on bread slice with kale.
7. Drizzle sesame seeds.
8. Serve and enjoy!

NUTRITIONAL INFORMATION

Calories Per Servings, 216 kcal, 17.36 g Fat, 8.43 g Total Carbs, 10.45 g Protein, 3.5 g Fiber

Tofu Scramble

Prep Time   20 min

Servings 2

INGREDIENTS

- 1 tablespoon olive oil
- 16 oz. block firm tofu
- 1 teaspoon salt
- 1/4 teaspoon turmeric
- 1/4 teaspoon garlic powder
- 2 tablespoons soy milk

DIRECTIONS

1. Heat the olive oil in a pan over medium heat. Mash the block of tofu right in the pan, with a potato masher or a fork.
2. Cook, stirring frequently, for 3-4 minutes until the water from the tofu is dried.
3. Add salt, turmeric and garlic powder. Cook and stir constantly for about 5 minutes.
4. Pour the milk into the pan, and stir to mix. Serve immediately.
5. Enjoy!

NUTRITIONAL INFORMATION

Calories Per Servings, 208 kcal, 15.44 g Fat, 5.45g Total Carbs, 15.2 g Protein, 0.6 g Fiber

Buckwheat Pancakes

Prep Time	20 min

Servings 3

INGREDIENTS

- 1 cup buckwheat flour
- 2 tbsps. dates syrup
- 1 cup soya milk
- 1 tbsps. olive oil

DIRECTIONS

1. Mix all ingredients in bowl.
2. Heat oil in pan over medium heat. Once oil is hot pour ¼ cup buckwheat batter and spread evenly.
3. Cook for 2-3 minutes until golden brown.
4. Flip and cook again.
5. Once cooked remove from heat.
6. Serve and enjoy!

NUTRITIONAL INFORMATION

Calories Per Servings, 197 kcal, 3.92 g Fat, 35.68 g Total Carbs, 7.73 g Protein, 4.43g Fiber

Waffle Sandwich

Prep Time   10 min

Servings 4

INGREDIENTS
- 1 1/2 cups buckwheat flour
- 2 teaspoons baking powder
- 1 teaspoon baking soda
- 1/4 teaspoon salt
- 1/4 teaspoon cinnamon, optional
- 1 1/2 cups soy milk,
- 1 tablespoon apple cider vinegar
- 1/8 cup olive oil

SERVING
- lettuce leaves
- cucumber slice

DIRECTIONS

1. Mix all ingredients in bowl until well incorporated.
2. Preheat a waffle iron and light grease with cooking spray. Cook waffles according to the manufacturer's instructions.
3. Serve with lettuce leaves and cucumber slice between two waffles.
4. Enjoy!

NUTRITIONAL INFORMATION

Calories Per Servings, 260 kcal, 10.27 g Fat, 38.37 g Total Carbs, 7.16 g Protein, 4.7 g Fiber

Buckwheat Porridge

Prep Time   10 min

Servings 4

INGREDIENTS

- 1 cup buckwheat groats
- 3 cups water
- 1 tablespoon walnut butter
- ½ tablespoon salt
- ½ cup soya milk
- 1 teaspoon dates syrup

DIRECTIONS

1. In a saucepan bring water to boil. Add uncooked buckwheat groats. Cover the pot and simmer for 10 minutes (or until water is absorbed).
2. Turn off heat, add the salt, dates syrup and let it sit for 10 more minutes.
3. Top with butter and serve warm in a savory dish, or as a porridge with milk and toppings.

NUTRITIONAL INFORMATION

Calories Per Servings, 188 kcal, 4.6 g Fat, 33.56 g Total Carbs, 5.85 g Protein, 4.2 g Fiber

Toast with Caramelized Apple

Prep Time   10 min

Servings 2

INGREDIENTS

- 2 slice buckwheat bread slices
- 2 oz. chocolate cream
- 1 cup apple
- 2 tbsps. dates syrup
- 1/2 cup water

DIRECTIONS

1. Grill bread for 2 minutes.
2. Heat water in a pan over medium heat.
3. Add dates syrup and apple and cook for 5-8 minutes until apples are soft and caramelize.
4. Spread chocolate cream over the grill bread slice.
5. Sprinkle caramelize apple on top.
6. Serve and enjoy!

NUTRITIONAL INFORMATION

Calories Per Servings, 168 kcal, 7.13 g Fat, 25.45 g Total Carbs, 2.44 g Protein, 2.9 g Fiber

Buckwheat Crepe with Apple

Prep Time   20 min

Servings 4

INGREDIENTS

- 1 cup buckwheat flour
- 2 tbsps. dates syrup
- 1 cup soy milk
- olive oil
- 2 oz. Caramelized apple

DIRECTIONS

1. Mix all ingredients in bowl.
2. Heat oil in pan over medium heat. Once oil is hot pour ¼ cup buckwheat batter and spread evenly.
3. Cook for 2-3 minutes until golden brown.
4. Flip and cook again.
5. Once cooked remove from heat.
6. Wrap with caramelized apple.
7. Serve and enjoy

NUTRITIONAL INFORMATION

Calories Per Servings, 121 kcal, 0.49 g Fat, 32.2 g Total Carbs, 0.85 g Protein, 5.3 g Fiber

Buckwheat & Apple Porridge

Prep Time   20 min

Servings 2

INGREDIENTS

- 1 cup buckwheat groats
- 2 cups soy milk
- pinch of salt
- 1 tsp cinnamon
- 1 sour apple
- Topping
- 1 apple, chopped
- 1 oz. walnuts

DIRECTIONS

1. Bring milk to a boil, season lightly with salt and add buckwheat groats.
2. Add cinnamon to taste, and a grated sour apple.
3. Cook for about 8 minutes, then low the heat and let the buckwheat rest in a covered pot for another 10 minutes.
4. Serve the buckwheat porridge with apple and walnuts topping.
5. Enjoy

NUTRITIONAL INFORMATION

Calories Per Servings, 292 kcal, 10.15 g Fat, 44 g Total Carbs, 10.7 g Protein, 6.2 g Fiber

Acai Berry Smoothie Bowl

Prep Time   5 min

Servings 1

INGREDIENTS

- 1/2 cup walnut milk
- 1 cup acai berry
- 1/4 tsp salt
- Fresh berries for topping

DIRECTIONS

1. Blend milk, berries salt, in a blender and blend on high speed.
2. Pour the smoothie in a bowl.
3. Top with raspberries, blueberries.
4. Serve cool and enjoy!

NUTRITIONAL INFORMATION

Calories Per Servings, 207 kcal, 10.43 g Fat, 27.1 g Total Carbs, 2.42 g Protein, 1.1 g Fiber

Buckwheat Salad Bowl

Prep Time   10 min

Servings 2

INGREDIENTS
- 1 cup buckwheat groats, cooked
- 1 red onion, sliced
- 1bunch parsley leaves
- I bunch arugula leaves.
- 2-3 tomatoes, sliced

DRESSING
- ¼ cup lemon juice
- 1 tbsp. olive oil
- Salt & pepper to taste
- 1 tsp garlic powder.

DIRECTIONS
1. Mix together dressing ingredients in bowl and set aside.
2. Chop veggies and arrange in bowl with cooked buckwheat.
3. Drizzle dressing over veggies.
4. Slightly mix.
5. Serve and enjoy!

NUTRITIONAL INFORMATION

Calories Per Servings, 188 kcal, 0.49 g Fat, 8.37 g Total Carbs, 6.98 g Protein, 5.5 g Fiber

Spinach Avocado Pomegranate Seeds

Prep Time   15 Min

Servings 2

INGREDIENTS

- 1 pack baby spinach
- ½ avocado, thinly sliced
- 4 oz. pomegranate seed

DRESSING

- 1 tbsp. olive oil
- 1 tbsp. lime juice
- 1 pinch salt and pepper

DIRECTIONS

1. Add all veggies in mixing bowl.
2. Mix dressing ingredients in bowl and pour over veggies.
3. Serve cold and enjoy!

NUTRITIONAL INFORMATION

Calories Per Servings, 237 kcal, 15.49 g Fat, 15.49 g Total Carbs, 7.3 g Protein, 9.7 g Fiber

Beetroot Salad with Spinach

Prep Time   15 Min

Servings 2

INGREDIENTS

- 1 pack baby spinach
- 1 beet root, sliced
- 1 oz. walnuts
- 4 oz. cranberries
- 1 oz. feta cheese crumbled

Dressing

- 1 tbsp. sesame oil
- 1 lime juice
- 1 pinch garlic salt

DIRECTIONS

1. Add all veggies in mixing bowl.
2. Mix dressing ingredients in bowl and pour over veggies.
3. Serve cold and enjoy!

NUTRITIONAL INFORMATION

Calories Per Servings, 121 kcal, 0.49 g Fat, 32.2 g Total Carbs, 0.85 g Protein, 5.3 g Fiber

Berries Salad with Spinach

Prep Time   15 Min

Servings 2

INGREDIENTS

1 pack arugula leaves
8 oz. strawberries, sliced
1 oz. walnuts
2 oz. smoked tofu

Dressing
1 tbsp. olive oil
1 lime juice
1 pinch garlic salt

DIRECTIONS

1. Add all veggies in mixing bowl.
2. Mix dressing ingredients in bowl and pour over veggies.
3. Serve cold and enjoy!

NUTRITIONAL INFORMATION

Calories Per Servings, 271 kcal, 22.09 g Fat, 15.48 g Total Carbs, 7.89 g Protein, 4.4 g Fiber

Pomegranate Salad with Spinach

Prep Time   15 Min

Servings 2

INGREDIENTS

- 1 pack baby spinach
- 1 cup pomegranate seeds
- 4-5 lettuce leaves, chopped

Dressing
- 1 tbsp. olive oil
- 1 lime juice
- 1 pinch garlic salt

DIRECTIONS

1. Add all veggies in mixing bowl.
2. Mix dressing ingredients in bowl and pour over veggies.
3. Serve cold and enjoy!

NUTRITIONAL INFORMATION

Calories Per Servings, 237 kcal, 9.35 g Fat, 37.15 g Total Carbs, 8.89 g Protein, 10.8 g Fiber

Hot & Spicy Tofu & Broccoli

Prep Time   20 min

Servings 2

INGREDIENTS

- 8 –12 oz. extra firm tofu
- 2 tbsps. olive oil
- ½ tsp. salt
- 1 tsp. garlic, minced
- 8 oz. broccoli, cut into florets
- 1 tsp. chili sauce and chili flakes
- 1 1/2 Soy Sauce
- 1 tbsp. toasted sesame seeds

DIRECTIONS

1. Heat oil in a large skillet over medium heat.
2. Once oil is hot, add broccoli and cook for 5 minutes.
3. Add salt, pepper and garlic, and cook for 1-2 minutes until the garlic is fragrant.
4. Mix the chili sauce, and soy sauce in a small bowl. Set aside.
5. Fry tofu in same pan for 4-5 minutes.
6. Serve tofu with broccoli.
7. Drizzle sesame seeds on top.
8. Serve and enjoy

NUTRITIONAL INFORMATION

Calories Per Servings, 273 kcal, 22.6 g Fat, 7.19 g Total Carbs, 15.62 g Protein, 4.3 g Fiber

Stir Fried Spinach

Prep Time   20 Min

Servings 2

INGREDIENTS
- 1 lb. spinach, trimmed
- 1 tbsp. paprika
- 1 tbsp. garlic, minced
- Salt and pepper, to taste
- 2-3 whole red pepper
- 2 tbsps. olive oil
- 2 cups vegetable broth

DIRECTIONS

Heat oil in a pan over medium heat.
Once the oil is hot, add garlic and sauté for 1 minute.
Add spinach in the same pan and cook for 4-5 minutes until spinach is welted.
Season with salt, pepper, and whole chili.
Add vegetable broth and cook for 5-10 minutes on medium heat.
Once cooked remove from heat.
Serve hot and enjoy!

NUTRITIONAL INFORMATION

Calories Per Servings, 242 kcal, 8.58 g Fat, 33.74 g Total Carbs, 14.28 g Protein, 9.2 g Fiber

Kale Stew

Prep Time   20 Min

Servings 2

INGREDIENTS
- 1 lb. kale trimmed and cut
- 1 tsp. cumin seeds
- 2 tbsps. dates syrup
- 1 tbsp. paprika
- 1 tbsp. garlic, roughly crushed
- Salt and pepper, to taste
- 2 tbsps. olive oil
- 1 cup vegetable broth

DIRECTIONS
Heat the oil in pan over medium heat.
Once the oil is hot, add garlic and sauté for 2-4 minutes.
Add kale and cook for 4-5 minutes.
Season with salt, pepper, red and dates
Add vegetable broth, garlic and cook for 5-10 minutes on medium heat.
Once cooked remove from heat.
Serve hot and enjoy!

NUTRITIONAL INFORMATION

Calories Per Servings, 161 kcal, 2.9 g Fat, 31.11 g Total Carbs, 11.15 g Protein, 10.6 g Fiber

Stir fry Tofu & Soba Noodles

Prep Time   20 min

Servings 2

INGREDIENTS
8 –12 oz. extra firm tofu
4 oz. soba noodles
2 tbsps. olive oil
½ tsp. salt
1 tsp. garlic, minced
8 oz. broccoli, cut into florets

DIRECTIONS

Boil noodles for 10 minutes in salted water. Drain and set aside.
Heat oil in a large skillet over medium heat.
Add broccoli and cook for 5 minutes until golden brown, over medium heat.
Add salt, pepper and garlic, and cook for another 1-2 minutes until the garlic is fragrant.
Fry tofu in same pan for 4-5 minutes.
For serving add broccoli tofu and noodles in bowl.
Serve and enjoy
NUTRITIONAL INFORMATION

Calories Per Servings, 321 kcal, 7.58 g Fat, 48.27 g Total Carbs, 23.05 g Protein, 3.5 g Fiber

Buckwheat Falafel Bowl

Prep Time 30 Min

Servings 8

INGREDIENTS
FALAFELS
1 onion, roughly chopped
1 tsp. garlic, minced
a large handful parsley
2 cups buckwheat flour
2 tsps. ground cumin
2 tsps. ground coriander
1/8 tsp, pepper & pepper
½ tsp baking powder
Olive oil for deep-frying

TO SERVE

Broccoli florets, stir fried
Brussel sprouts
Cucumber, sliced
Baby Spinach
Arugula leaves
2 lemons, sliced

DIRECTIONS

Add falafel ingredient in food processor and mix well. Add water to make paste
Roll mixture into small falafels the size of walnuts.
Heat oil in pan and cook the falafels, in batches, for 1-2 minutes or until golden.
Remove with a slotted spoon and drain on kitchen paper.

Serve falafel with broccoli, Brussel sprout, cucumber, and veggies. Enjoy!

NUTRITIONAL INFORMATION

Calories Per Servings, 150 kcal, 1.59 g Fat, 30.79 g Total Carbs, 7.52 g Protein, 6 g Fiber

Kale Stew

Prep Time   10 min

Servings 2

INGREDIENTS

l bunch kale, chopped
1 tsp garlic, Minced
3 oz. avocado oil
3 cups vegetables stock
1 tsp Salt
1 tsp Pepper
1 tbsp. Parsley chopped

DIRECTIONS

Sauté the garlic over low heat until they are beginning to turn into brown.
Add kale and rest of ingredients.
Simmer on low to medium heat for 8 Minutes. Once cooked remove from heat.
Stir through the salt, pepper and parsley.
Adjust seasoning to taste.
Enjoy!

NUTRITIONAL INFORMATION

Calories Per Servings, 191 kcal, 8.41 g Fat, 26.19 g Total Carbs, 11.15 g Protein, 11.4 g Fiber

Broccoli Soup

Prep Time   10 min

Servings 2

INGREDIENTS
- 1 medium broccoli florets
- 1 tsp garlic, Minced
- 1 tbsp. olive oil
- 3 cups vegetables stock
- 1 tsp Salt
- 1 tsp Pepper
- 1 tbsp. Parsley chopped

DIRECTIONS

Sauté the broccoli with garlic over low heat until they are beginning to turn into brown.
Add rest of the ingredients.
Simmer on low to medium heat for 8 minutes. Once broccoli is cooked and soft remove from heat.
Carefully blend the soup until no lumps are remaining.
Stir through the salt, pepper and parsley.
Adjust seasoning to taste.
Enjoy!

NUTRITIONAL INFORMATION

Calories Per Servings, 193 kcal, 9.1 g Fat, 23.86 g Total Carbs, 11.31 g Protein, 8.5 g Fiber

Buckwheat Noodles Soup

Prep Time   40 Min

Servings 4

INGREDIENTS
- 1 large onion-diced
- 1 tsp. garlic, minced
- 1–2 tbsps. olive oil
- 1 cup spinach leaves
- 4 cups veggie stock
- 4 cups water
- 6– 8 oz. soba noodles

DIRECTIONS

Sauté the onion for about 2-3 minutes in oil over medium heat, until tender. Turn heat to medium, add the garlic and continue cook onions until they are deeply golden brown.
Add the veggie stock, water, spinach, noodles and bring to a simmer.
Simmer for 25-30 minutes uncovered on med heat.
Fill bowls with cooked noodles and broth.
Serve immediately.
Enjoy!

NUTRITIONAL INFORMATION

Calories Per Servings, 209 kcal, 1.16 g Fat, 45.53 g Total Carbs, 9.14 g Protein, 2.1 g Fiber

Buckwheat Tortilla

Prep Time   10 min

Servings 6

INGREDIENTS

- 100 grams Buckwheat (soba) flour
- 1 dash Salt
- 1 tbsp. olive oil
- 120 ml to 150 ml Lukewarm water

DIRECTIONS

Combine the buckwheat flour, and salt in a bowl.
Add the water, and form into a ball.
Wrap the dough, and let sit for a while.
Divide the dough into 6 parts
Flatten out into thin, round pancakes, then grill both sides in a frying pan.
Enjoy!

NUTRITIONAL INFORMATION

Calories Per Servings, 76 kcal, 02.77 g Fat, 11.77 g Total Carbs, 2.1 g Protein, 1.7 g Fiber

Sautee Tofu & Kale

Prep Time   10 min

Servings 2

INGREDIENTS

8 –12 oz. extra firm tofu
2 tbsps. olive oil
½ tsp. salt & pepper
1 tsp. garlic, minced
1 bunch kale, chopped

DIRECTIONS

Heat oil in a large skillet over medium heat.
Fry tofu in pan for 4-5 minutes.
Add kale and stir fry for 3-4 minutes until kale is soft.
Add salt, pepper and garlic, and cook for another 1-2 minutes until the garlic is fragrant.
Drizzle sesame seeds on top.
Serve and enjoy!

NUTRITIONAL INFORMATION

Calories Per Servings, 280 kcal, 21.17 g Fat, 12.72 g Total Carbs, 16.17 g Protein, 4.6 g Fiber

Stir Fried Green Beans

Prep Time   10 Min

Servings 2

INGREDIENTS

2 lb. green beans, ends trimmed
1 tbsp. extra-virgin olive oil
2 large garlic cloves, minced
1 tsp. red pepper flakes
1 tbsp. lemon zest
Salt and freshly ground black pepper

DIRECTIONS

Blanch green beans for about 2-4 minutes in a salted boiling water until bright green in color and tender crisp.
Drain and shock in a bowl of ice water to stop from cooking.
Heat a large heavy skillet over medium heat. Add the oil, once oil is hot, add the garlic and red pepper flakes and sauté until fragrant, about 30 seconds.
Add lemon zest and season with salt and pepper.
Serve and enjoy!

NUTRITIONAL INFORMATION

Calories Per Servings, 134 kcal, 5.12 g Fat, 21.21 g Total Carbs, 5.34 g Protein, 8.7 g Fiber

Baked Asparagus

Prep Time   30 Min

Servings 2

INGREDIENTS

1 bunch thin asparagus spears, trimmed
3 tbsps. olive oil
1 clove garlic, minced
1 tsp. oregano
1 tsp. sea salt
½ tsp. ground black pepper
1 tbsp. lemon juice

DIRECTIONS
Preheat an oven to 425 degrees F (220 degrees C).
Place the asparagus into a mixing bowl, and drizzle with the olive oil. Toss to coat the spears, then sprinkle with garlic, salt, oregano, and pepper.

Arrange the asparagus onto a baking sheet in a single layer.
Bake in the preheated oven until just tender, 12 to 15 minutes depending on thickness.
Sprinkle with lemon juice just before serving.

NUTRITIONAL INFORMATION
Calories Per Servings, 234 kcal, 20.59 g Fat, 11.23 g Total Carbs, 5.38 g Protein, 5.2 g Fiber

Broccoli with Olive Tahini

Prep Time   30 Min

Servings   2

INGREDIENTS
1 bunch baby broccoli, trimmed
1 tbsp. olive oil
salt and pepper to taste

OLIVE TAHINI SAUCE
3/4 cup water
3 tbsps. lemon juice
2 tbsps. olive oil
2 garlic cloves
2–3 slices jalapeno
1/4 tsp. salt
¼ cup olives

DIRECTIONS
Brush broccoli with olive oil and sprinkle with salt and pepper.
Place on a parchment lined sheet pan in the oven, to roast until fork tender about 20-25 minutes.

Meanwhile, place all the tahini ingredients in the blender, and blend until combined.
Adjust seasoning according to taste.
Arrange the broccoli with tahini sauce in plate.
Drizzle some olive oil and olives on top.
Enjoy!

NUTRITIONAL INFORMATION
Calories Per Servings, 180 kcal, 9.91 g Fat, 15.96 g Total Carbs, 9.4 g Protein, 7.3 g Fiber

Apple & Walnuts Pie

Prep Time   50 Min

Servings   16

INGREDIENTS
- 8 cups sliced peeled tart apples
- 1 cup dates syrup
- 2 cups walnuts milk
- 2 teaspoons ground cinnamon
- 1 cup walnut butter, softened
- 2 cups buckwheat flour
- 1 cup finely chopped walnuts, divided

DIRECTIONS

Place apples in a greased 13x9-in. baking dish.
Sprinkle with cinnamon. In a bowl, mix flour, milk, syrup and walnuts. in bowl.
Spread mixture over apples. Sprinkle with remaining walnuts.
Bake at 350° for 45-55 minutes or until the apples are tender.
Serve and enjoy!

NUTRITIONAL INFORMATION

Calories Per Servings, 293 kcal, 16.37 g Fat, 36.89 g Total Carbs, 3.89 g Protein, 3.3 g Fiber

Baked Walnut Bars

Prep Time   30 Min

Servings   16

INGREDIENTS
4 tablespoons walnuts butter
3/4 cup buckwheat flour
1/2 teaspoon salt
3/4 teaspoon baking powder
1/8 teaspoon baking soda
1 cup dates chopped
¼ cup dates syrup
1 cup walnuts (chopped)
1 cup dark chocolate melted

DIRECTIONS
Preheat oven to 350 F. Grease and flour an 8-inch square baking pan.
In a medium bowl, mix the flour with salt, baking soda, and baking powder. Whisk or stir to blend thoroughly.
Mix the dates, melted butter, dates and walnuts in blender.
Stir in flour mixture until well blended.
Spoon the thick batter into the prepared baking pan and spread it evenly with a spatula.
Bake in the preheated oven for about 20 to 24 minutes, or until browned and the top has formed a crust.
Drizzle melted chocolate on top. Serve cold and enjoy!

NUTRITIONAL INFORMATION
Calories Per Servings, 170 kcal, 6.57 g Fat, 27.85 g Total Carbs, 2.12 g Protein, 2.1 g Fiber

Coco & Walnuts Milkshake

Prep Time   10 Min

Servings   1

INGREDIENTS

- 1 cup soy milk
- 1 tsp dates syrup
- 1/2 oz. walnuts
- 1 tbsps. coco powder
- 1/2 cup ice cubes

DIRECTIONS
Add all ingredients in high speed blender.
Blend until all ingredients are incorporated.
Serve and enjoy!

NUTRITIONAL INFORMATION
Calories Per Servings, 262 kcal, 17.25 g Fat, 16.09 g Total Carbs, 9.85 g Protein, 1 g Fiber

Walnut Butter Cake

Prep Time   40 Min

Servings   10

INGREDIENTS

- 4 oz. buckwheat flour
- 1 teaspoon baking powder
- 4 oz. walnut butter
- ¼ cup dates syrup
- 1 cup soy milk
- 2 oz. walnut, chopped

DIRECTIONS
Grease cake pan with oil.
Sift the flour and baking powder, set aside.
Add dates syrup sugar and rest of ingredients in it.
Transfer the batter into the greased pan, shake gently to level off the batter.
Bake at a pre-heated oven at 180C (350F) for about 30-35 minutes or until a cake tester inserted into the walnut butter cake comes out clean.
NUTRITIONAL INFORMATION
Calories Per Servings, 195 kcal, 14.06 g Fat, 16.51 g Total Carbs, 3.16 g Protein, 1.5 g Fiber

Walnuts Bits

Prep Time   40 Min

Servings   20

INGREDIENTS
- 1/2 cup walnut butter softened
- 8 oz. walnut cream
- 1/2 cup dates, finely chopped
- cup walnuts, chopped
- 1/2 cup mini chocolate chips
- tbsps.sesame seeds

DIRECTIONS

Line a baking sheet with a silicone mat or parchment paper. Set aside.
In a large bowl, mix all ingredienst except sesame seeds.
Use a cookie scoop to make 20 even bites and place onto prepared cookie sheet.
Roll on sesame seeds.
Place in fridge for 30 minutes - 1 hour, or until firm.
Serve and enjoy!

NUTRITIONAL INFORMATION
Calories Per Servings, 185 kcal, 17.04 g Fat, 7.47 g Total Carbs, 2.92 g Protein, 1.9 g Fiber

Walnuts Muffins

Prep Time   40 Min

Servings   12

INGREDIENTS

- 1/2 cup dates sugar
- 2 cups buckwheat flour
- 2 teaspoons baking powder
- 1/2 teaspoon salt
- 2/3 cup soy milk
- 1/2 cup walnut butter, melted, cooled
- 1 cup dark chocolate, melted
- 1/2 cup California walnuts, chopped

DIRECTIONS
Preheat oven to 400°F. Grease or line 12 large muffin cups.
In large bowl mix, sugars, fnuts, lour, baking powder and salt. In medium bowl combine milk, butter, cgocolate and blend well.
Mix dry ingredients with wet ingredeints.
Pour batter into greased muffin cups.
Bake for 15 to 20 minutes or until cooked.
Serve hot and enjoy!

NUTRITIONAL INFORMATION
Calories Per Servings, 271 kcal, 18.37 g Fat, 23.85 g Total Carbs, 5.51 g Protein, 4.7 g Fiber

Buckwheat Cinnamon Roll

Prep Time   30 Min

Servings   8

INGREDIENTS

- 14-16 oz. buckwheat dough
- 1 cup dates syrup
- 2 tbsps. cinnamon powder,
- 2 tbsps. walnut butter, melted

DIRECTIONS

Preheat oven to 400 degrees F.
Roll dough into a rectangle about 10 X 14 inches.
Mix syrup and cinnamon powder in mixing bowl.
Spread this mixture over rolled dough.
Roll dough in a circle.

Slice dough with knife or pizza cutter into 1-inch pieces. Place rolls on prepared sheets.
Quickly brush butter over rolls.

Bake rolls for about 15 minutes or until lightly brown and rolls are cooked through.

NUTRITIONAL INFORMATION
Calories Per Servings, 170 kcal, 0.41 g Fat, 43.33 g Total Carbs, 1.8 g Protein, 1.4 g Fiber

DOUBLE LAYER NO BAKE CAKE

Prep Time   10 min
Servings   16

INGREDIENTS

- 1 cup walnuts crushed
- 2 cups walnuts cream
- 1 cup chocolate melted
- 4 cups raspberries
- 2 cups walnuts cream

DIRECTIONS

Add walnuts, cream, and chocolate in a bowl and mix well.
Pour mixture in heart shape baking mold and freeze for about 2 hours until set.
Blend raspberries and cream in a blender and pour it over chocolate mixture.
Again, freeze for overnight.
Serve and enjoy.

NUTRITIONAL INFORMATION

Calories Per Servings, 274 kcal, 16.59 g Fat, 30.58 g Total Carbs, 4.73 g Protein, 4.3 g Fiber

Fudgy Brownies

Prep Time   40 Min

Servings   12

INGREDIENTS

- 2 cups buckwheat flour
- ¼ cup dates syrup
- 1 tsp. baking powder
- 1 tsp. sea salt
- ½ cup walnut butter, melted
- ½ cup walnut milk
- 1/2 cup cocoa powder

DIRECTIONS

Preheat oven to 350°.
In a large bowl mix dry ingredient and mix wet ingredients in another bowl.
Mix ingredients until well incorporated.
Pour brownies mixture in lined brownies mold.
Bake in preheated oven for about 25-30 minutes until cooked.
Slice it and drizzle chocolate syrup on top.
Serve and enjoy!

NUTRITIONAL INFORMATION

Calories Per serving 156 Cal, Fats 8.97 g, Protein 3.66 g, Total Carbs 19 g, Fiber 3.3 g

Chocolate Pudding With Berries

Prep Time   5 min
Servings   4

INGREDIENTS

- 2 cups walnut milk
- 2 tbsps. chai seeds
- 2 tbsps. coco powder
- 1 tsp dates syrup
- fresh berries, coconut flake for topping

DIRECTIONS

Mix together milk with dates syrup, chia seeds and coco powder in bowl and mix well.
Pour in serving jar and let it stand overnight in fridge.
In morning top pudding with berries.
Serve and enjoy!

NUTRITIONAL INFORMATION

Calories Per serving 136 Cal, Fats 13.05 g, Protein 3.05 g, Total Carbs 4.11 g, Fiber 1.3 g

Chocolate Chip Cookies

Prep Time   30 min

Servings   12

INGREDIENTS

- 1/4 cup olive oil
- 2 tbsps. walnut cream
- 2 cup buckwheat flour
- 1 pinch. sea salt
- 1 tbsps. dates syrup
- 3/4 cup dark chocolate chips

DIRECTIONS

Preheat the oven to 350°.
Mix all ingredients in bowl.
Carefully add chocolate chips into the cookie dough.
Divide the dough into 15 equal balls.
Shape ball and flatten the balls on a greased baking tray.
Bake cookies for about 15-20 minutes in the preheated oven until cooked and golden brown.
Serve and enjoy!

NUTRITIONAL INFORMATION

Calories Per serving 194 Cal, Fats 11.26 g, Protein 3.68 g, Total Carbs 21.08 g, Fiber 3.6 g

WEEK-1 SIRTFOOD MEAL PLAN

MONDAY

BREAKFAST – Spinach Green Juice 181 kcal

LUNCH – Hot & Spicy Tofu & Broccoli 273 kcal

MID DAY SNACK – Berries Green Juice 121 kcal

DINNER – Broccoli Green Juice 187 kcal

TUESDAY

BREAKFAST – Mix Green Juice 146 kcal

LUNCH – Stir Fried Spinach 242 kcal

MID DAY SNACK – Celery Green Juice 118 kcal

DINNER – Kale Green Juice 171 kcal

WEDNESDAY

BREAKFAST – Spinach & Apple Juice 178 kcal

LUNCH – Sautee Tofu & Kale 208 kcal

MID DAY SNACK – Cucumber Green Juice 124 kcal

DINNER – Creamy Spinach Juice 184 kcal

THURSDAY

BREAKFAST - Spinach Green Juice 181 kcal

LUNCH - Pomegranate Salad with Spinach 237 kcal

MID DAY SNACK - Berries Green Juice 121 kcal

DINNER - Kale Stew 191 kcal

FRIDAY

BREAKFAST - Mix Green Juice 146 kcal

LUNCH - Stir fry Tofu & Soba Noodles 321 kcal

MID DAY SNACK - Celery Green Juice 118 kcal

DINNER - Broccoli Soup 193 kcal

SATURDAY

BREAKFAST - Spinach & Apple Juice 178 kcal

LUNCH - Stir Fried Green Beans 134 Kcal

MID DAY SNACK - Cucumber Green Juice 124 kcal

DINNER - Buckwheat Noodles 209 kcal

SUNDAY

BREAKFAST - Spinach Green Juice 181 kcal

LUNCH - Berries Salad with Spinach 271 kcal

MID DAY SNACK - Berries Green Juice 121 kcal

DINNER - Broccoli with Olive Tahini 180kcal

WEEK-2 SIRTFOOD MEAL PLAN

MONDAY

Morning Juice - Berries Green Juice 121 kcal

Breakfast - Apple Porridge 277 kcal

LUNCH - Spinach Avocado Pomegranate Seeds 237 kcal

DINNER - Sautee Tofu & Kale 280 kcal

TUESDAY

Morning Juice - Celery Green Juice 118 kcal

Breakfast - Spinach Omelet 283 kcal

LUNCH - Beetroot Salad with Spinach 121 kcal

DINNER - Stir Fried Green Beans 134 kcal

WEDNESDAY

Morning Juice - Cucumber Green Juice 124 kcal

Breakfast - Tofu & Kale Toast 216 kcal

LUNCH - Berries Salad with Spinach 231 kcal

DINNER - Baked Asparagus 234 kcal

THURSDAY

Morning Juice - Spinach Green Juice 181 kcal

Breakfast - Tofu Scramble 208 kcal

LUNCH - Pomegranate Salad with Spinach 237 kcal

DINNER - Broccoli with Olive Tahini 180 kcal

FRIDAY

Morning Juice - Broccoli Green Juice 187 kcal

Breakfast - Buckwheat Pancakes 197 kcal

LUNCH - Buckwheat Salad Bowl 188 kcal

DINNER - Broccoli Soup 193 kcal

SATURDAY

Morning Juice - Kale Green Juice 171 kcal

Breakfast - Waffle Sandwich 260 kcal

LUNCH - Stir Fried Spinach 242 kcal

DINNER - Buckwheat Noodles 209 kcal

SUNDAY

Morning Juice - Creamy Spinach Juice 184 kcal

Breakfast - Toast with Caramelized Apple 168 kcal

LUNCH - Buckwheat Falafel Bowl 150 kcal

DINNER - Broccoli with Olive Tahini 180kcal

Green Juice with Lime & parsley

Prep Time   10 min

Servings   1

INGREDIENTS

- 1 bunch parsley
- 1 bunch spinach
- 1/2 green apple
- 1 tbsp. lime juice
- 1 tsp. matcha green tea

DIRECTIONS

Extract the juice of spinach, apple and parsley
Pour a Half juice into a glass, then add the matcha, lemon juice and mix well with fork.
Once the matcha is dissolved add the
remaining of the juice.
Mix well.
Pour some water on top.
Enjoy!

NUTRITIONAL INFORMATION

Calories Per Servings, 151 kcal, 1.97 g Fat, 11.82 g Protein, 29.98 g Total Carbs, 1.7 g Fiber

Green Juice with Basil & Strawberries

Prep Time   10 min

Servings   1

INGREDIENTS

- 1 bunch basil leaves
- ¼ cup strawberries
- 1/8 tsp. ginger, paste
- half a lemon, juiced
- 1 tsp. matcha green tea

DIRECTIONS

Extract the juice of basil & strawberries
Pour a Half juice into a glass, then add the matcha, lemon juice, ginger paste and mix well with fork.
Once the matcha is dissolved add the
remaining of the juice.
Mix well.
Pour some water on top.
Enjoy!

NUTRITIONAL INFORMATION

Calories Per Servings, 23 kcal, 0.32 g Fat, 1.1 g Protein, 5.11 g Total Carbs, 1.2 g Fiber

Lettuce Green Juice

Prep Time   10 min

Servings   1

INGREDIENTS
- 1 bunch spinach
- 1 bunch lettuce leaves
- ½ green apple
- 1/8 tsp ginger
- half a lemon, juiced
- 1 tsp. matcha green tea

DIRECTIONS

Extract the juice of spinach, apple and lettuce leaves.
Pour a Half juice into a glass, then add the matcha, lemon juice, ginger paste and mix well with fork.
Once the matcha is dissolved add the
remaining of the juice.
Mix well.
Pour some water on top.
Enjoy

NUTRITIONAL INFORMATION

Calories Per Servings, 94 kcal, 1.49 g Fat, 10.47 g Protein, 16.19 g Total Carbs, 8.4 g Fiber

Broccoli & Kiwi Juice

Prep Time   10 min

Servings   1

INGREDIENTS
- 2 cups broccoli
- 1 kiwi
- 1 apple
- half a lemon, juiced
- 1 tsp. matcha green tea
- 1 tsp. flaxseeds

DIRECTIONS

Extract the juice of broccoli, apple & kiwi
Pour a Half juice into a glass, then add the matcha, lemon juice and mix well with fork.
Once the matcha is dissolved add the
remaining of the juice.
Mix well.
Pour some water and flax seeds on top.
Enjoy!

NUTRITIONAL INFORMATION

Calories Per Servings, 136 kcal, 2.19 g Fat, 3.72 g Protein, 30.05 g Total Carbs, 7.5 g Fiber

Mix Green Juice

Prep Time   10 min

Servings   1

INGREDIENTS
- 1 cucumber
- 1 bunch parsley
- 1 cup rosemary
- 1 cup broccoli
- ½ apple
- half a lemon, juiced
- 1 tsp. matcha green tea

DIRECTIONS

Extract the juice all veggies
Pour a Half juice into a glass, then add the matcha, lemon juice and mix well with fork.
Once the matcha is dissolved add the
remaining of the juice.
Mix well.
Pour some water on top.
Enjoy!

NUTRITIONAL INFORMATION

Calories Per Servings, 121 kcal, 2.32 g Fat, 3.68 g Protein, 25.34 g Total Carbs, 8.6 g Fiber

Basil Juice with Walnuts

Prep Time   10 min

Servings   1

INGREDIENTS
- 2 cups basil leaves
- ½ cup strawberries
- 2 stalk celery with leaves
- ½ cup walnut milk
- 1/8 tsp. ginger, paste
- half a lemon, juiced
- 1 tsp. matcha green tea

DIRECTIONS

Extract the juice of basil, celery, and strawberries
Pour a Half juice into a glass, then add the matcha, lemon juice, ginger and mix well with fork.
Once the matcha is dissolved add the
remaining of the juice.
Mix well.
Pour milk on top.
Enjoy!

NUTRITIONAL INFORMATION

Calories Per Servings, 106 kcal, 3.06 g Fat, 6.35 g Protein, 15.38 g Total Carbs, 2.8 g Fiber

Kiwi & Cucumber Juice

Prep Time   10 min

Servings   1

INGREDIENTS

- 1 bunch parsley
- 1 cucumber
- 1 kiwi
- ½ green apple
- half a lemon, juiced
- 1 tsp. matcha green tea

DIRECTIONS

Extract the juice of kiwi, apple, cucumber and parsley.
Pour a Half juice into a glass, then add the matcha, lemon juice and mix well with fork.
Once the matcha is dissolved add the
remaining of the juice.
Mix well.
Pour some water on top.
Enjoy!

NUTRITIONAL INFORMATION

Calories Per Servings, 142 kcal, 1.96 g Fat, 6.86 g Protein, 29.96 g Total Carbs, 9.6 g Fiber

Cucumber & Apple Green Juice

Prep Time   10 min

Servings   1

INGREDIENTS
- 1 cucumber
- 1 green apple
- 1 bunch kale
- 1 kiwi
- half a lemon, juiced
- 1 tsp. matcha green tea

DIRECTIONS

Extract the juice of veggies & fruits
Pour a Half juice into a glass, then add the matcha, lemon juice and mix well with fork.
Once the matcha is dissolved add the
remaining of the juice.
Mix well.
Pour some water on top.
Enjoy!

NUTRITIONAL INFORMATION

Calories Per Servings, 190 kcal, 1.93 g Fat, 7.49 g Protein, 42.86 g Total Carbs, 10.7 g Fiber

Broccoli & Basil Juice

Prep Time   10 min

Servings   1

INGREDIENTS
- 1 bunch basil
- 1 cucumber
- 1 cup broccoli
- half a medium green apple
- half a lemon, juiced
- 1 tsp. matcha green tea

DIRECTIONS

Extract the juice of basil, apple, cucumber and broccoli.
Pour a Half juice into a glass, then add the matcha, lemon juice and mix well with fork.
Once the matcha is dissolved add the
remaining of the juice.
Mix well.
Pour some water on top.
Enjoy!

NUTRITIONAL INFORMATION
Calories Per Servings, 102 kcal, 1.19 g Fat, 5.05 g Protein, 21.26 g Total Carbs, 5.9 g Fiber

Rocket Green Juice

Prep Time   10 min

Servings   1

INGREDIENTS
- 1 bunch rocket leaves
- large stalks green celery, including leaves
- half a medium green apple
- half a lemon, juiced
- 1 tsp. matcha green tea
- 1 tsp. chia seeds

DIRECTIONS

Extract the juice of rocket leaves, apple, and celery
Pour a Half juice into a glass, then add the matcha, lemon juice and mix well with fork.
Once the matcha is dissolved add the
remaining of the juice.
Mix well.
Pour some water and chia seeds on top.
Enjoy!

NUTRITIONAL INFORMATION

Calories Per Servings, 76 kcal, 0.77 g Fat, 2.55 g Protein, 17.65 g Total Carbs, 3.8 g Fiber

Walnuts Porridge

Prep Time   20 Min

Servings   2

INGREDIENTS
1 cup soy milk
1 date, chopped
2 tbsps. buckwheat flakes
1 tsp. walnut butter
1 green apple slices
2 oz. pomegranate seeds
1/2 oz. walnuts

DIRECTIONS

Place the milk and dates in pan over medium heat.
Add the buckwheat flakes, walnuts and cook for 10 minutes.
Once porridge is cooked remove from heat.
Serve with apple slice, pomegranate seeds and walnuts on top.
Enjoy!

NUTRITIONAL INFORMATION

Ca Calories Per Servings, 278 kcal, 11.39 g Fat, 7.28 g Protein, 41.29 g Total Carbs, 5.7 g Fiber

Apple Pancakes

Prep Time   20 min
Servings   4

INGREDIENTS

- 2 apples, puree
- 1 cup, buckwheat flour
- 2 tsp baking powder
- 2 tbsps. dates syrup
- ¼ teaspoon salt
- 1 tbsp. olive oil
- 1 cup blueberries
- 2-3 strawberries, sliced

DIRECTIONS

Mix apple puree, flour, baking powder, dates syrup, and salt to the blender and blend for 2 minutes.
Pour the mixture to a large bowl and fold in half of blueberries.
Heat your skillet over medium heat and grease it with olive oil
Pour ¼ cup pancake batter in skillet and spread it slightly.
Cook pancake for 2-3 minutes per side, until cooked through.
Serve with berries.
Enjoy

NUTRITIONAL INFORMATION

Calories Per Servings, 211 kcal, 4.62 g Fat, 4.43 g Protein, 42.34 g Total Carbs, 6.5 g Fiber

Morning Parfait

Prep Time   10 min

Servings   2

INGREDIENTS
- 1 cup soy yogurt
- 1 cup cranberries
- 1 tbsp. dates syrup
- Mint leaves
- 1 tbsp. walnuts, chopped

DIRECTIONS

Pour 2 tbsps. soy yogurt in serving glass. then layer with cranberries.

Repeat with layer.

Top with dates syrup, mint leaves and walnuts.

Serve cold and enjoy!

NUTRITIONAL INFORMATION

Calories Per Servings, 196 kcal, 2.84 g Fat, 12.48 g Protein, 33.05 g Total Carbs, 1.2 g Fiber

Chocolate Pancakes

Prep Time   20 min

Servings   4

INGREDIENTS
- 1 cup buckwheat flour
- 2 tbsps. cocoa powder
- 1 tsp baking powder
- 2 tbsp. dates syrup
- 3/4 cup soy milk
- 1 tsp. olive oil

DIRECTIONS

Mix buckwheat flour, baking powder, and cocoa powder in mixing bowl.
Add dates syrup, milk and oil and mix well.
Heat nonstick griddle over medium heat, and grease with cooking spray.
Pour ¼ batter in griddle and Let It cook for 2-3 minutes until cooked.
Flip and cook for another 2-3 minutes until cooked through.
Stack the pancakes, drizzle chocolate syrup on top and banana slice.
Enjoy!

NUTRITIONAL INFORMATION

Calories Per Servings, 169 kcal, 3.57 g Fat, 5.23 g Protein, 31.81 g Total Carbs, 3 g Fiber

Spinach Muffins

Prep Time   30 min

Servings   12

INGREDIENTS

2 cups buckwheat flour
¼ cup ground flaxseed
2 tsp. baking powder
½ tsp salt
½ cup soy milk
1 tsp ground cinnamon
½ cup dates syrup
2 cups spinach, chopped
¼ cup walnuts butter

DIRECTIONS

Preheat oven to 375 degrees F.
Mix dry ingredients in bowl and mix well.
Mix wet ingredients in bowl and mix well.
Mix wet ingredients to dry mixture and stir to combine.
Carefully mix chopped spinach in batter.
Pour batter in lined and greased muffin tins.
Bake muffins for about 20-25 minutes or until toothpick comes out clean.
Serve hot with green tea and enjoy!

NUTRITIONAL INFORMATION

Calories Per Servings, 166 kcal, 6.19 g Fat, 3.52 g Protein, 26.94 g Total Carbs, 3.2 g Fiber

Tofu Toast

Prep Time   10 min

Servings   4

INGREDIENTS
- ½ lb. tofu
- 2 onions, sliced
- 1 tsp. garlic, chopped
- 1 tsp of ground turmeric
- 1/8 tsp. pepper & salt
- 2 tbsps. olive oil
- 4 slice buckwheat bread
- chopped parsley for topping

DIRECTIONS

Heat oil in pan over medium heat, once oil is hot, add garlic and fry.
Stir and cook, until it softens.
Add onions and fry on low-medium heat until softened.
Add tofu and mash it with a fork.
Sprinkle with turmeric, salt and pepper and mix well.
Grill buckwheat bread slice on electric grill.
Pour tofu scramble onto warm toast, sprinkle chopped parsley on top.
Serve and enjoy!

NUTRITIONAL INFORMATION

Calories Per Servings, 263 kcal, 18.6 g Fat, 11.78 g Protein, 16.48 g Total Carbs, 4.1 g Fiber

Buckwheat Bread Loaf

Prep Time   60 min

Servings   12

INGREDIENTS

- 1/4 cup melted walnut butter
- 2 apples, puree
- 1/4 cup pure dates syrup
- 2 cups buckwheat flour
- 2 tsps. baking powder

DIRECTIONS

Preheat the oven to 350 degrees F.
Grease 8-inch loaf pan with coconut oil and set aside.
Mix apple, dates syrup and butter in a blender and blend.
Pour the mixture in mix bowl.
Add flour and baking powder in bowl and mix well.
Pour the batter in greased baking loaf pan.
Bake for 40-60 Minutes, or until cooked through.
Allow to cool before cutting.
Enjoy!

NUTRITIONAL INFORMATION

Calories Per Servings, 134 kcal, 4.51 g Fat, 2.65 g Protein, 22.71 g Total Carbs, 2.7 g Fiber

Broccoli Muffins

Prep Time   40 min

Servings   12

INGREDIENTS

- 2 cups buckwheat flour
- ¾ cup soy milk
- ¼ cup walnut butter
- 1 cup broccoli, roughly chopped
- 4-8 strawberries, sliced
- ¼ cup chopped walnuts
- 1 tsp. cinnamon powder

DIRECTIONS

Mix buckwheat flour, walnuts and cinnamon powder in bowl.
Mix milk, butter, strawberries and broccoli in another bowl,
Gently pour the wet ingredients into the bowl containing the dry ingredients.
Preheat the oven to 200 degrees Celsius.
Line muffin tray with paper liners.
Pour batter into each muffin cup in the tray

Bake for about 20-25 minutes.
Once cooked remove from oven.
Serve and enjoy!

NUTRITIONAL INFORMATION
Calories Per Servings, 122 kcal, 5.89 g Fat, 3.22 g Protein, 15.89 g Total Carbs, 2.4 g Fiber

Buckwheat Waffles

Prep Time   20 min

Servings   4

INGREDIENTS

- 1 cup buckwheat flour
- ¼ cup walnut butter
- 1/2 cup soy milk
- ¼ tsp. cinnamon powder
- 2 tbsps. dates syrup
- 1 tsp. baking powder

DIRECTIONS

Turn your waffle maker and set it on medium.
Mix together all recipe ingredients in bowl and mix well.
Pour this batter into your waffle maker and cook until the waffle are cooked and crispy.
Gently remove the waffles from machine.
Serve with walnuts butter on top

NUTRITIONAL INFORMATION

Calories Per Servings, 231 kcal, 13.46 g Fat, 4.96 g Protein, 25.45 g Total Carbs, 3.4 g Fiber

Eggless Pudding

Prep Time   30 min

Servings   6

INGREDIENTS

8 slice buckwheat bread
1 ½ cups soy milk
2 tbsps. dates syrup
3 tbsps. dates sugar
1 tbsps. walnut butter

DIRECTIONS

Blend bread, milk and dates syrup in blender.
Add sugar with butter in a pan and place it on medium to high heat.
Allow sugar to melt and turn golden.
Transfer the caramel into an oven safe soufflé dish and fill the dish with the bread mixture.
Cover with an aluminum wrap and steam for 25 minutes on low to medium flame.
Once cooked remove from dish.
Refrigerate for at least 2 hours.
Serve and enjoy!

NUTRITIONAL INFORMATION
Calories Per Servings, 239 kcal, 3.17 g Fat, 8.63 g Protein, 48.19 g Total Carbs, 6.1 g Fiber

Turmeric Tea

Prep Time   5 min
Servings   2

INGREDIENTS

2 cups water

1 tsp freshly grated turmeric root

1 tsp freshly grated ginger root

1/2 tsp ground cinnamon

1 tbsp. dates syrup

DIRECTIONS

Place water in a saucepan and heat over medium.
Add the turmeric root, ginger, ground cinnamon and dates syrup and cook for 10 minutes.
Once cooked pour in glass.
Enjoy!

NUTRITIONAL INFORMATION

Calories Per Servings, 38 kcal, 0.09 g Fat, 0.19 g Protein, 10.16 g Total Carbs, 0.7 g Fiber

Green Juicy Salad Bowl

Prep Time   10 min

Servings   2

INGREDIENTS

1 bag, baby spinach

1 cucumber, sliced

16 oz. broccoli, florets

1 bunch lettuce leaves

4 oz. tofu, fried.

2-3 tomatoes, sliced

DRESSING

2 tbsps. raw apple cider vinegar
1 tbsp. olive
2 garlic cloves, minced
2 tbsps. lemon juice
1 tsp dijon mustard
1/4 tsp salt
2 tbsps. water optional

DIRECTIONS

Mix together dressing ingredients in bowl and set aside.
Fry tofu in pan until brown.
Steam broccoli in microwave with some water.

Chop veggies and arrange in bowl with tofu and broccoli.
Drizzle dressing over veggies.
Slightly mix.
Serve and enjoy!

NUTRITIONAL INFORMATION
Calories Per Servings, 229 kcal, 13.26 g Fat, 17.61 g Protein, 17.93 g Total Carbs, 9 g Fiber

Green Salad with Flaxseed

Prep Time   15 Min

Servings   2

INGREDIENTS

1 pack arugula leaves

1 cucumber sliced

1 red bell pepper, sliced

2-3 tomatoes, sliced

1 tsp. flaxseeds

Dressing

1 tbsp. Italian seasoning
1 tbsp. olive oil
4 tbsps. red wine vinegar
½ tsp salt
¼ tsp ground black pepper
1 tbsp. Dijon mustard

DIRECTIONS
Add all veggies in mixing bowl.
Mix dressing ingredients in bowl and pour over veggies.
Serve cold and enjoy!
NUTRITIONAL INFORMATION

Calories Per Servings, 110 kcal, 8.08 g Fat, 2.29 g Protein, 7.86 g Total Carbs, 2.5 g Fiber

Beetroot Salad with Spinach

Prep Time   15 Min

Servings   2

INGREDIENTS

1 pack lettuce leaves, chopped

1 cucumber, sliced

8 oz. strawberries, sliced

1 tsp. flaxseeds

Dressing

1 tbsp. olive oil

3/4 cup apple cider vinegar

1/4 cup prepared mustard

1 tbsp. soy sauce

1 tbsp. Splenda

4 cloves garlic, minced

1 tsp. kosher salt

1 tsp. ground black pepper

DIRECTIONS

Cup and slice all veggies and arrange in serving plate.
Mix dressing ingredients in bowl and pour over veggies.
Drizzle flax seeds on top.
Serve cold and enjoy!

NUTRITIONAL INFORMATION

Calories Per Servings, 183 kcal, 10.41 g Fat, 3.61 g Protein, 17.66 g Total Carbs, 5 g Fiber

Tabbouleh with Lime Dressing

Prep Time   15 Min

Servings   2

INGREDIENTS

1 cucumber, finely chopped

8 oz. spinach, finely chopped

1 red onion finely chopped

1 cup buckwheat groats, cooked

8 oz. parsley, finely chopped

8 oz. strawberries, chopped

Dressing

3 cloves garlic, finely minced

1 ½ tsps. anchovy paste

1 tsp. Worcestershire sauce

2 tbsps. fresh lemon juice

1 ½ tsps. Dijon mustard

Salt and Pepper to taste

DIRECTIONS

Add all chopped veggies and buckwheat in mixing bowl and mix well.

Mix dressing ingredients in bowl and pour over veggies.
Serve cold and enjoy!

NUTRITIONAL INFORMATION

Calories Per Servings, 238 kcal, 2.84 g Fat, 12.96 g Protein, 49.7 g Total Carbs, 12.1 g Fiber

Salad Wrap with Walnut Cream

Prep Time   15 Min

Servings   2

INGREDIENTS

2 buckwheat tortilla

1 cucumber, chopped

4-6 strawberries, chopped

2 lettuce leaves

2 oz. walnut cream

DIRECTIONS

Toss tortilla on griddle until heat up.
Lay tortilla on plate.
Place lettuce leave over it.
Then strawberries and spread walnut cream over it.
Roll tortilla like roll.
Serve with lettuce leaves.

NUTRITIONAL INFORMATION

Calories Per Servings, 223 kcal, 18.84 g Fat, 5.68 g Protein, 11.71 g Total Carbs, 3.7 g Fiber

Buffalo Broccoli Bites

Prep Time   40 min

Servings   4

INGREDIENTS

1 head of broccoli, cut into bite sized florets
1 cup buckwheat flour
3/4 cup soy milk
2 tsps. garlic powder
1 1/2 tsps. paprika powder
salt &black pepper
1 tsp. oregano
3/4 cup breadcrumbs
1 cup spicy BBQ sauce

DIRECTIONS

Mix flour, soy milk, water, garlic power, paprika powder, salt, and black pepper in mixing bowl.
Dip the florets into the batter until they are coated well.
Roll florets over the breadcrumbs.
Arrange the florets over baking tray and bake for 25 minutes at 350 °F.
Transfer the cooked broccoli bits to a bowl and coat BBQ sauce over it and bake again for 20 minutes at 350 °F.

NUTRITIONAL INFORMATION

Calories Per Servings, 161 kcal, 2.77 g Fat, 7.62 g Protein, 30.1 g Total Carbs, 5.5 g Fiber

Creamy Spinach Curry

Prep Time   20 Min

Servings   4

INGREDIENTS

1 lb. spinach, chopped
1 tsp. ginger garlic paste
salt & pepper to taste
1 tsp. paprika powder
1 tsp. cumin seeds
1 tsp red chilli powder
1/2 tsp. turmeric powder
1 tbsp. olive oil
½ cup walnut cream

DIRECTIONS

Heat the oil in a pan over medium heat.
Once oil is hot, add ginger garlic paste and cook for a minute.
Add chopped spinach in pan and cook for 4-5 minutes until spinach is welted.
Add rest of the spices and mix well.
Blender spinach in blender for 1 minutes.
Pour spinach in a pan again, add walnut cream and cook on low heat for about 4-5 minutes.
Once cooked remove from heat, drizzle cream on top.
Enjoy!

NUTRITIONAL INFORMATION

Calories Per Servings, 125 kcal, 9.84 g Fat, 4.51 g Protein, 7.47 g Total Carbs, 3.1 g Fiber

Broccoli Olives Pizza

Prep Time   30 min

Servings   8

INGREDIENTS

1 lb. buckwheat pizza dough

2 tbsp. olive oil

1 bunch broccoli, cut into florets.

1 red onion, sliced

1 tsp minced garlic

salt & pepper to taste

1 oz. BBQ sauce

2 oz. olives

6 oz. tofu, sliced

DIRECTIONS

Heat oil in skillet over medium heat.
Once oil is hot, sauté onion and garlic for 2-3 minutes.
Season with spices and mix well.
Add broccoli in skillet and cook for about 5 minutes.
Preheat oven to 400.
Set buckwheat pizza dough over greased pizza pan.

Cover dough with BBQ sauce. Layer with tofu sliced, cooked broccoli, and broccoli.
Bake for about 10 minutes.
Serve hot and enjoy!

NUTRITIONAL INFORMATION

Calories Per Servings, 296 kcal, 10.7 g Fat, 11.44 g Protein, 44.03 g Total Carbs, 6.9 g Fiber

Spinach Soup

Prep Time   20 Min

Servings   4

INGREDIENTS

1 lb. spinach, chopped

1 tsp. ginger garlic paste

salt & pepper to taste

1 tsp. paprika powder

1 tsp. cumin seeds

1 tsp red chilli powder

1/2 tsp. turmeric powder

1 tbsp. olive oil

3 cups vegetable broth

DIRECTIONS

Heat the oil in a pan over medium heat.
Once oil is hot, add ginger garlic paste and cook for a minute.
Add chopped spinach in pan and cook for 4-5 minutes until spinach is welted.
Add rest of the spices and mix well.
Blender spinach in blender for 1 minutes.

Pour spinach in a pan again, add broth and cook on low heat for about 4-5 minutes.
Once cooked remove from heat, drizzle cream on top.
Enjoy

NUTRITIONAL INFORMATION

Calories Per Servings, 67 kcal, 4.05 g Fat, 3.7 g Protein, 6.37 g Total Carbs, 3.1 g Fiber

Chilli Tofu

Prep Time   20 Min
Servings   4

INGREDIENTS

8 oz. tofu cut into cubs

1 tbsp. extra-virgin olive oil

2 large garlic cloves, minced

1 tsp. chilli flakes

salt & pepper

1 red chilli, cut into rings

2 tbsps. green onion

Salt and freshly ground black pepper

DIRECTIONS

Heat a large heavy skillet over medium heat. Add the oil, once oil is hot, add the tofu with garlic cook for 5-8 minutes until brown.
Season with spices and add red chilli rings.
Drizzle green onion on top.
Serve and enjoy!

NUTRITIONAL INFORMATION

Calories Per Servings, 174 kcal, 12.99 g Fat, 10.02 g Protein, 7.56 g Total Carbs, 2.5 g Fiber

Spicy Spinach Fillet

Prep Time 20 min

Servings 4

INGREDIENTS

1 cup buckwheat Flour

2 cups spinach, chopped

1/2 cup Onions, chopped

1 tsp. red chilli

1/2 cup Kale, chopped

2 tsp. Basil

2 tsp. Oregano

½ cup water

Olive Oil for frying

DIRECTIONS

Mix together all seasonings and vegetables in a large bowl.
Add flour and spicy in same bowl with seasoning and mix together.
Add water in this mixture and mix.
The mixture should be thick enough to make petties.
Heat oil in skillet over medium heat.
Once oil is hot, cook petties in skillet for about 2-3 minutes.
Flip and cook for another 2-3 minutes until both sides are brown.

Serve with tomatoes slice and enjoy.

NUTRITIONAL INFORMATION

Calories Per Servings, 119 kcal, 1.07 g Fat, 4.75 g Protein, 25.11 g Total Carbs, 4.1 g Fiber

Broccoli Patties

Prep Time   20 min

Servings   4

INGREDIENTS

1 cup buckwheat Flour

1 cup broccoli, chopped

1/2 cup Onions, chopped

1/2 cup Green Peppers, chopped

1/2 cup Kale, chopped

2 tsp. Basil

2 tsp. Oregano

2 tsp. Onion Powder

1/2 tsp. Ginger Powder

½ cup water

Olive Oil for frying

DIRECTIONS

Mix together all seasonings and vegetables in a large bowl.
Add flour and broccoli in same bowl with seasoning and mix together.
Add water in this mixture and mix.
The mixture should be thick enough to make petties.
Heat oil in skillet over medium heat.

Once oil is hot, cook petties in skillet for about 2-3 minutes. Flip and cook for another 2-3 minutes until both sides are brown. Serve hot and enjoy!

NUTRITIONAL INFORMATION

Calories Per Servings, 117 kcal, 1.06 g Fat, 4.63 g Protein, 24.85 g Total Carbs, 4.1 g Fiber

Spinach & Tofu Pizza

Prep Time   40 Min

Servings   8

INGREDIENTS

1/2 lb. spinach, trimmed

1 lb. buckwheat pizza dough.

16 oz. tofu, cut into cubes

salt & pepper to taste

1 tsp oregano

1 tsp. chilli powder

1 tbsp. olive oil

1 oz. walnut cream

DIRECTIONS

Preheat the oven to 400°F.
Sautee spinach in a skillet over medium heat, for about 10 minutes until spinach in wilted.
Season with spices and mix well.
Set pizza dough over greased pizza pan.
Spread the walnut cream over pizza dough then spread spinach.
Top with tofu bites.
Bake pizza for 20 about minutes in preheated oven.

Once cooked remove from oven.
Serve and enjoy.

NUTRITIONAL INFORMATION

Calories Per Servings, 254 kcal, 15.93 g Fat, 13.17 g Protein, 19.63 g Total Carbs, 4.8 g Fiber

Broccoli Flatbread Pizza

Prep Time   30 min

Servings   8

INGREDIENTS

1 lb. buckwheat dough

2 tbsp. olive oil

1 bunch broccoli, cut into florets.

1 red onion, sliced

1 tsp minced garlic

salt & pepper to taste

1 oz. walnut cream

DIRECTIONS

Heat oil in skillet over medium heat.
Once oil is hot, sauté onion and garlic for 2-3 minutes.
Season with spices and mix well.
Add broccoli in skillet and cook for about 5 minutes.
Preheat oven to 400.
Set buckwheat dough over greased pizza pan.
Cover dough with walnut cream. Layer with cooked broccoli.
Bake for about 10 minutes.
Serve hot and enjoy!

NUTRITIONAL INFORMATION

Calories Per Servings, 112 kcal, 6.13 g Fat, 3.08 g Protein, 12.97 g Total Carbs, 2.3 g Fiber

Turmeric Spinach Patties

Prep Time   20 min

Servings   4

INGREDIENTS

1 cup buckwheat Flour

2 cups spinach, chopped

1/2 cup Onions, chopped

1 tbsp. turmeric

1/2 cup Kale, chopped

2 tsp. Basil

2 tsp. Oregano

2 tsp. Onion Powder

1/2 tsp. Ginger Powder

½ cup spring water

olive Oil for frying
DIRECTIONS
Mix together all seasonings and vegetables in a large bowl.
Add flour and spinach in same bowl with seasoning and mix together.
Add water in this mixture and mix.
The mixture should be thick enough to make petties.
Heat oil in skillet over medium heat.
Once oil is hot, cook petties in skillet for about 2-3 minutes.
Flip and cook for another 2-3 minutes until both sides are brown.
Serve hot and enjoy!

NUTRITIONAL INFORMATION

Calories Per Servings, 124 kcal, 1.13 g Fat, 4.86 g Protein, 26.16 g Total Carbs, 4.6 g Fiber

Stir Fried Broccoli & Tofu

Prep Time   20 Min
Servings   4

INGREDIENTS

8 oz. tofu cut into cubes

16 oz. broccoli cut into

1 tbsp. extra-virgin olive oil

2 large garlic cloves, minced

Salt and freshly ground black pepper

2 oz. walnut cream

Spinach leaves

DIRECTIONS

Heat a large heavy skillet over medium heat. Add the oil, once oil is hot, add broccoli with garlic and cook for 4-8 minutes until cooked.
Transfer cooked broccoli in plate.
Add the tofu cook for another 5-8 minutes until brown.
Transfer cooked tofu with broccoli and assemble spinach with them.
Drizzle walnut cream, salt and pepper on top.
Serve and enjoy!

NUTRITIONAL INFORMATION

Calories Per Servings, 287 kcal, 22.75 g Fat, 15.81 g Protein, 11.62 g Total Carbs, 6.3 g Fiber

Wilted Spinach with Onion

Prep Time   40 Min

Servings   2

INGREDIENTS

4 red onions, cut into rings

1/4 cup olive oil

2 1lb. spinach with stems

Salt and freshly ground pepper

DIRECTIONS

Heat oil in large pan over medium heat.
Add the onion rings and cook for about 10-15 minutes over low heat until i=onion is caramelized.
Transfer onion to plate.
Add spinach in same pan and cook for about 5-10 minutes until about to wilted.
 Transfer spinach to plate.
Top with caramelized onion.
Drizzle salt & pepper on top.
Serve and enjoy!

NUTRITIONAL INFORMATION

Calories Per Servings, 300 kcal, 22.79 g Fat, 13.6 g Protein, 18.13 g Total Carbs, 11.1 g Fiber

Broccoli with Garlic sauce

Prep Time   30 Min

Servings   2

INGREDIENTS

1/3 cup minced fresh garlic

2 tablespoons olive oil

1 heat broccoli cut into florets with stems

1 cup vegetable broth

1 tsp. turmeric

salt & pepper to taste

1 tbsp. buckwheat flour

DIRECTIONS
Heat oil in skillet over medium he
Add broccoli florets and cook for 4-5 minutes. Set aside.
Add minced garlic in same skillet and cook for 3 - 5 minutes, until garlic begins to brown.
Add broth salt & pepper and flour and mix well.
Pour broccoli in skillet again and cook for another 4-5 minutes until broccoli is soft and sauce is thick.
Serve hot and enjoy!

NUTRITIONAL INFORMATION

Calories Per Servings, 282 kcal, 14.95 g Fat, 11.07 g Protein, 33.39 g Total Carbs, 9.4 g Fiber

Hot & Sour Spinach

Prep Time   40 Min

Servings   2

INGREDIENTS

1 red onion, minced

1/2 cup sherry vinegar

1 thyme sprig

1 tablespoon dates syrup

2 1lb. spinach

3 tablespoons extra-virgin olive oil

Salt and freshly ground pepper

1 cup vegetable broth

DIRECTIONS

Heat oil in pan over medium heat.
Add the onion and cook for about 2-3 minutes over low heat.
Add the vinegar and thyme sprig and bring to a boil.
Simmer over low heat until the vinegar is reduced.
Add dates syrup and mix well.

Add broth in pan, bring to a boil.
Add the spinach and cook until wilted.
Season with salt and pepper and cook for about 5 minutes.
Transfer the spinach to a platter with some broth.
Serve and enjoy!

NUTRITIONAL INFORMATION

Calories Per Servings, 296 kcal, 11.86 g Fat, 15.79 g Protein, 37.91 g Total Carbs, 12.3 g Fiber

Spinach & Tofu Curry

Prep Time   30 Min

Servings   4

INGREDIENTS

2 cups, tofu cubes

2 cups spinach, chopped

2 cloves

1 cardamom

2 tbsps. olive oil

1 green chili, chopped

1 onion, chopped

1 cup walnut milk

½ tsp. ginger-garlic paste

1 tsp. cumin seeds

Salt to taste

DIRECTIONS

Heat oil in a pan over medium heat. once oil is hot, add tofu cubes and cook for 2-3 minutes.
Transfer fried tofu in plate.
Add the clove, cardamom, cinnamon, and cumin seeds and onion in pan and cook for 2-3 minutes.

Add spinach, milk, salt and ginger-garlic paste.
Stir-fry for 10-15 minutes over medium heat
Add fried tofu stir and combine well.
Once cooked remove from heat.
Serve and enjoy!

NUTRITIONAL INFORMATION

Calories Per Servings, 237 kcal, 11.31 g Fat, 7.34 g Protein, 27.12 g Total Carbs, 1.1 g Fiber

Easy Walnut Milk

Prep Time   5 Min

Servings   4

INGREDIENTS

1 cup walnuts

3 cups filtered water

1/4 tsp cinnamon

DIRECTIONS

Soak walnuts in water for 8 hours or overnight.
 night for at least 8 hours.
In morning strain, the walnuts and place walnuts with filtered water and cinnamon in blender.
Blend for 1-2 minutes.
Strain milk and store in fridge for 3-4 days.
Serve and enjoy!

NUTRITIONAL INFORMATION

Calories Per Servings, 131 kcal, 13.04 g Fat, 3.05 g Protein, 2.88 g Total Carbs, 1.4 g Fiber

Strawberries & Walnut Smoothie

Prep Time   10 Min

Servings   1

INGREDIENTS

1 cup walnuts milk

1 tsp dates syrup

2 oz. strawberries

1 pinch cinnamon

DIRECTIONS

Add all ingredients in high speed blender.
Blend until all ingredients are incorporated.
Serve and enjoy!

NUTRITIONAL INFORMATION

Calories Per Servings, 169 kcal, 13.23 g Fat, 3.43 g Protein, 12.55 g Total Carbs, 2.5 g Fiber

Walnut Cream

Prep Time   10 Min

Servings   4

INGREDIENTS

2 cups California walnuts
1 cup water
DIRECTIONS

Blend walnuts and water in a high-power blender or food processor until very smooth and light and fluffy.
Store in airtight jar and use in desserts.

NUTRITIONAL INFORMATION
Calories Per Servings, 262 kcal, 26.08 g Fat, 6.08 g Protein, 5.48 g Total Carbs, 2.7 g Fiber

Walnut Butter

Prep Time   30 Min
Servings   4

INGREDIENTS

1 1/2 cups walnuts

DIRECTIONS

Roast the walnuts in preheated oven for about 12 minutes until golden brown but not burnt.
Blend the walnut sin food processor for 1-2 minutes.
Scrape and blend for another 1-3 minutes
Store in airtight container and use in desserts.

NUTRITIONAL INFORMATION

Calories Per Servings, 196 kcal, 19.56 g Fat, 4.57 g Protein, 4.11 g Total Carbs, 2 g Fiber

Dark Chocolate Bites

Prep Time   15 min

Servings   8

INGREDIENTS

½ cup walnuts

¼ cup dark chocolate

1 cup Medjool dates, pitted

1 tbsp. cocoa powder

1 tbsp. ground turmeric

1 tbsp. extra virgin olive oil

water

DIRECTIONS
Place the all the ingredients in food processor and mix well.
Add water if required. Mixture should not be sticky.
Form walnut sized balls with your hands and roll over coco powder.
Freeze balls in freezer.

NUTRITIONAL INFORMATION
Calories Per Servings, 95 kcal, 7.16 g Fat, 1.61 g Protein, 7.37 g Total Carbs, 1.8 g Fiber

Walnut & Berries Ice-cream

Prep Time   10 min

Servings   2

INGREDIENTS

1 cup walnut cream

1 cup blueberries

DIRECTIONS
Pour walnut cream and half blueberries in blender and mix well.
Pour batter in silicon molds and freeze in freezer for 2- 4 hours until set and firm.
Serve with fresh berries.

NUTRITIONAL INFORMATION
Calories per serving 173 Cal, Fats 13.29 g, Protein 3.59 g, Total Carbs 13.46 g, Fiber 3.1 g

Smoothie with Kiwi

Prep Time   10 min

Servings   2

INGREDIENTS

1 kiwi

1 cup fresh blueberries

2 tbsps. chia seed

1 cup soy milk

¼ cup berries for topping

1 kiwi, slice for topping

DIRECTIONS

Pour kiwi, blueberries in electric high speed blender and blend.
Pour chia seeds in milk and mix well.
Set kiwi slice on the wall of glass and pour milk.
Top with blackberries mixture and fresh blackberries.

NUTRITIONAL INFORMATION
Calories per serving 178 Cal, Fats 2.16 g, Protein 3.78 g, Total Carbs 38.77 g, Fiber 1.8 g

Blueberries Smoothie

Prep Time   10 min
Servings   1

INGREDIENTS
4-5 strawberries
1/2 cup frozen blueberries
½ cup soy milk
1 cup ice cubes

DIRECTIONS
Mix all the ingredients into a blender, blend until thick and creamy Pour smoothie in serving glass and top with fresh blueberries and strawberries slice.

NUTRITIONAL INFORMATION
Calories per serving 113 Cal, Fats 3.1 g, Protein 2.64 g, Total Carbs 20.04 g, Fiber 3.2 g

Chinese Chocolate Truffles

Prep Time   20 Min

Servings   20

INGREDIENTS

16 oz. chocolate

1 cup walnut cream

1 tbsp. Chinese Five Spice Powder

I cup cocoa powder for rolling

DIRECTIONS

Mix together all ingredients in bowl.

Let the mixture sit for 15 minutes.

Freeze the mixture for 2 hours until firm.

Scoop or spoon the mixture into small balls and roll on coco powder.

Refrigerate the rolled truffles for 2 hours.

NUTRITIONAL INFORMATION

Calories per serving 359 Cal, Fats 26.04 g, Protein 14.5 g, Total Carbs 22.31 g, Fiber 10.1 g

Sirt Food Diet Recipes 2020

Meal Plans and Recipes for Beginners to Activate Anti-Aging Effects and Your Skinny Gene. Get Lean and Healthy with Simple and Tasty Food Plans

ASHLEY GOSLING

Copyright © 2020 Ashley Gosling

All rights reserved.

INTRODUCTION

The Sirtfood Diet is a weight loss program based on a type of protein called "sirtuins". These proteins are found in all living things and can mimic the effects of fasting and exercise by burning fat, building muscle and fighting disease.

Sirtuin occurs naturally in a variety of foods that we eat. We start with the two most notable members of the sirt food diet: red wine and chocolate. Other foods that are rich in sirtuins are kale, green tea, and apples.

If you focus on sirtuin foods (called "sirt foods" by dieters), you may be able to stimulate the lean genes that help you lose weight quickly - or at least that's the idea.

According to the inventors of the special diet, Aidan Goggins and Glen Matten, who, as nutrition experts and authors of the ordering nutritional guide "The SIRT Food Diet", have intensively dealt with the role of certain enzymes in the body, one does not take conscious Sirtfood nutrition only lose up to three kilograms a week, but also strengthens the immune system and muscles. In addition, the cell metabolism should decrease, which in turn slows down the aging process. Of course, an additional supportive sports program lets the pounds melt even faster.

SPECIAL DISCLAIMER

All the informations included in this book are given for instructive, informational and entertainment purposes, the author can claim to share very good quality recipes but is not headed for the perfect data and uses of the mentioned recipes, in fact the informations are not intent to provide dietary advice without a medical consultancy.

The author do not hold any responsibility for errors, omissions or contrary interpretation of the content in this book.

It is recommended to consult a medical practitioner before to approach any kind of diet, especially if you have a particular health situation, the author isn't headed for the responsibility of these situations and everything is under the responsibility of the reader, the author strongly recommend to preserve the health taking all precautions to ensure ingredients are fully cooked.

All the trademarks and brands used in this book are only mentioned to clarify the sources of the informations and to describe better a topic. All the trademarks and brands mentioned own their copyrights and they are not related in any way to this document and to the author.

This document is written to clarify all the informations of publishing purposes and cover any possible issue. This document is under copyright and it is not possible to reproduce any part of this content in every kind of digital or printable document. All rights reserved.

INTRODUCTION OF THE SIRTFOOD DIET

WHAT IS SIRT FOOD?

The new magic word in the diet jungle is "Sirtfood". A wide range of special foods should help you slim down, build muscle at the same time and also strengthen the immune system. Even luxury foods such as chocolate and red wine are allowed. Stilpalast reveals the secret of this trendy weight loss method.

The "Sirtfoods" are foods which, in combination with a restricted calorie intake, are supposed to influence the activity of the so-called sirtuins. Sirtuins are a group of enzymes that can affect, among other things, the metabolism, inflammatory processes and various factors of aging.

Certain foods are particularly rich in substances that are said to increase the activity of these enzymes. The assumptions of the inventors of the sirt food diet lie in the fact that a high consumption of these sirtuin foods (short: sirt foods) has a positive influence on the metabolism and the aging of the participants. At the same time, people who eat on the basis of the sirt food diet pay attention to a calorie deficit.

Sirtuin describes a certain protein, i.e. a protein building block. In various guides that exist on the subject of sirt food, this is also touted as a "slim gene" or "super protein". This protein helps build muscle as well as burning fat - up to three kilos a week. And sirtuins, of which we humans have seven, do not just build muscles and fat from - they can still more: Sirtuine strengthen the immune system, protect the body from disease and inflammation and work off. They also prevent cravings and slow down the aging process. Another plus: Thanks to the many vitamins and minerals in the food, not only is the immune system pushed, you also feel healthier and fitter thanks to "Sirtfood".

HOW DOES THE SIRT FOOD DIET WORK?

Every diet is different and each promises to drop several kilos within a short time. Unfortunately, this often involves a very one-sided diet that is anything but healthy in the long run. The Sirtfood Diet is said to be different, because it not only promises weight loss, but is supposed to be healthy and keep the user young and fresh. So what more do you want?

While the famous low-carb diet is full of proteins and excludes carbohydrates, the latest weight loss cure focuses on sirtuins. These are enzymes in the body that, through their special activity, namely the reduction in the production of free radicals, protect the cells in the body from stress. If the body absorbs enough sirtuins from food, they also burn fat.

The advantage: Sirtuins are contained in a number of many foods and beverages, including luxury foods, and thus enable a varied diet that is not very restrictive. The only task during this diet is to eat as many foods as possible that are rich in said sirtuins.

The crux of this method is therefore not the sparse choice of dishes, but rather the total amount of calories that are "allowed" per day: In the first three days of the diet, there are just 1,000 calories a day (mainly vegetables), after that 1,500 per day. In the long run, the sirtuin-rich foods should be included in the menu as often as possible to keep the weight and not fall prey to the yo-yo effect. Healthy drinks in the form of green smoothies are also part of the conscious diet.

The 3 phases of the Sirtfood Diet

The sirt food diet is divided into three phases. In order to detoxify the body and prepare the metabolism for the change in diet and weight loss, you start with a daily calorie intake of 1000 kilocalories in the form of juices.

The first phase is to reprogram the metabolism to "lean". This works, for example, with sirtuin-rich green juices that detoxify the body. That means:

1000 calories a day in the form of three juices and a main meal. In the second phase, the number of calories is increased to 1500. For example: two healthy juices, two main dishes. And phase three is used to stabilize the new weight; there are still many sirt foods on the menu, but more calories again.

Phase 1: 1000 kcal daily. Three green juices and a main meal, all rich in sirtuin foods. The body is programmed to "lose weight". This first phase should last three days. Juices from sirtuin-containing foods such as arugula, apples, celery or parsley as well as an additional main meal are on the menu list.

Phase 2: The first and most difficult phase has been completed. In phase two, the calorie intake is increased to 1500 calories. There are now two green juices and two main meals a day. Two juices and two main meals from sirtuin-rich foods are consumed during this time. However, the "miracle ingredients" are also combined with other "normal" foods in order to slowly get used to it again. Once the desired weight has been reached, this phase can be ended.

Phase 3: In the third or maintenance phase, everything is actually allowed as long as you have as many sirt foods on the menu as possible and eat around 1800 calories. There are three main meals a day; this is to be consolidated with 1800 kilocalories per day. It is important to be careful not to fall into old habits and to ensure a high protein intake.

If you want to reduce your weight, you should consistently stick to sirtuin-rich foods during the sirt food diet. You can find an overview of the most important sirt foods below - including, for example, apples, arugula, strawberries, green tea and spices such as chili or turmeric. There is also a piece of dark chocolate in it every day. Particularly practical: the slimming products not only boost fat burning, they also help build muscle. Because if you also exercise on a diet, you will achieve better results. Better not: Use fast food and the like again after the diet, otherwise the famous yo yo effect threatens!

Sirt food diet: You can eat these foods

The taste does not tell you what foods Sirtuin contains - it is found in both bitter fruits and vegetables and in sweets. That is why we have created a small overview with foods that contain sirtuin:

- ➢ Arugula

Arugula or rocket not only tastes great as a salad, but also with other sirt foods to make a green smoothie. Our recipe suggestion: chop 2 handfuls of uncooked kale, 1 handful of arugula, two to three stalks of celery, half a handful of flat-leaf parsley and lovage leaves in a blender. Add half a teaspoon of matcha powder and fill with apple juice, done!

- Red onions

In combination with sirtuins, red onions are the perfect slender vegetable! Why? Like all onions, they have a certain degree of heat, which can be attributed to the high content of isoalliin. The resulting amino acid taurine causes the pituitary gland to release hormones. These accelerate fat loss.

- Strawberries

Compared to other fruits, strawberries contain little sugar (a little more than 5 g per 100 g), but plenty of fiber. These swell in the stomach and fill you up faster.

- Red wine

The polyphenol resveratrol contained in red wine (especially in Pinot Noir) activates the sirtuin enzymes in the body.

- Chili

The chilli-enhancer capsaicin increases the heat production in the body by up to 25 percent. To compensate for this rise in temperature, the body begins to sweat. That uses a lot of energy.

- Olive oil

Olive oil contains valuable unsaturated fatty acids. The oil also has a high phenol content, which boosts fat burning. Rule of thumb: the more natural the aromatic oil, the greater the slimming power.

- Walnuts

Vitamin B 6, which is largely contained in walnuts, improves concentration, makes you more alert and prevents cravings.

- Coffee and green tea

Both coffee and green tea ensures that the metabolism is in full swing. Some studies even show that caffeine also increases fat burning.

➤ Dark chocolate

A piece of dark chocolate with a cocoa content of at least 85% is also allowed in the sirt food diet.

Of course, you do not only need to feed on the following food list. The aim is only to incorporate the treats containing sirtuin as often as possible into the menu. The following applies to luxury foods such as coffee, chocolate or red wine: Always enjoy with sensibility and do not eat or drink in abundance.

And we still have some others food listed below containing sirtuin

- Kale
- Celery
- Ruccola
- Radicchio
- Shrimp
- Spices: turmeric, chilli, parsley
- Apples
- Citrus fruits (e.g. oranges)
- Blueberries
- Soy products
- Walnuts
- Buckwheat

You should avoid these foods

In principle, all foods listed below that are rich in sirtuins can be consumed without hesitation. Foods that are completely free of these enzymes, such as potatoes or legumes, should only be used as a combination and should not be the main component of the meal.

Note:

Even if you do not stick to the recommendation of the very low daily calorie intake: The increased incorporation of sirtuin-rich foods into a balanced and nutrient-rich menu certainly does no harm and leaves - if not so quickly - one or the other in combination with sporting activities Melt down pounds (you can find a simple workout program for each type of figure here). Because the more muscles there are, the more calories are burned. Practical: Sirtuin-rich foods also inhibit cravings.

The Sirt Food: Lean and healthy thanks to proteins

Similar to a low-carb diet, the Sirtfood diet also relies on proteins or a very specific protein: Sirtuin. This belongs to the group of proteins and helps to build muscle and burn fat. As if that weren't enough, sirtuins strengthen the immune system and protect the body from diseases and inflammation. They are also said to help reduce stress, prevent cravings and slow down the aging process. A real super protein!

In order for the body to enjoy the positive effect of these enzymes, foods and spices containing sirtuin must be consumed daily. These are, for example, chilli, soy products, buckwheat, shrimp, blueberries, strawberries, green apples, citrus fruits, walnuts, kale, capers, turmeric, parsley, ginger, celery, green tea, coffee, dark chocolate (from 85% cocoa content), Olive oil and red wine.

HOW SIRTFOOD DIET CAN HELP IN LOSING OF WEIGHT AND BURNING OF FAT

You might be wondering: can the sirtfood diet really help us lose weight and burn fat?

The diet claims that eating foods that increase the amount of sirtuins, such as those rich in polyphenols, will activate a 'skinny gene' pathway generally induced by exercise and fasting. One of the statements they make is that you will lose 3 kilos in seven days; and of course, rapid weight loss is always attractive.

Sounds great, but does it have a solid scientific basis? The short answer is no. Despite some preliminary studies, a sirtuin-activating diet for weight loss is not yet scientifically proven.

This plan sounds appealing, but there is actually little research to back up these claims. Rapid weight loss at the beginning of the diet plan may have more to do with calorie restriction than sirtuins.

But we all know that rapid weight loss is neither healthy nor sustainable; experts recommend reducing almost a kilo a week. That way, you're more likely to lose fat instead of water and lean muscle, and less likely to be exposed to nutritional deficiencies.

The name already reveals what the diet is basically based on: so-called sirt foods are all those foods that stimulate the fat-burning enzyme sirtuin and reduce the extra pounds.

The basis of the sirt food diet is the scientific knowledge that certain plant substances stimulate the activity of the body's own sirtuins as well as fasting. Aidan Goggins and Glen Metten, the nutritionists and authors of the diet bestseller of the same name, are convinced that a diet based on the sirtuin principle not only leads to a dream figure, but also with enjoyment. As long as you combine the relevant foods in a targeted manner and outwit your metabolism in this way.

Examples of the secondary plant substances that are considered to be sirtuin activators are allicin, which gives garlic its typical aroma, capsaicin, which is mainly found in chillies, or curcumin, to which turmeric owes its yellow color.

Sirtfoods not only boost fat burning effectively, they also protect the organism from cell damage, heart or cancer diseases and slow down the general aging process. Sirtuins also prevent typical cravings, support muscle building and cellular fitness and strengthen the immune system. What makes a sirtuin diet so much easier: Sirtfoods are neither particularly unusual nor boring. These are everyday foods, especially fruits and vegetables. By the way, red wine and chocolate are also allowed.

THE MOST IMPORTANT SIRT FOODS FOR LOSING WEIGHT

The basis first: All foods are plant-based in the Sirtfood diet. The valuable sirtuins provide fruit and vegetables, but also spices and herbs. Typical sirt foods include apples, blueberries, raspberries and citrus fruits as well as broccoli, kale, tomatoes, arugula, onions, celery, garlic, parsley, chilli, turmeric, walnuts and cashew nuts. Sirtuins are also contained in dark chocolate with 85 percent cocoa and in red wine. These foods are supplemented with proven protein sources known from the low carb diet: soy products, white meat or eggs.

The sirt diet is supposed to boost your metabolism and thus accelerate weight loss

Sirtfood develops its effects via secondary plant substances, which form the plant's immune system. The antibodies are supposed to trigger the following reactions in the human body: optimized metabolism, improved immune defense, cancer protection, life extension.

HOW TO ACTIVATE YOUR METABOLISM AND YOUR SKINNY GENE

1. Activate a lot of drinking for metabolism

With water you support your digestion and increase your basic metabolism. The German Society for Nutrition (DGE) recommends taking in about 2.7 liters of water a day, of which about 1.5 liters from drinks. According to a research series by the Berlin Charité, 500 milliliters of water already increase energy consumption by 24 percent for the next 60 minutes.

If you drink water instead of sugary drinks, you automatically absorb fewer calories and are more likely to maintain or reach a healthy weight. If you drink water about half an hour before eating, you also eat less because you feel fuller. According to a study, this even led to 44 percent more weight loss during a diet (e.g. the metabolic diet).

The drinking of water can therefore provide the stimulation of the metabolism. Cold water is even more effective for stimulating the metabolism because the body has to use more energy to warm it up to body temperature.

Also Green Tea and coffee are known fat burner and can boost your metabolism. Green tea helps convert the fat in the body into free fatty acids, thereby increasing fat burning by ten to 17 percent.

This effect is also believed to be coffee, but it works more in slim people than in obese people, as a study showed.

NOTE!

Drink a lot of water! This can stimulate the metabolism and help you lose weight. Green tea or coffee can also effectively boost metabolism.

2. Eating spicy and protein-rich stimulates the metabolism

Eating can push your metabolism for a few hours. This effect is called TEF, the Thermic Effect of Food, and refers to the additional energy that the body has to spend to digest and process the nutrients of a meal.

The body needs the most energy for proteins, so you can boost your metabolism by 15 to 30 percent. Carbohydrates have a low nutrient density and, on the other hand, only stimulate metabolism by five to ten percent, fat only by zero to three percent.

Proteins are generally recommended during a weight loss phase because they fill you up, counteract the loss of muscle.

NOTE!

The body needs more energy to process proteins than it provides itself - proteins also keep you full for a long time and prevent muscle mass from being lost.

3. Stimulate the metabolism with coconut oil

Coconut oil contains more medium chain fatty acids than most oils. Medium-chain fatty acids can stimulate the metabolism more than long-chain fats (e.g. in butter). According to a study, the basal metabolic rate is even increased by twelve percent, while long-chain fats could only stimulate it by four percent. According to these studies, it may be beneficial to use coconut oil more often.

Nevertheless, coconut oil should only be enjoyed in moderation, since the ratio of fatty acids in it is unfavorable: the proportion of saturated fatty acids is 90 percent. These can increase the risk of fat metabolism disorders, cardiovascular diseases and even breast cancer.

NOTE!

According to some studies, coconut oil can stimulate the metabolism. However, since it contains a lot of saturated fatty acids, it should only be consumed in moderation.

4. Sport boosts metabolism and skinny gene

Exercise can increase your basal metabolic rate. With increasing muscles, the basal metabolic rate and energy consumption also increase. Since both fat mass and muscle mass are lost when you lose weight, it is all the more important to compensate for this through exercise. The DGE recommends about 30 to 60 minutes of exercise a day.

Do not only do endurance sports, but also strength training, because the lean muscle mass is crucial for losing weight. Some studies have shown that strength training is one of the most effective types of training to build muscle and optimize metabolism. The best results are achieved when endurance and strength training are combined. Studies have now shown that a HIIT workout (high-intensity interval training) is particularly good for the metabolism, since the after burn effect is strongest here in comparison to other sports. This means that even after training, the metabolism remains elevated. In addition, HIIT training, which alternates between training at the highest intensity and short, relaxing intervals, promotes fat burning and thus the tumbling of the kilos.

In a twelve-week research series, the male subjects who regularly did HIIT workouts lost two kilograms of body weight and 17 percent of belly fat. Even small changes can have an effect. Instead of sitting at work all day, you should always get up or work standing up. According to a study, a "seasoned afternoon" can burn up to 174 kilocalories (kcal) extra.

NOTE!

Exercise increases basal metabolism. A mix of strength and endurance training is most effective for losing weight. This tells you how many kilocalories you can burn with which sport. Is your favorite sport included?

5. Sleep is good for your metabolism

Sleep has a positive effect on the metabolism. Here the deep, coherent sleep is most important in the first three hours of the night's rest. A disturbed or too short sleep can lead to obesity and generally has a negative effect on the metabolism.

Poor sleep behavior has been shown to increase blood sugar levels and insulin resistance. Both can lead to diabetes disease lead.

Sufficient sleep is also important for athletes because the muscles that have been exposed to a stimulus during exercise are regenerated during sleep.

Poor sleep can also stimulate the hunger hormone ghrelin while reducing the satiety hormone leptin. This could explain why people who lack sleep are often hungry and have difficulty losing weight.

6. Eat enough healthy fats

Did you know that your daily food intake should consist of 30 percent healthy fats?

So, don't demonize fat in your diet. For example, go for avocado, linseed oil, almonds, walnuts, olive oil, linseed and salmon. Instead, avoid trans fatty acids - the so-called bad fat. It is in cookies, fries, chips and crackers - in everything that has been baked and fried for a long time.

EASY EXERCISES TO OPTIMIZE YOUR FAT BURNING

1. Go on foot:

Since our society has developed so that physically heavy work can be done by machines, most jobs are limited to mental activities in front of a screen.

This makes it difficult for most people to reach the often recommended 6,000 to 10,000 steps a day. For many, however, these steps are simply not possible because it forces work to sit. Taking short walks or actively choosing a slightly longer way to work can help to at least increase the steps.

Choosing a more active everyday life can already lead to more calories being burned throughout the day, which increases the chance of successfully burning fat.

2. Endurance training - low intensity, long duration:

Classic cardio training is probably the best known and most popular exercise for burning fat. It is easy to understand and can be carried out several times a week due to the low load.

The usual cardio machines in the gym are ideal for this, but also cycling and jogging.

Note: Even though this type of fat burning is relatively easy to regenerate, it does not mean that you can start jogging for 1 hour as an absolute beginner.

Give your body time to get used to the stress.

3. Strength training:

Strength training has two important factors that will help you burn fat. For one, strength training is work and already consumes calories in itself. A training session of approx. 2 hours can burn around 200-600 calories, depending on the intensity and your own body weight.

But strength training also ensures that the muscles are preserved and, in some cases, for example as a beginner or as a very overweight, even muscle can be built up.

These muscles are important for burning fat because they contribute a little to your calorie consumption.

The more muscles you have, the higher your basal metabolism. This effect is small, but it is there.

So, strength training is an important factor in burning fat and shouldn't be left out.

Supplement - strength training finisher:

In addition to strength training, a whole-body workout, known as a finisher, can be introduced after the workout.

Joe DeFranco describes this finisher as an additional full-body cardio that is supposed to help his athletes lose weight.

4. Dead weight complex

The easiest way to train the whole body again is with your own weight exercises.

These should be carried out one after the other. Depending on the level of performance, this complex can be repeated after a few minutes.

- 30 mountain climbers
- 20 pushups
- 10 Groiners
- 5 burpees

For advanced - barbell complex:

For something more advanced, there is a complex with the barbell, you need a barbell and, depending on the level of performance, weight plates.

- 10 deadlifts

- 10 oars
- 10 hang clean
- 10 push press
- 10 squats

Note:

Since there is no break between exercises, a weight is selected for each exercise. For most of them this means choosing the weight with which the Hang cleans can be easily carried out. It is advisable to start with the empty bar and then increase in upcoming training sessions.

5. Interval training:

In addition to normal cardio, there is also time-efficient interval training or also known as HIIT.

HIIT stands for High Intensity Interval Training and initially only describes that one type of movement alternates with extremely high intensity and low intensity.

For example, it can mean sprinting as fast as you can for 1 minute and then relaxing for 30 seconds. This type of cardio can burn the same as a longer static cardio, but is a major problem for regeneration due to the high intensity.

For this reason, it is recommended to do some kind of interval training at most 2-3 times a week.

6. Tabata jumping rope:

Jumping rope only requires rope and can actually be done anywhere. In order to be able to do rope jumping in tabata style, you need a watch or your mobile phone.

There are also some Tabata clock apps.

Jump 20 seconds as fast as you can rope, followed by 10 seconds of complete pause. Repeat 8-10 times.

7. Interval sprints:

Interval sprints can be run anywhere. Some cardio treadmills already offer an interval function. Aim for approximately 200-400 meters of sprints, followed by 60 seconds of easy walking.

Depending on how good your condition is, you can repeat these sprints several times.

8. Hill sprints:

Hill sprints are, as the name suggests, sprints on a hill. The downhill path is used for an active break and when you reach the bottom, the hill is sprinted up again.

Of course, this only works if you have a hill in your area. Find only a very small and short hill at the beginning and try to sprint for about 15 minutes and then slowly jog down again. Depending on the level of performance, a steeper and / or longer hill can then be selected.

WHAT YOU NEED TO KNOW BEFORE TO START (PRO & CONS)

WHAT IS IT ABOUT THE SIRT FOOD DIET?

Opinions differ on how successful a sirt food diet really is. It is positive that the diet plan allows a certain degree of freedom of design. Even allergy sufferers and vegans get their money's worth. The groceries can easily be bought in the supermarket; the preparation of the recipes is mostly simple and takes no longer than 20-30 minutes. The concept also includes all food groups and does not allow the effect. At the same time, great importance is attached to health.

Opponents of the diet question the effect of the sirt foods and attribute the weight loss to the limited calorie intake. Especially since only 1,000 calories are consumed in the first three days, then 1,500 calories afterwards.

CRITICISM OF THE SIRTFOOD DIET

So far, there is no evidence of the effectiveness of the sirt food diet. Sensible scientific studies are completely lacking. Only the inventors themselves tested their diet in the context of their book with 39 participants. The loss success of the participants is most likely due to the large calorie deficit of 1000 kilocalories per day.

During this time, the participants lost an average of 3.2 kilograms of body weight. Anyone who chooses to consume fewer calories can lose a lot of weight in the short term. Regarding weight loss, it doesn't matter which foods are eaten here, the decisive factor is the calorie deficit. But the 3.2 kilograms are not just body fat. At the beginning of every diet, it is often stored water that is released when the body uses energy reserves in the form of glycogen.

If you eat more after the diet, the glycogen stores replenish and new water is bound. Thus the weight increases again.

Over a period of several weeks, a high calorie deficit (1000+ calories per day) can cause your metabolism to drop. The body switches to a low flame and thus lowers its energy requirements. If, after the diet is completed, old eating patterns are resumed, the weight rises because the body gets more energy than it needs. The dreaded effect sets in.

Of course, the Sirtfoods are extremely healthy foods. Due to their high nutrient and antioxidant content, they are an important part of a healthy diet and should be eaten regularly. At this point it must be said that chocolate and red wine contain antioxidants, but they can prevent excess weight loss. The motto here is: enjoy everything in moderation.

However, the activity of the sirtuins does not affect humans. Rather, it appears to be the calorie deficit that affects the sirtuins. Sirt foods without a calorie deficit only have an effect on bacteria and not on mammals.

When it comes to long-term fat loss, avoiding side effect and keeping the body healthy and slowing aging processes, the only thing that is required is a long-term dietary change. There is a high probability that short-term diet success will quickly lead to a side effect after completing the diet.

NOTE

The Sirtfood Diet is suitable for short-term weight loss. However, it is not designed for long-term weight loss.

Who is the diet suitable for?

The Sirtfood Diet is suitable for:

- People with perseverance and discipline
- Nutrition-loving people with background knowledge

The Sirtfood Diet is not suitable for:

- People who have a hard time consuming only a few calories every day

Many advisors reveal which other foods are suitable for the sirt food diet and which other foods are combined with them. These can be helpful in order to better plan daily food preparation and thus make it easier. Because a comprehensive knowledge of sirtuins, their effects and how to best integrate them into your daily diet increases your stamina.

Relaxation is also an essential part of the sirt food diet. In stressful situations, the hormone cortisol is released, which, together with insulin, stimulates blood sugar levels and causes the body to feel hungry during periods of rest . Mainly due to the calorie reduction, one should avoid stressful situations in everyday life as much as possible. Small activities to balance out like a little walk in the fresh air can work wonders.

NOTE!

In order to keep up with the Sirtfood Diet in the long term, advice can be helpful. It is also important to avoid stress.

CONCLUSION

In the end, everyone who has a long-term diet of 1500 kcal a day and mostly vegetables will lose weight. But there is also a risk of starvation, because this amount is simply very, very little.

Nevertheless, the sirt food diet also provides valuable insights into the role of certain enzymes in the body. In fact, sirtuins can stimulate fat metabolism and contribute to increasing antioxidant enzymes. Sirtuin-rich foods can therefore still be on the menu more often, even if you do not fully adhere to the sirtfood concept.

The lasting success of the Sirtfood Plan is questionable, but the food for thought is certainly valuable. In the end, you can draw at least a small part of every wisdom for yourself. It seems to be the same with this brand-new diet.

SIRT FOOD RECIPES

SUMMARY

The sirt food diet is all about the so-called sirtuins. The enzymes that influence the metabolism and are said to have a positive effect on our body, in particular on the aging process, are activated with the help of some foods such as chilli, arugula, walnuts or buckwheat.

The body is to undergo a long-term dietary change within three phases. It starts with a calorie intake of 1000 kilocalories, which increases over 1500 to 1800 kilocalories (phases 1 to 3).

So far, there is no scientific evidence of an actual positive effect of the sirtuins, which is why this diet is very controversial.

It is advantageous to get an overview of sirtuins and their effects with advice before choosing this diet for yourself.

GREEN TAGLIATELLE WITH PISTACHIO GREMOLATA

Ingredients for 2 portions

- 1 Organic juice orange
- 1 Tablespoons pistachios (roasted, chopped)
- Garlic (chopped)
- 0.5 Tbsp thyme leaves (chopped)
- 1 Tablespoons chopped parsley
- Pepper (freshly ground)
- 50 Grams (green soybean pasta,
- salt
- 150 Grams of pepper (green, halved lengthways, cored)
- 3rd Spring onions (in rings)
- 1 Tablespoons of olive oil
- 1 Beef tomato (chopped)
- 1 Tablespoons balsamic vinegar (white)
- 1Tablespoons chili sauce (sweet and spicy)

Preparation

Cooking time: 30 minutes

Difficulty: light

- For the pistachio gremolata, rinse the orange hot, dry and grate 1 tbsp. orange peel. Mix with the pistachios, garlic, thyme and parsley. Season the gremolata vigorously with pepper. Squeeze the orange and set the juice aside.
- Cook the noodles in salted water, braise onions and green peppers in olive oil.
- Add tomatoes and melt briefly. Salt and pepper. Add orange juice and vinegar and boil.
- Drain the noodles, mix with peppers and chili sauce and serve with the gremolata.

Nutritional info

Per serving:

- 455 kcal,
- 22g fat,
- 30g carbohydrates,
- 28g protein

CHICKEN TAGINE WITH FENNEL AND HARISS CREAM

Ingredients for 2 portions

- 80 Grams of whole grain rice
- salt
- 70 Grams of tomato (fresh or canned, chopped)
- 1 red onion (in eighth)
- 0.25 Tsp turmeric (ground)
- 3rd Peppercorns
- 0.5 Tsp fennel (fennel seed)
- 1 Organic chicken drumstick (340 g)
- 150 Grams of fennel bulb (in large pieces)
- 100 Grams of carrot (in 2 cm slices)
- 1 TL Harissa (paste)
- 2nd Tablespoons plain yogurt (3.8% fat)
- 2nd Tablespoons goat cream cheese
- 0.5 Handful of coriander leaves

Preparation

Cooking time: 60 minutes

Difficulty: light

- Rinse rice cold in a colander. Bring to a boil in a saucepan with 200 ml of salted water, stir once and cover and swell over a low heat for 20–30 minutes until the water is completely absorbed. Let cool overnight. Divide into 2 portions.
- Boil 400 ml water, tomato, onion, salt and spices. Put the chicken drumsticks in it and cook covered for 20 minutes. Add vegetables and cook over medium heat for 10-15 minutes.
- Take out the chicken drumsticks, make it withour skin and bones (approx. 160 g) and divide into 2 portions. Divide one portion into coarse pieces, pluck the rest into fine pieces and chill with 1 portion of rice for the next day. Collect broth.
- Mix 1 cup of hot cooking stock, harissa, yoghurt and cream cheese for the haris cream.
- Arrange the chicken, rice, vegetables and hariss cream and sprinkle with coriander.

Nutritional info

Per serving:
- 350 kcal,
- 10g fat,
- 32g carbohydrates,
- 28g protein

TUNA BALLS ON ZUCCHINI SALAD

Ingredients for 2 Servings

- 100 Grams of sheep's cheese
- 1 Tin of tuna (tuna salad, 160 g)
- Pepper (freshly ground)
- 1 Clove of garlic
- 1 Juice orange
- 4th Tsp olive oil
- 1 Tablespoons apple cider vinegar (mild)
- 1 Tsp Dijon mustard
- 2nd Tablespoons pumpkin seeds
- 0.5 Lettuce (125 g)
- 150 Grams of carrot
- 150 Grams of zucchini
- Basil leaves

Preparation

Cooking time: 20 minutes

Difficulty: light

- Chop the sheep's cheese into small pieces, mix with the tuna salad and pepper well. Cut small cams from the mass or roll them into balls with moistened hands.
- Peel and crush garlic. Squeeze orange. Mix the orange juice, garlic, olive oil, vinegar, mustard and pepper.
- Roast the pumpkin seeds then clean lettuce, rinse and cut into strips. Peel the carrot, rinse the zucchini, dry and grate into long strips. Mix all the ingredients.
- Arrange the lettuce and tuna balls on 2 plates, sprinkle pumpkin seeds over them and sprinkle with basil leaves if necessary.

Nutritional info

Per serving:

- 400 kcal,
- 27g fat,
- 17g carbohydrates,
- 21g protein

ZUCCHINI AND BEAN SALAD WITH SPINACH FLAN

Ingredients for 2 servings

- 2nd (cooked spinach flans, see tip)
- 150 Grams of legumes (TL-legume mixture)
- 150 Grams of zucchini (in fine strips)
- salt
- 6 Tablespoons of lemon juice
- 1 Tablespoons of balsamic vinegar
- 1 Clove of garlic (chopped)
- 1 Tablespoons acacia honey (liquid)
- Pepper (freshly ground)
- 2nd Tablespoons of olive oil
- 2nd Tsp. linseed oil
- 1 red onion (in fine rings)
- 2nd Sticks of celery (in thin slices)
- 1 Handful of mint (fresh leaves)

Preparation

Cooking time: 35 minutes

Difficulty: light

- Prepare frozen legumes, drain and let cool.
- Salt the zucchini strips a little. Mix the lemon juice, vinegar, garlic, honey and pepper. Fold in olive oil and linseed oil with a fork.
- Mix legume mix, onion, celery, zucchini with liquid, mint and vinaigrette and arrange with both spinach flans on deep plates or in bowls.

Nutritional info

Per serving:

- ❖ 460 kcal,
- ❖ 28g fat,
- ❖ 29g carbohydrates,
- ❖ 20g protein

PAPAYA BOWL WITH TUNA

Ingredients for 2 portions

- 40 Grams of iceberg lettuce (cut)
- 1 Tin of tuna (tuna salad, 160 g,
- 140 Grams of papaya (papaya pulp, sliced)
- 1 Tbsp papaya (papaya seeds)
- 100 Grams of cucumber (sliced)
- 0.5 red peppers (finely sliced)
- 2nd Tablespoons of lime juice
- 1 Tsp camelina oil
- Pepper (freshly ground)
- Salt
- 40 Grams of bread

Preparation

Cooking time: 15 minutes

Difficulty: light

- Fill iceberg lettuce, tuna salad, papaya, papaya seeds, cucumber and bell pepper into a storage box or lunch box.

- Mix lime juice, camelina oil, pepper, salt and 1-2 teaspoons of water and drizzle over the vegetables. Close the can. Pack the bread strips separately.

Nutritional info

Per serving:

- 470 kcal,
- 26g fat,
- 34g carbohydrates,
- 22g protein

SPICY MUESLI WITH SHEEP'S CHEESE

Ingredients for 2 portions

- 150 Grams of kefir
- 1 Tsp tomato paste
- 1 Tablespoons acacia honey (or rosemary honey)
- 1 Tsp soy sauce
- Cayenne pepper
- 50 Grams of sheep's cheese
- 150 Grams of cucumber (in cubes)
- 1 Kiwi (gold kiwi, sliced)
- 3rd Tablespoons of muesli

Preparation

Cooking time: 10 minutes

Difficulty: light

- Mix the kefir, tomato paste, honey and soy sauce and season with cayenne pepper.
- Roughly crumble sheep's cheese. First put kefir, then cucumber, kiwi and sheep's cheese in a transport container and sprinkle with muesli

Nutritional info

Per serving:

- 445 kcal,
- 15g fat,
- 51g carbohydrates,
- 20g protein

CHICKEN PINEAPPLE SALAD

Ingredient for 2 servings

- 40 Grams of whole grain rice
- 80 Grams of chicken (see recipe "Chicken Tagine with Fennel")
- 2nd Spring onions (in rings)
- 1 Carrot (grated)
- 150 Grams of pineapple (in pieces)
- 150 Grams of red cabbage (finely sliced)
- 2nd Tbsp. apple cider vinegar
- 1 Tablespoons orange jam (bitter)
- 3rd Tablespoons of orange juice
- 3rd Tablespoons chicken broth (bouillon)
- 1 TL curry powder (medium hot)
- Cayenne pepper
- 5 Tsp. linseed oil (or rapeseed oil)
- salt
- 2nd Tbsp cashew nuts (roasted)

Preparation

Cooking time: 30 minutes

Difficulty: light

- Mix the rice, chicken, spring onions, carrot, pineapple and red cabbage loosely.
- Mix together apple cider vinegar, jam, orange juice, stock, curry and cayenne pepper. Fold in linseed oil with a fork and mix the dressing with the rice salad and season with salt.
- Divide the salad into 2 portions. Put one half in a glass and arrange the other half on a plate. Chill the salad in a glass and eat the next day.

Nutritional info

Per serving:

- 410 kcal,
- 17g fat,
- 46g carbohydrates,
- 15g protein

PUMPERNICKEL SANDWICH

Ingredients for 2 portions

- 60 Grams of sour milk cheese (Harzer, Mainzer)
- Pepper (freshly ground)
- 2nd Pumpernickel slices (80 g)
- 1 Tablespoons of tomato paste
- 40 Grams of arugula
- 2nd Pickled gherkins (sliced)
- 1 Apple (half in thin slices, half whole)
- 1 Teaspoons of lemon juice
- 1 Tsp mustard (sweet)

Preparation

Cooking time: 10 minutes

Difficulty: light

- Cut the cheese into four slices and pepper. Spread a slice of bread with tomato paste and top with rocket, cheese and pickled cucumbers.

- Drizzle lemon slices and the whole half of the cut surface with lemon juice. Spread the slices over the cucumbers. Brush the other slice of bread with mustard and cover the apple slices. Eat the remaining apple

Nutritional info

Per serving:

- ❖ 350 kcal,
- ❖ 3g fat,
- ❖ 50g carbohydrates,
- ❖ 24g protein

HAZELNUT PORRIDGE WITH PEAR

Ingredients for 2 portions

- 1 Tsp camelina oil
- 1 Tbsp maple syrup
- 2nd Knife sp. Cardamom (ground)
- 3rd Tablespoons of orange juice
- 3rd Tablespoons of oatmeal
- salt
- 1 Tablespoons flaxseed
- 150 Grams of pear (in columns)
- 3rd Tablespoons hazelnut leaves (roasted)
- 1 Passion fruit (passion fruit)

Preparation

Cooking time: 15 minutes

Difficulty: light

- Mix the camelina oil, maple syrup, cardamom and orange juice.
- Boil 150 ml of water. Add oatmeal, a pinch of salt and flaxseed and cook everything with a whisk for 2-3 minutes.

- Arrange porridge with pears, hazelnuts, the juicy seeds of the passion fruit and orange syrup.

Nutritional info

Per serving:

- ❖ 405 kcal,
- ❖ 16g fat,
- ❖ 53g carbohydrates,
- ❖ 8g protein

PORRIDGE WITH PINEAPPLE

Ingredients for 2 portions

- 70 Milliliters of oat milk
- 2nd Pinch of turmeric (ground)
- 2nd Pinch of coriander (ground)
- 40 Grams of millet (millet-buckwheat porridge, or oatmeal)
- 100 Grams of pineapple (in cubes)
- 1 Tsp rapeseed oil
- 50 Grams of frozen blueberries
- 1 Tsp ginger syrup
- 2nd Tbsp walnuts (chopped)

Preparation

Cooking time: 10 minutes

Difficulty: light

- Boil 50 ml water, oat drink, spices and millet-buckwheat mixture according to the package instructions.

- Roast pineapple cubes in rapeseed oil. Add blueberries, ginger syrup, walnuts, arrange the porridge with the fruits.

Nutritional info

Per serving:

- ❖ 420 kcal,
- ❖ 16g fat,
- ❖ 56g carbohydrates,
- ❖ 7g protein

FLAX SEED CURD WITH APPLE AND CUCUMBER

Ingredients for 4 servings

- 150 Grams of herb curd ("Almased vital food")
- 150 Grams of cream cheese ("Buko with Skyr")
- 1 Tablespoons linseed oil
- 3rd Tablespoons of lemon juice
- 2nd Tablespoons flaxseed (crushed, see merchandise knowledge)
- 30th Grams
- Seasoned Salt
- Pepper (freshly ground)
- 3rd Tablespoons chives (rolls, fresh or frozen)
- 1 Apple (150 g)
- 1 Mini cucumber (80 g)
- Linseed (for sprinkling)
- Chives (for sprinkling)

Preparation

Cooking time: 10 minutes

Difficulty: light

- Mix the herb curd, "Buko with Skyr", linseed oil, lemon juice, linseed and "Almased" and season with herb salt and pepper. Stir in chives.
- Rinse the apple and cucumber hot and grate dry. Quarter the apple, core it and cut it into thick slices, cucumber into long sticks.
- Arrange the quark, apple and cucumber and sprinkle with flax seeds and chives.

Nutritional info

Per serving:

- ❖ 345 kcal,
- ❖ 17g fat,
- ❖ 22g carbohydrates,
- ❖ 26g protein

BREAD TOPPED WITH HERRING, EGG AND MUSTARD CREAM

Ingredients for 4 portions

- 1 Tbsp mustard (sweet)
- 2nd Tsp mustard (spicy)
- 2nd Tablespoons of orange juice
- 2nd EL low-fat curd
- 1 Teaspoon quark
- 1 Tablespoons chives (rolls, fresh or frozen)
- Pepper (freshly ground)
- salt
- 1 Slice of bread ("Brigitte Balance Bread", 50 g)
- 0.5 Handful of lettuce (e.g. radicchio, in strips)
- 1 Bismarck herring (approx. 100 g)
- 40 Grams of pickled onion (sliced)
- 1 Organic egg (hard-boiled, size M)

Preparation

Cooking time: 15 minutes

Difficulty: light

- Mix both types of mustard, orange juice, 2 tbsp curd cheese and chives and season the cream with pepper and salt.
- Spread 1 teaspoon of curd on the bread slice, add the salad on a plate, herring and onions. Pour a dollop of mustard cream over it, arrange the remaining cream and the halved egg.

Nutritional info

Per serving:

- ❖ 487 kcal,
- ❖ 21g fat,
- ❖ 36g carbohydrates,
- ❖ 36g protein

STALL WITH PIMENTO CHEESE AND ZUCCHINI

Ingredients for 2 portions

- 2nd Tsp olive oil
- 2nd Knife sp. cumin
- 120 Grams of zucchini (sliced lengthways)
- 1 Slice of bread (BRIGITTE balance bread, 60 g)
- 40 Grams of sour milk cheese (e.g. Harzer, Mainzer)
- 2nd Spring onions (in rings)
- Paprika powder (spicy)
- 40 Grams of low fat curd
- 1 Teaspoons of orange juice
- 0.25 Tsp black pepper
- 0.5 Handful of lettuce (e.g. lettuce)
- 30th Grams of tomato (pickled, semi-dried, from a glass, in strips)

Preparation

Cooking time: 15 minutes

Difficulty: easy

- Heat a pan. Add olive oil and cumin. Add zucchini and fry briefly on both sides. Take out and let cool. Toasting bread.
- Dice the cheese and mix with spring onions, paprika powder, curd cheese, orange juice and pepper.
- Top the bread slice with the salad and pimento cheese and serve with zucchini and tomatoes.

Nutritional info

Per serving:

- ❖ 435 kcal,
- ❖ 14g fat,
- ❖ 43g carbohydrates,
- ❖ 29g protein

FISH BALLS, PAK CHOI AND LEMON KEFIR

Ingredients for 4 portions

- 250 Grams of cod fillet (skinless)
- 2nd Tbsp. hemp seeds (peeled)
- 0.5 Tsp. fish spice (eg "Ahoi" from Herbaria)
- 3rd Tablespoons corn (canned corn kernels)
- 2nd Spring onions (finely chopped)
- 1 Organic lemon
- 4th tsp. rapeseed oil
- 200 Grams of pak choi (halved lengthways)
- 150 Milliliters of vegetable broth
- 75 Grams of beetroot (pre-cooked, vacuum-packed or glass, in pieces)
- 80 Grams of kefir (or plain yogurt)
- 1 Tbsp. mustard (sweet)
- salt

Preparation

Cooking time: 40 minutes

Difficulty: light

- Pat well chilled fish fillet dry and dice. Puree the fish, hemp and spice mixture. Stir in the corn kernels, spring onions and 1–2 teaspoons of grated lemon zest. Then shape 6 bulbs with wet hands and chill for 10 minutes.
- Spread the bottom of a hot, coated pan with 2 teaspoons of rapeseed oil. Briefly fry the pak choi with the cut side down, turn and add 4–6 tablespoons of vegetable stock. Cover and cook Pak Choi covered for 4–5 minutes. Add the beetroot and heat briefly.
- Fry the cutlets in another pan in 2 teaspoons of hot rapeseed oil for 3 minutes over medium heat.
- Mix the kefir, mustard, 1 pinch of salt, 4 tablespoons of vegetable broth, 2 teaspoons of grated lemon peel and 1–2 tablespoons of lemon juice.
- Arrange three fish buns with pak choi, lemon kefir and lemon slices. Eat or freeze the remaining cutlets the next day.

Nutritional info

Per serving:

- 475 kcal,
- 25g fat,
- 25g carbohydrates,
- 35g protein

ARTICHOKE SALAD WITH CAPER AND EGG SAUCE

Ingredients for 2 portions

- A Glass of artichokes
- 4th Handful of leaf lettuce (seasonal leaf lettuce, e.g. lettuce and endive salad)
- 2nd Peppers (grilled peppers, glass, 100 g)
- 2nd Tablespoons chives (rolls)
- 60 Grams (whole grain chips)
- CAPER EGG SAUCE
- 3rd Organic eggs
- 2nd Tablespoons capers (fine, glass)
- 2nd Tarragon mustard
- 2nd Tablespoons salad cream (organic)
- 1 Tablespoons apple cider vinegar (mild)
- Cayenne pepper
- Lemon juice
- salt

Preparation

Cooking time: 30 minutes

Difficulty: light

- Drain the artichokes and collect the oil. Clean salad, rinse, dry, pluck into pieces. Dry and dice the grilled peppers.

FOR THE SAUCE

- Boil the eggs for 7–9 minutes. Drain the capers.
- Rinse eggs cold, peel, halve, separate protein and yellow. Dice the egg whites, mash the egg yolks with a fork, mix with the mustard, lettuce cream, 2 tablespoons artichoke oil and vinegar. Add 2-3 tablespoons of water after consistency. Stir in the capers, season with cayenne, possibly lemon juice and salt.
- Arrange the leaf lettuce, artichokes, peppers and egg whites then pass in chips.

Nutritional info

Per serving:

- ❖ 350 kcal,
- ❖ 17g fat,
- ❖ 25g carbohydrates,
- ❖ 21g protein

SIRT FOOD SMOOTHIE AFTER GOGGINS AND MATS

Ingredients For one serving

- 100g unsweetened Greek yogurt
- 6 walnut halves
- 8-10 medium-sized strawberries
- a handful of kale leaves without woody parts
- 20g dark chocolate (at least 85% cocoa)
- 1 date
- 1/2 teaspoon of turmeric
- 1 to 2 mm from a Thai chili, finely chopped
- 200ml unsweetened almond milk

Preparation

Cooking time: 25 minutes

Difficulty: light

- If you want it vegan, use soy yogurt instead of Greek yogurt.
- Put everything in a blender or blender and mix until a smoother smoothie is made.

- Tip: if I have parsley stalks left over, I still add them, chop them roughly beforehand.
- More smoothies that go well with the sirt food diet or that you can drink.

Nutritional info
1 serving approx.:

- ❖ 380 kcal
- ❖ 41 g protein
- ❖ 17 g fat
- ❖ 12 g carbohydrates

SIRTFOOD GREEN JUICE

Ingredients for 2 servings

- 2 big hands of kale
- A large handful of arugula
- A very small hand of flat-leaf parsley
- a very small hand lovage leaves
- 2-3 stalks of celery, including the leaves
- 1/2 small green apple - e.g. Granny Smith
- Lemon Juice from Half of a lemon
- Half of teaspoon of matcha powder

Preparation

Cooking time: 15 minutes

Difficulty: light

- First mix the kale, rocket, parsley and lovage and add to the juicer. About 50ml should come out. Then they recommend juicing the apple and celery stalks and squeezing half the lemon by hand. Then you should have about 250ml of liquid.

- Add a small amount of this to the glass from which you will later drink and dissolve the matcha powder in it. Once it has dissolved, add the rest of the liquid.

Nutritional info

1 serving approx.:

- ❖ 270 kcal
- ❖ 9 g protein
- ❖ 18 g fat
- ❖ 12 g carbohydrates

SPINACH FLAN WITH TOMATO RAGOUT

Ingredients for 4 servings

FLAN

- 250 Grams of frozen leaf spinach (thawed)
- 1 Clove of garlic (crushed)
- 1 Tsp olive oil
- 3rd Organic eggs (size M, separated)
- salt
- 2nd Tbsp hemp seeds (or flax seeds)
- 150 Milliliters (hemp drink or milk)
- Pepper (freshly ground)
- Nutmeg (freshly grated)
- (Baking spray oil)

RAGOUT

- 1 Onion (in cubes)
- 4th Tsp olive oil
- 1 Tsp marjoram (shredded)
- 200 Grams of mushrooms (sliced)
- 200 Grams of smoked tofu (cubes)
- 200 Grams of tomato (chopped, fresh or canned)
- sugar
- 3rd Tablespoons parsley (chopped, fresh or frozen)

Preparation

Cooking time: 60 minutes

Difficulty: light

FLAN

- Squeeze and stir up the spinach. Braise with garlic in a teaspoon of oil in a pan for about 4 minutes. Take out and let cool.
- Preheat the oven to 160 degrees, convection 140 degrees, gas level 2. Beat egg whites and a pinch of salt until stiff. Mix egg yolk, hemp seeds, hemp drink and spinach, season with pepper, nutmeg and salt. Carefully fold in the egg whites.
- Fill the drip pan of the oven on the middle shelf approximately 2 cm high with hot water. Spray 4 cups with spray oil, distribute the spinach mixture in it. Let it set in the oven water bath for 25-30 minutes. Take out, let cool completely on a wire rack.

RAGOUT

- Braise the onions in oil. Add marjoram, mushrooms and tofu and braise. Add tomatoes then cook for about 8 minutes.
- Season with pepper, 2 pinches of sugar, salt. Mix in the parsley. Arrange ragout sprinkled with 2 flans and hemp seeds.

Nutritional info

Per serving:

- ❖ 445 kcal,
- ❖ 31g fat,
- ❖ 11g carbohydrates,
- ❖ 30g protein

ENERGY CUTS WITH WALNUT CREAM

Ingredients for 4 servings

- 1 Bread mix package
- 100 Grams of frozen peas (thawed)
- 40 Grams of walnuts
- 4th EL low-fat curd
- 3rd Tsp walnut oil (or olive oil)
- 2nd Tablespoons horseradish (grated, glass)
- 1 Tsp white wine vinegar
- white pepper (freshly ground)
- salt
- 80 Grams of cherry tomato
- Basil leaves

Preparation

Cooking time: 120 minutes

Difficulty: light

- Bake energy bread then let it cool.
- Puree the peas, walnuts (take 4 kernels for later), quark, oil, horseradish and white wine vinegar.

- Season the cream with salt and pepper. Pour 1/2 of the cream into a screw-top jar and chill.
- Cut 2 slices (approx. 50 g each) of energy bread and brush with the remaining cream. Arrange with 2 walnut kernels, half of quartered tomatoes and basil. The second serving z. B. eat the next day.

Nutritional info

Per serving:

- ❖ 470 kcal,
- ❖ 32g fat,
- ❖ 23g carbohydrates,
- ❖ 18g protein

PUMPKIN SOUP WITH PASTRAMI

Ingredients for 2 servings

- 2nd Sticks of celery (in cubes)
- 200 Grams of sweet potato (in cubes)
- 3rd dried apricots (in cubes)
- 1 Tablespoons of rapeseed oil
- 300 Grams of pumpkin (frozen organic pumpkin)
- 1 Tablespoons spice mixture (eg "Querbeet" from Herbaria)
- 1 Tsp thyme (grated)
- Pepper (freshly ground)
- 2nd Tablespoons of lemon juice
- salt
- 2nd Tablespoons pumpkin seeds
- 2nd Teaspoon sour cream
- 2nd Tablespoons horseradish (freshly grated)
- 60 Grams of pastrami (salted and smoked sausage in cold cuts)
- 2nd Tsp pumpkin seed oil (to drizzle)

Preparation

Cooking time: 40 minutes

Difficulty: light

- Braise the celery, sweet potatoes and apricots in rapeseed oil. Add the pumpkin, spice mixture, thyme and 500 ml of boiling water, cook on an low heat for 20 minutes.
- Puree the soup and season with salt, pepper and lemon juice.
- Roast the pumpkin seeds in a pan without fat.
- Arrange soup with a dollop of sour cream, horseradish, pumpkin seeds and pastrami slices and drizzle with pumpkin seed oil.

Nutritional info

Per serving:

- ❖ 445 kcal,
- ❖ 20g fat,
- ❖ 45g carbohydrates,
- ❖ 17g protein

TORTILLA WITH HERB TOMATOES

Ingredients for 4 servings

- 180 Grams of chilli pepper (green, or 1 green bell pepper, in thin slices)
- 2nd red onion (in rings)
- 250 Grams of mushrooms (sliced)
- 1 Tablespoons of rapeseed oil
- 60 Grams of smoked tofu (finely chopped)
- 1 Tablespoons of thyme leaves
- Pepper (freshly ground)
- Seasoned Salt
- Oil (baking oil for the mold)
- 5 Organic eggs (size M)
- 5 Tablespoons milk
- 1 Clove of garlic (crushed)
- 100 Grams of tomato (chopped)
- 2nd Tablespoons herbal mixture (fresh or frozen, chopped)

Preparation

Cooking time: 35 minutes

Difficulty: light

- Preheat the oven to 180 degrees.
- Braise the peppers, onions and mushrooms in rapeseed oil for 3-4 minutes. Mix in the smoked tofu and thyme. Pepper vigorously and salt a little. Spray a rectangular, ovenproof dish (26 x 4 x 17 cm) with baking oil. Lightly whisk eggs, milk and garlic. Mix egg mass and vegetables and pour everything into the mold and smooth out. Bake the tortilla in the oven for 25 minutes.
- Mix tomatoes with herb salt and herbs. Take out the tortilla, let it cool slightly, cut half into cubes and arrange herb tomatoes with half.

Nutritional info

Per serving:

- ❖ 425 kcal,
- ❖ 27g fat,
- ❖ 15g carbohydrates,
- ❖ 31g protein

SALAD WITH LENTILS, PASTRAMI AND PEPPER BANANA

Ingredients for 4 portions

- 250 Milliliters of chicken broth
- 0.5 tsp. turmeric
- 1 Star anise
- 1 Bay leaf
- 80 Grams of red lentils
- 4th Tablespoons plain yogurt (3.8% fat)
- 2nd Tablespoons chives (rolls, fresh or frozen)
- 1 lime
- 2nd Bananas (200 g, peeled)
- 1 Tablespoons of olive oil
- 1 Teaspoons of agave syrup
- Pepper (coarse, colored)
- 1 green peppers (sliced into rings)
- 1 Chicory (red, in strips)
- 60 Grams of pastrami (cured and smoked beef brisket in cold cuts)

Preparation

Cooking time: 35 minutes

Difficulty: light

- Bring 150 ml of bouillon, turmeric, star anise and laurel to the boil. Add the lentils and cook until firm for 7–10 minutes. Let the lentils cool.
- Mix the yogurt with chives and 1 tablespoon of grated lime zest.
- Briefly fry the bananas in a small pan in the olive oil on both sides, add the agave syrup. Cover the bananas with the broth and pepper. Remove the bananas from the pan. Bring the roasting broth to the boil with 100 ml of chicken stock and 2-3 tablespoons of lime juice. Mix salad dressing, lentils and bell pepper.
- Arrange the lentils with chicory, bananas and pastrami and drizzle with yoghurt.

Nutritional info

Per serving:

- ❖ 440 kcal,
- ❖ 12g fat,
- ❖ 59g carbohydrates,
- ❖ 22g protein

GOAT CHEESE OMELET WITH CLEMENTINE

Ingredient for 1 portion

- 2nd Organic proteins
- salt
- 3rd Tablespoons parmesan (freshly grated)
- Pepper (freshly ground)
- 2nd Spring onions (in fine rings)
- 0.5 Tablespoons of olive oil
- 40 Grams soft goat cheese (in thin slices)
- 1 Clementine (in pieces)
- 6 Slices of cucumber

Preparation

Cooking time: 20 minutes

Difficulty: light

- Mix the egg whites and salt in a plate until very foamy. Add the parmesan and pepper the omelette.
- Sauté half of the spring onions in a small pan in olive oil. Put the omelette mixture on top and fry until crispy from the bottom.
- Spread the goat's cheese slices on the omelet and cook for 2 minutes over a low heat.
- Sprinkle the other onions on the cheese omelet and serve with clemetines and cucumber.

Nutritional info

Per serving:

- ❖ 435 kcal,
- ❖ 31g fat,
- ❖ 15g carbohydrates,
- ❖ 23g protein

TILAPIA FISH STEW WITH SAVOY CABBAGE

Ingredients for 4 servings

- 300 Grams of tilapia fish fillet (back fillets)
- 1 Lime (juice)
- 2nd TL (yellow mustard seed)
- 1 Onion (in cubes)
- 2nd Sticks of celery (finely chopped)
- 2nd Cloves of garlic (finely chopped)
- 1 Tbsp curry powder (mild)
- 1 Tablespoons of rapeseed oil
- 500 Milliliter fish stock (or vegetable stock)
- 2nd Tomatoes (diced)
- 250 Grams of savoy cabbage (in 2-3 cm pieces)
- 5 Tablespoons brown lentils (can, drained)
- 100 Grams of cream yogurt (10% fat)
- 2nd Tablespoons granular mustard
- 1 Tsp fish sauce
- salt

Preparation

Cooking time: 35 minutes

Difficulty: light

- Rinse fish cold, dry and cut into 3–4 cm pieces.
- Braise mustard seeds, onions, celery (keep the green for later), garlic and curry in hot rapeseed oil while stirring. Add the fish stock, tomatoes and savoy cabbage, bring to the boil, cook over a low heat for about 10 minutes.
- Add fish anf lentils and cook for 6 minutes over a low heat. Mix yogurt and mustard.
- Season the stew with 2-3 tablespoons of lime juice, fish sauce and possibly salt and serve with yogurt and celery green.

Nutritional info

Per serving:

- ❖ 390 kcal,
- ❖ 15g fat,
- ❖ 19g carbohydrates,
- ❖ 42g protein

LIME PASTA WITH SAITHE

Ingredients for 4 portions

- 0.5 Limes
- 100 Grams of pollack fillet (skinless)
- 1 tsp. sesame oil
- salt
- 1 tsp. rapeseed oil
- 4th Spring onions (cut diagonally into rings)
- 50 Grams of mushrooms (roughly chopped)
- 100 Grams of savoy cabbage (or pointed cabbage, in strips)
- 100 Grams of fennel (in strips, put tender green aside)
- 100 Grams of spelled spaghetti (cooked spelled or buckwheat spaghetti, halved)
- 3rd EL (vegetable dressing, e.g. "Chi Chlorella" from SpiceNerds)
- Pepper (freshly ground)
- 1 tsp. sesame (toasted)

Preparation

Cooking time: 30 minutes

Difficulty: light

Rinse the lime, dry and grate 2 teaspoons of peel, squeeze out 2 teaspoons of juice. Rinse fish fillet, dry, roughly dice and mix with lime zest, sesame oil and 1 pinch of salt.

Heat rapeseed oil in a wok or in a pan. Put the vegetables in the pan and stir-fry for 7 minutes. Add the fish cubes, lime juice and pasta then fry for 3 minutes.

Heat the vegetable dressing in a saucepan. Season the fish paste with pepper and salt. Arrange on the dressing and sprinkle with sesame seeds and fennel green.

Nutritional info

Per serving:

- ❖ 465 kcal,
- ❖ 17g fat,
- ❖ 42g carbohydrates,
- ❖ 31g protein

WHOLE GRAIN PILAF WITH KALE

Ingredients for 2 portions

- 40 Grams of whole grain rice
- 2nd Allspice
- 0.5 Tsp thyme (grated)
- salt
- 1 Clementine
- 125 Grams of zucchini (in large cubes)
- 1 red bell pepper (in thick strips)
- 1 Clove of garlic (crushed)
- 0.5 Chili peppers (chopped)
- 1 Tablespoons of olive oil
- 2nd Handful of kale (finely plucked, 100 g)
- 0.5 Tsp paprika powder (Pimentón de la Vera, sweetly smoked paprika powder)
- 1 Tsp balsamic vinegar
- 2nd Tablespoons cream yogurt (10% fat)

Preparation

Cooking time: 45 minutes

Difficulty: light

- Rinse rice cold in a colander. Bring to a boil in a saucepan with 250 ml of cold water, allspice, thyme and salt, stir once and cover and swell over low heat for 20–30 minutes until the water is completely absorbed. Let cool overnight.
- Peel the clementine and dice the pulp, catching the juice.
- Braise zucchini, bell pepper, garlic and chilli in olive oil. Stir in the kale and stir-fry everything for about 4–5 minutes.
- Add rice and smoked peppers and heat briefly. Season the pilaf with balsamic vinegar and salt and serve with clementine cubes, clementine juice and yoghurt.

Nutritional info

Per serving:

- ❖ 455 kcal,
- ❖ 19g fat,
- ❖ 54g carbohydrates,
- ❖ 14g protein

PUMPKIN BOBOTIE

Ingredients for 4 portions

- 150 Grams of pumpkin (frozen organic pumpkin)
- 100 Grams of leek (in thick rings)
- 3rd Teaspoon ginger (frozen)
- 1 Tsp rapeseed oil
- 1 EL Garam Masala (or curry powder)
- 2nd Tsp tomato paste
- 1 Tomato (75 g, chopped)
- 0.5 cinnamon sticks
- 1 Tablespoons fruit spread (fig fruit spread)
- Pepper (freshly ground)
- salt
- 100 Milliliters of kefir (or milk)
- 1 Organic egg (size M)
- 2nd Knife sp. Chilli flakes
- 50 Grams of frozen peas
- 2nd Teaspoon hemp seeds (peeled)
- (Baking oil, e.g. from Byodo)

Preparation

Cooking time: 45 minutes

Difficulty: light

- Preheat the oven to 200 degrees, gas level 4 and fan over 180 degrees.
- Stew the frozen pumpkin, leek and ginger in rapeseed oil for 3-4 minutes in a saucepan. Add Garam Masala and tomato paste and sauté briefly. Add the tomato, cinnamon stick, fruit spread and 150 ml water. After the vegetables have reached the boil add pepper and salt.
- Place the vegetables in a flat, ovenproof dish (content 500 ml). Whisk the kefir, egg, 1 pinch of salt and chilli and pour over the vegetables. Sprinkle with frozen peas, hemp seeds and some chilli and dust with a little spray oil. Bake in the oven for 25 minutes.

Nutritional info

Per serving:

- ❖ 445 kcal,
- ❖ 21g fat,
- ❖ 37g carbohydrates,
- ❖ 23g protein

PARMESAN CHICORY ZUPPA

Ingredients for 4 portions

- A Onion (chopped)
- 60 Grams of celery (in fine cubes)
- 200 Grams of parsnip (sliced)
- 1 Tablespoons of olive oil
- 2 Tablespoons spice mixture
- 1 Tsp rosemary (rosemary needles, freshly chopped, or 0.5 tsp dried)
- 2nd Chicory (approx. 250 g, in strips)
- 100 Grams of chickpeas (can)
- 1 Tbsp mustard (spicy)
- 3rd Tablespoons milk
- 5 Tablespoons parmesan (freshly grated)
- 2nd Organic egg yolks
- 0.5 Juice oranges
- Pepper (freshly ground)

Preparation

Cooking time: 35 minutes

Difficulty: light

- Braise the onion, celery and parsnips in olive oil. Add the spice mixture, rosemary and chicory (take a few vegetable strips for later) and add 600–800 ml of boiling water and cook over a medium heat for 8 minutes. Add drained chickpeas and heat in the soup for 5 minutes.
- Mix the mustard, milk, 3 tablespoons of Parmesan cheese and egg yolk and alloy (bind) the soup with the mixture. Do not let the soup boil anymore and season with a few splashes of orange juice and pepper.
- Arrange the soup and sprinkle with chicory and 1 tablespoon of Parmesan cheese.

Nutritional info

Per serving:

- 385 kcal,
- 8g fat,
- 49g carbohydrates,
- 23g protein

DEER SHREDS WITH SAVOY CABBAGE

Ingredients for 2 portions

- 150 Milliliter chicken broth (clear)
- 2nd Allspice
- 1 Tsp thyme leaves (or 0.5 tsp grated thyme)
- 60 Grams of potato (in cubes)
- 200 Grams of savoy cabbage (in strips)
- 2nd Tsp goat cream cheese (or cream cheese)
- Pepper (freshly ground)
- salt
- 140 Grams of deer meat (deer medallions)
- 3rd Tsp olive oil
- 0.5 TL Ras el Hanout
- 100 Grams of mushrooms (sliced)
- 1 Tsp honey (forest honey)
- 1 Tsp balsamic vinegar

Preparation

Cooking time: 35 minutes

Difficulty: light

- Bring the chicken stock, allspice, thyme and potatoes to the boil. Add savoy cabbage and cook over low heat for 12–15 minutes. Mix in the goat's cream cheese and season with pepper and salt.
- Cut medallions into strips. Mix with 2 teaspoons of olive oil, Ras el Hanout and 1-2 pinches of salt.
- Heat a coated pan and stir-fry the meat strips in it for 2 minutes. Add a teaspoon of olive oil and mushrooms and fry for 1 minute and a half. Season with honey and vinegar.
- Arrange shreds of deer and mushrooms with savoy cabbage and sprinkle with pepper.

Nutritional info

Per serving:

- ❖ 455 kcal,
- ❖ 21g fat,
- ❖ 25g carbohydrates,
- ❖ 39g protein

TURKEY KEBAB WITH CHAKALAKA

Ingredients for 4 portions

- 100 Gram of organic turkey breast fillet
- 3rd Tsp olive oil
- 1 TL (BBQ Rub spice mix)
- 80 Grams of papaya (in large pieces)
- 1 Onion (finely chopped)
- 1 Clove of garlic (finely chopped)
- 1 Tsp curry powder (mild)
- 1 Teaspoon ginger (frozen)
- 1 TL chilli (TK)
- 200 Grams of carrot (grated)
- 0.5 green peppers (diced)
- 1 Tsp agave syrup
- 0.5 Tsp cumin
- salt
- 2nd Tsp tomato paste
- 150 Grams of tomatoes (in cubes)
- 100 Grams of legumes (frozen mixture, e.g. Mexican)
- 1 EL papaya (kernels)
- 2nd Tablespoons plain yogurt (3.8% fat)

Preparation

Cooking time: 35 minutes

Difficulty: light

- Preheat the oven to 180 degrees, convection 160 degrees, gas level 3.
- Dice the meat and mix with 1 teaspoon of olive oil and BBQ rub. Put the meat and papaya on wooden skewers and place on a baking sheet lined with baking paper.
- For the chakalaka, braise the onion, garlic, curry, ginger and chili in 2 teaspoons of olive oil. Add carrots and peppers and stir-fry for 2-3 minutes. Season with agave syrup, cumin and salt. Add the tomato paste, tomatoes and frozen legumes and cook over a medium heat for 10–12 minutes.
- Meanwhile, fry the skewers in the oven on the middle rail for 5 minutes on each side. Arrange with half of the chakalaka, garnish with yoghurt and papaya seeds. The rest of the chakalaka should be eaten the next day with fish, omelet or whole grain rice.

Nutritional info

Per serving:

- ❖ 465 kcal,
- ❖ 13g fat,
- ❖ 43g carbohydrates,
- ❖ 39g protein

FENNEL CREAM CHEESE FRITTATA WITH SALSA

Ingredients for 4 servings

- 4th Organic eggs
- salt
- Cayenne pepper
- 2nd Fennel bulbs (250 g each)
- 1 Red onion
- 2nd Garlic cloves
- 1 Tablespoons of olive oil
- 150 Grams of cream cheese (granular)
- 100 Grams of red bell pepper (roasted, glass)
- 2nd tomatoes
- 1 Chili pepper
- 100 Gram of organic cucumber
- 1 Tablespoons of lime juice
- 1 Tablespoons of red wine vinegar
- Pepper (freshly ground)
- 8th Basil leaves

Preparation

Cooking time: 35 minutes

Difficulty: light

- Preheat the oven to 200 degrees, fan oven 180 degrees, gas level 4.
- Whisk eggs, 80 ml water, salt, cayenne. Clean the fennel, cut into fine strips. Peel the onion and garlic, dice finely.
- Heat the oil in a coated ovenproof pan (Ø 24 cm). Fry the fennel, onion and garlic for 3-4 minutes. Place cream cheese on top as a blob. Pour the egg mixture over it, let it set for 3 minutes. Bake in the oven on a medium rack for about 10 minutes. Drain the paprika, dice finely.
- Clean tomatoes, chilli, cucumber, rinse, finely dice. Mix with lime juice, vinegar, salt and pepper. Pluck the basil smaller, stir in. Arrange everything.

Nutritional info

Per serving:

- ❖ 420 kcal,
- ❖ 23g fat,
- ❖ 19g carbohydrates,
- ❖ 33g protein

CHICKEN AVOCADO TAGLIATA WITH COLORED BEANS

Ingredients for 1 portion

- 1 Piece of organic chicken breast fillet (without skin, 150g)
- sea-salt
- 1.5 Tsp olive oil
- 2.5 Tablespoons of sangrita (or tomato juice)
- 1 Red onion
- 150 Grams of frozen princess beans
- 4th Tablespoons corn (canned grains)
- 60 Grams of cherry tomato
- 0.5 Avocados (the pulp, approx. 60g)
- 0.5 Organic lemons

Preparation

Cooking time: 30 minutes

Difficulty: light

- Preheat the oven with an ovenproof dish to 140 degrees, convection 120 degrees, gas level 1/2-1.
- Lightly salt the meat, brush thinly on the top with 1/2 teaspoon of oil and sear on the oiled side in a small coated pan for 2 minutes. Turn and fry for a minute.
- Finish cooking in the oven for 12-15 minutes.
- Sauté the onion cubes in a table spoon olive oil in the pan. Add beans and corn, season with salt and sear. Add sangrita, tomatoes and 2 tablespoons of water and cook covered for 3 minutes.
- Take out the meat and cut it into fine slices. Arrange the tagliata, colored beans and avocado slices, drizzle with lemon juice and sprinkle with lemon zest.

Nutritional info

Per serving:

- ❖ 465 kcal,
- ❖ 23g fat,
- ❖ 21g carbohydrates, 44g protein

STEAMED POTATOES WITH CUCUMBER AND VEGETABLES

Ingredients for 2 portions

- 250 Grams of potato (peeled and rinsed)
- 1 Tablespoons cumin
- 0.5 Organic lemons (rinsed off)
- 100 Grams of fresh goat cheese
- 100 Grams of whole milk yogurt
- 1 Tsp garam masala (or bombay curry powder)
- salt
- Cayenne pepper
- 100 Grams of cherry tomato
- 0.5 Organic cucumbers (or 2 mini cucumbers)
- 2nd Spring onions (in fine rings)
- 1 Tablespoons of rapeseed oil
- 3rd Tablespoons pistachios (roasted)

Preparation

Cooking time: 35 minutes

Difficulty: light

- Halve the potatoes, place them in a steamer and sprinkle with cumin. Place in a suitable pot with 1–2 cm of water. Bring to the boil, steam with lid for 18–20 minutes.

- Grate the lemon zest, squeeze out the juice. Mix the cheese, yogurt, Garam Masala, 1-2 teaspoons of lemon juice, season with salt and cayenne pepper.

- Rinse tomatoes and cucumber. Dice the cucumber 1 cm. Set aside 1 tablespoon of spring onions. Fry the cucumber in the oil for 2 minutes. Add the pistachios, spring onions and tomatoes and steam briefly.

- Sprinkle potatoes, dip and vegetables with lemon peel and remaining spring onion rings.

Nutritional info

Per serving:

- 435 kcal,
- 25g fat,
- 35g carbohydrates,
- 15g protein

FETA MEDALLIONS WITH BELL PEPPER SALSA

Ingredients for 4 servings

- 1 Artichoke can (240 g drained weight, drained)
- 150 Grams of jacket potato (cooked)
- 2nd Spring onions (finely chopped)
- 1 Clove of garlic (crushed)
- 100 Grams of feta
- 2nd Tablespoons dill tips (fresh or frozen)
- 2nd Tablespoons parsley (chopped, fresh or frozen)
- 2nd Tablespoons of yeast flakes
- 1 Protein (size M)
- Pepper (freshly ground)
- salt
- 1 Tablespoons of olive oil
- 320 Grams of bell pepper (grilled peppers in oil, glass)
- 1 Tablespoons (paprika oil, glass)
- 4th Tablespoons capers (glass)
- 1 Handful of corn salad (or rocket, 80 g)

- ❖ 3rd Tablespoons parmesan (freshly grated)

Preparation

Cooking time: 40 minutes

Difficulty: light

- Preheat the oven to 180 degrees, fan oven 160 degrees, gas level 3.
- Squeeze and chop artichokes gently. Peel the potatoes and coarsely with a fork. Process both with spring onions, garlic, crumbled feta, herbs, yeast flakes and egg white into a dough. Season with pepper and salt. Form 6 medallions from the mass.
- Heat 1 tablespoon of olive oil in a medium sized pan. Fry medallions in each side for 2 minutes. Then place on a tray lined with baking paper and finish cooking in the oven on the middle shelf for another 13–15 minutes.
- Only puree the paprika, paprika oil and 1–2 pinches of salt. Stir in the capers.
- Fill the pepper salsa into a deep plate, arrange with lamb's lettuce and 3 medallions and sprinkle with parmesan. Eat the second serving the next day.

Nutritional info

Per serving:

- ❖ 450 kcal,
- ❖ 27g fat,
- ❖ 24g carbohydrates,
- ❖ 26g protein

SALAD WITH EGG, RADICCHIO AND POTATO PASTE

Ingredients for 2 servings

- 4th tsp. olive oil
- 300 Grams of sweet potato (in cubes)
- 2nd Cloves of garlic (chopped)
- 1 tsp. spice mix (eg "Wilde Hilde" from Herbaria)
- 2nd Organic eggs (hard-boiled, size M)
- 75 Grams (tomato and pepper in a mild infusion (glass), in pieces)
- 1 Tablespoons of lemon juice
- 100 Grams of radicchio (in strips)
- 3rd Spring onions (chopped)
- 150 Grams of tomato (halved)
- 40 Grams of green olives (without stone, halved)
- 2nd Tablespoons sunflower seeds (roasted)

Preparation

Cooking time: 35 minutes

Difficulty: light

- Heat a pan, add 3 teaspoons of oil, sweet potatoes and garlic and stir-fry for about 2 minutes. Pour in 140 ml of water, bring to the boil and cover and simmer for 10-15 minutes. Remove 2 tablespoons of cooking water at the end and mix with the spice mixture. Chop the eggs.
- Puree the sweet potatoes, tomato peppers and the mixed spice mixture and season the paste with 1 teaspoon of oil and lemon juice.
- Pour half of the paste into a large screw-top jar and set aside. Spread the other half on a plate, spread half of the salad ingredients and sunflower seeds on top and sprinkle with the spice mixture if necessary.
- Fill the cooled paste in the glass as well, chill and eat the next day.

Nutritional info

Per serving:

- ❖ 465 kcal,
- ❖ 23g fat,
- ❖ 49g carbohydrates,
- ❖ 14g protein

CUCUMBER AND PINEAPPLE SALAD WITH MACKEREL

Ingredients for 2 servings

SAUCE

- 2nd Tablespoons of lime juice
- 1 Tablespoons fish sauce
- 1 Tsp cane sugar
- 2nd Tablespoons of rapeseed oil

SALAD

- 2nd Spring onions
- 100 Grams of chicory (red, Treviso, or radicchio salad)
- 200 Gram of organic cucumber
- 1 Baby pineapple (330 g)
- 2nd Handful of baby chard (or spinach leaves)
- 150 Grams of mackerel fillet (smoked, without skin)
- 40 Grams of peanuts (toasted)
- Chilli flakes

Preparation

Cooking time: 20 minutes

Difficulty: light

FOR THE SAUCE

- Mix the lime juice, fish sauce, sugar, oil and 2 tablespoons of hot water.

FOR THE SALAD

- Clean the spring onions, chicory, cucumber and pineapple or peel if necessary. Cut the spring onions into rings and cut the chicory into fine strips. Dice the cucumber and pineapple 1 cm. Read the chard, rinse it, spin dry. Cut the mackerel into pieces.
- Mix the spring onions, cucumber and pineapple with half of the salad dressing. Put the chard and chicory in a flat bowl. First pour cucumber and pineapple cubes over it, then spread mackerel, peanuts and chili flakes over it. Drizzle with the remaining salad dressing.

Nutritional info

Per serving:

- ❖ 470 kcal,
- ❖ 32g fat,
- ❖ 22g carbohydrates,
- ❖ 23g protein

HUMMUS WITH COLESLAW

Ingredients for 4 servings

- 1 Clove of garlic
- 1 Tin of chickpeas (160 g drained weight)
- 250 Grams of sauerkraut (fresh sauerkraut, see tips)
- 2nd EL Tahini (sesame paste)
- 1 Tsp oregano (dried)
- 0.5 Tsp paprika powder (smoked, dulce / sweet)
- salt
- 3rd Tablespoons of olive oil
- 1 lemon
- Cayenne pepper
- 2nd Stems of mint
- 2nd Stems of coriander
- 1 Spring onions
- 1 Mini cucumber
- 4th radish
- 1 Tsp sesame (toasted)

Preparation

Cooking time: 30 minutes

Difficulty: light

- Peel off the garlic. Puree the chickpeas with liquid, garlic, 125 g sauerkraut, tahini, oregano, bell pepper, 1/2 tsp salt and 2 tbsp oil. Gradually add the juice of 1/2 lemon. Season the hummus with salt, cayenne pepper and lemon juice.
- Rinse herbs and vegetables, dry. Chop the herb leaves, spring onions and 125 g sauerkraut. Cut the cucumber and radishes into small pieces. Mix the salad ingredients and season with a few sprinkles of lemon juice and salt.
- Spread the hummus smoothly on 2 flat plates with a spoon, sprinkle with lettuce and sesame. Drizzle in the remaining oil.

Nutritional info

Per serving:

- ❖ 435 kcal,
- ❖ 22g fat,
- ❖ 42g carbohydrates,
- ❖ 13g protein

EGG IN SERRANO HAM CASSEROLE

Ingredients for 4 servings

- ❖ 2 Egg
- ❖ 2 Serrano ham slices
- ❖ 50g Onion
- ❖ 50g Mozzarella Cheese
- ❖ Fresh parsley
- ❖ Salt
- ❖ Ground black pepper
- ❖ Muffin or cupcake molds

Preparation

Cooking time: 15 minutes

Difficulty: light

- We grease each mold with butter and roll up a slice of Serrano ham in each one.
- Chop the onion, a couple of branches of parsley and the mozzarella cheese.
- We beat the eggs in a container and add the onion, parsley and cheese. Salt and pepper to taste.

- Fill each mold with this mixture in such a way that it reaches the top of the mold and completely fills it.
- Finally we place the molds in the hot oven at 180ºC for about 20 minutes. Once ready, remove from the oven and serve.

Nutritional info

1 person approx.:

- ❖ 290 kcal
- ❖ 26 g protein
- ❖ 10 g fat
- ❖ 21 g carbohydrates

BAKED EGGS OVER AVOCADO WITH GOAT CHEESE OR BACON

Ingredients for 4 servings

- ❖ 1 medium-large avocado at its point,
- ❖ 2 eggs
- ❖ 2 tablespoons of goat cheese or bacon
- ❖ sweet or spicy paprika,
- ❖ ground cumin,
- ❖ granulated garlic, black pepper,
- ❖ Salt
- ❖ Extra virgin olive oil.

Preparation

Cooking time: 25 minutes

Difficulty: light

- Preheat the oven to 200ºC; preferably have the avocado and eggs at room temperature.

- Cut the avocado in half. Carefully remove the bone. With a spoon, enlarge the cavity of each one a little so that the egg fits easily.
- Add salt and pepper a day and put a little cheese inside each avocado or bacon previously cooked.
- Carefully break the eggs and put them inside. Add spices to taste, salt and pepper
- Bake for about 15-20 minutes
- Serve with the rest of the crumbled cheese and add a splash of good extra virgin olive oil.

Nutritional info

1 serving approx.:

- 350 kcal
- 14 g protein
- 13 g fat
- 41 g carbohydrates

CHICKEN SALAD WITH AVOCADO

Ingredients for 4 servings

- ❖ 2 chicken breast
- ❖ 2 ripe avocado
- ❖ 30 mayonnaise
- ❖ 15 ml lemon juice
- ❖ 1 jalapeño or serrano pepper
- ❖ Fine herbs
- ❖ Salt
- ❖ Ground black pepper

Preparation

Cooking time: 45 minutes

Difficulty: light

- We are going to heat the olive oil in a frying pan and roast the chicken breasts over medium heat.

- Season with the fine herbs, salt and pepper, slightly lower the fire and leave them for about 25 minutes, turning them from time to time.
- Once ready, remove them from the pan, let cool for about 10 minutes and cut into pieces.
- Peel the avocados, remove the bone and cut into pieces similar in size to chicken.
- We place the chicken and the avocado on a plate to which we add the mayonnaise and the lemon juice. Add the chopped chili and stir. Let cool about 20 minutes before serving.

Nutritional info

1 person approx.:

- ❖ 200 kcal
- ❖ 1680 kJ
- ❖ 11 g protein
- ❖ 14 g fat
- ❖ 15 g carbohydrates

TURKEY CURRY

Ingredients for 4 servings

- 500 g turkey sirloin
- 80 g onion
- 250 g plain yogurt
- 50 g cream cheese
- 50 ml evaporated milk
- 15 g ground curry (2 tablespoons)
- 12 fresh coriander leaves
- Salt
- Sesame seeds

Preparation

Cooking time: 15 minutes

Difficulty: light

- Cut the sirloin into strips of approximately 1 x 4 centimeters and season.

- Peel and cut the onion
- In a microwave steamer, mix the plain yogurt together with the cream cheese, the evaporated milk, the ground curry and the chopped fresh coriander leaves.
- Season and stir with a few rods until all the ingredients are integrated into a single mixture,
- Add the turkey and onion to the steamer mixture and stir well so that no pieces are left unmarinated.
- Cover and place in a microwave oven, where we cook at 800w for five minutes.
- Once the cooking time has elapsed, we remove the steamer from the oven and let it rest for five minutes, without removing the lid.

Nutritional info

1 serving approx.:

- ❖ 280 kcal
- ❖ 14 g protein
- ❖ 16 g fat
- ❖ 16 g carbohydrates

CLOUD BREAD

Ingredients for 9 units

- 3 eggs
- 100 g Cream cheese (Philadelphia type)
- 1/4 teaspoon baking soda

Preparation/ Cooking time: 25 minutes / Difficulty: light

- As a first point we preheat the oven to 150ºC.
- We separate the whites from the yolks of eggs.
- We beat the yolks with the cream cheese until obtaining a homogeneous and smooth mass.
- In a separate bowl, beat the egg whites until stiff with the baking soda.
- We mix both masses with the help of a spatula, making enveloping movements.
- We place a sheet of baking paper on a baking sheet and on it we distribute 9 piles of dough, forming circles.
- Bake 20 minutes, the bread cloud or cloud can be made salty (adding rosemary, chopped garlic, salt, pepper or spices) or sweet (adding cocoa). An excellent option is adding york ham or serrano ham.

Nutritional info

1 person approx .:230 kcal, 12 g protein, 15 g fat, 10 g carbohydrates

FURIOUSLY DELICIOUS CAULIFLOWER SOUP

Ingredients for 4 servings

- ❖ 2 cans (425 ml each) Chickpeas
- ❖ large cauliflower
- ❖ 6 tbsp olive oil
- ❖ Curry powder, ground coriander, salt, pepper
- ❖ 1 tsp Vegetable broth (instant)
- ❖ 50 g Baby spinach
- ❖ lemon
- ❖ 150 g Greek yogurt (10% fat)
- ❖ Baking paper

Preparation

Cooking time: 50 minutes

Difficulty: very light

- Preheat the oven (electric stove: 200 ° C / convection: 180 ° C / gas: see manufacturer). Line a sheet of baking paper. Drain the chickpeas. Clean cauliflower, cut into florets, washes.

- Mix both with oil, 3 tbsp. curry and 1⁄2 tsp coriander, salt and pepper. Spread on the baking sheet and bake in the oven for about 30 minutes.

- Approx. set aside 1⁄4 of the cauliflower-chickpea mix. Bring the rest to the boil in a large saucepan with 1 1⁄2 l of water, stir in the broth. Simmer covered soup for approx. 5 minutes.

- Read out the spinach, wash and shake dry. Puree the soup. Season with salt, pepper and the lemon juice. Heat the remaining cauliflower mix briefly in the soup. Arrange with yogurt and spinach.

Nutritional info

1 serving approx.:

- ❖ 270 kcal
- ❖ 9 g protein
- ❖ 20 g fat
- ❖ 12 g carbohydrate

RELAXED MEDALLIONS WITH SWEET AND SPICY SAUCE

Ingredients for 4 servings

- 1 piece (approx. 2 cm each) ginger
- 600 g pork tenderloin
- 400 g Baby Pak Choi
- 400 g Carrots
- 2nd Spring onions
- red chili pepper
- tbsp Soy sauce
- 1-2 tsp Liquid honey
- 8-10 stems Asian herbs (e.g. coriander, Vietnamese mint or Thai basil)
- 2-3 tbsp oil
- salt
- 6 tbsp roasted, salted peanuts

Preparation

Cooking time: 40 minutes

Difficulty: light

- Peel and finely grate the ginger. Squeeze the limes. Pat the pork fillet dry and cut into medallions. Mix with ginger and 4 tablespoons of lime juice, marinate for about 15 minutes.

- In the meantime, clean, wash and cut Pak Choi into strips. Peel and wash the carrots and cut lengthways into strips. Clean, wash and cut leek onions diagonally into rings.

- For the sauce, clean the chilli, cut lengthways, core, wash and finely chop. Mix the rest of the lime juice, chilli, soy sauce, honey and 3 tablespoons of water. Wash herbs, shake dry, pluck leaves.

- Heat oil in a large pan. Fry the meat in portions from each side for 1-2 minutes. Salt and take out. Add the carrots, pak choi and 2 tablespoons of water to the pan and cook for about 3 minutes. Braise the spring onions and meat for 1 minute. Season with salt. Arrange vegetables and meat, sprinkle with nuts and herbs. Drizzle with sauce.

Nutritional info

1 serving approx.:

- ❖ 380 kcal
- ❖ 41 g protein
- ❖ 17 g fat
- ❖ 12 g carbohydrates

JERKY LETTUCE WITH LENTILS

Ingredients for 4 servings

- 4th Carrots
- 1 cauliflower
- Salt and pepper
- 200 g green beans
- 2 cans Lentils (425 ml each)
- 75 g arugula
- Clove of garlic
- tbsp Tahin (sesame paste; glass)
- 1-2 tsp Maple syrup
- tbsp Lemon juice
- 2 tbsp olive oil

Preparation

Cooking time: 40 minutes

Difficulty: very light

- Peel, wash and quarter the carrots. Clean the cauliflower, cut into florets and wash. Cook vegetables in a large saucepan in salted water for about 8-10 minutes. In the meantime, clean and wash the beans, halve lengthways and cook for the last approx. 4 minutes. Drain the vegetables, chill them cold and let them drain.

- In the meantime, rinse the lentils in the sieve and let them drain well. Read out the arugula, wash and shake dry.

- Peel and finely chop the clove of garlic. Mix with tahini, maple syrup, lemon juice, oil and approx. 4 tablespoons water to a salad dressing, season with salt and pepper. Mix the prepared ingredients, arrange and drizzle with the Tahin salad dressing.

Nutritional info

1 serving approx.:

- 240 kcal
- 11 g protein
- 11 g fat
- 22 g carbohydrates

VEGGIE BOWL WITH FRIED EGG

Ingredients for 4 servings

- 400 g Champignons
- 1 zucchini
- 200 g Long grain rice
- salt
- 3-4 tbsp olive oil
- 4 tbsp Soy sauce
- 2 tbsp Sriracha sauce (hot chili sauce)
- 1 tbsp sesame oil
- 50 g Pea or mung bean sprouts
- 1-2 red chili peppers
- 4th Eggs
- 1 box red shiso cress

Preparation

Cooking time: 35 minutes

Difficulty: light

- Clean mushrooms and wash if necessary. Clean zucchini, wash, quarter lengthways, cut into pieces. Prepare rice in approx. 400 ml of boiling salted water according to the package instructions.

- In the meantime, heat 2–3 tablespoons of oil in a large pan. Fry the mushrooms in it. Add zucchini and fry for about 4 minutes. Stir in the soy and sriracha sauce, sesame oil and 3 tablespoons of water, bring to the boil briefly. Take off the stove and keep warm.

- Read sprouts, rinse and drain. Clean and wash the chilli and cut into rings with seeds. Heat 1 tablespoon of oil in another pan. Fry the eggs to fried eggs, salt. Cut the cress from the bed. Arrange rice and vegetables in bowls. Spread the fried eggs and sprouts on top, sprinkle with cress. Sprinkle chilli over it as desired.

Nutritional info

1 serving approx.:

- ❖ 400 kcal
- ❖ 16 g protein
- ❖ 17 g fat
- ❖ 44 g carbohydrates

FILLED HOT PEPPER PEPPERS

Ingredients for 4 servings

- ❖ 3rd Spring onions
- ❖ 125 g couscous
- ❖ 1/2 tsp Vegetable broth (instant)
- ❖ 2 can (s) (425 ml each) chunky tomatoes
- ❖ 1 can (s) (425 ml each) Chickpeas
- ❖ 250 g Cherry tomatoes
- ❖ 150 g small mushrooms
- ❖ Salt, pepper, sugar, dried oregano
- ❖ 1 tsp Sambal Oelek
- ❖ 4th red pointed peppers (approx. 150 g each)
- ❖ 2 tbsp Lemon juice
- ❖ 2 tbsp olive oil
- ❖ 75 g Parmesan (piece)

Preparation

Cooking time: 50 minutes

Difficulty: very light

- Preheat the oven (electric stove: 200 ° C / convection: 180 ° C / gas: see manufacturer). Boil 175 ml of water. Clean and wash spring onions, cut into rings. Mix the couscous and broth in a bowl, add the spring onions. Pour boiling water over the couscous mix, cover and let swell for approx. 5 minutes.
- Rinse and drain the chickpeas. Wash and halve cherry tomatoes. Clean the mushrooms. Place half of the chickpeas, cherry tomatoes and mushrooms with chunky tomatoes in a baking dish. Season with salt, pepper, 1 teaspoon sugar, 2 teaspoon oregano and Sambal Oelek. Put in the oven.
- Cut a rectangle lengthwise from each bell pepper and dice finely. Core and wash the peppers. Add the paprika cubes, lemon juice, oil and the rest of the chickpeas to the couscous, mix. Season with salt and pepper and pour into the peppers.
- Put the stuffed peppers on the vegetables. Finely grate the cheese. Bake in the hot oven for about 30 minutes.

Nutritional info

1 serving approx.:

- ❖ 390 kcal
- ❖ 15 g protein
- ❖ 16 g fat
- ❖ 44 g carbohydrates

5 SPICES AND READY FILLET WITH PAK CHOI

Ingredients for 4 servings

- 400 g pork tenderloin
- 5-spice powder
- 3 tbsp Almonds (without skin)
- carrot
- 2nd Garlic cloves
- 1 piece (approx. 2 cm) ginger
- 500 g Baby Pak Choi
- 100 g sugar snap
- 75 g Mung bean sprouts
- 2-3 tbsp oil
- tbsp Lime juice
- 6 tbsp Soy sauce
- 2nd tbsp sweet chili sauce

Preparation

Cooking time: 30 minutes

Difficulty: light

- Pat the fillet dry, cut into thin slices and mix with 1 tsp 5-spice powder. Chop the almonds. Peel and wash the carrot, cut into fine strips. Peel and chop garlic and ginger.
- Clean, wash and cut the Pak Choi in half lengthways. Clean and wash sugar snap peas. Read sprouts, wash and drain.
- Heat oil in a large pan. Fry the fillet in portions over high heat, remove. Braise carrots, garlic and ginger in hot frying fat.
- Add the pak choi, lime juice, 2 tbsp water, soy and chili sauce, bring to the boil, continue cooking for approx. 2 minutes. Fold in the fillet and sugar snap peas, heat for approx. 1 minute. Sprinkle with the almonds and sprouts. In addition, rice noodles taste great.

Nutritional info

1 serving approx.:

- 280 kcal
- 29 g protein
- 13 g fat
- 9 g carbohydrates

KOHLRABI SCHNITZEL WITH YOGHURT HERB DIP

Ingredients for 4 servings

- 800 g Kohlrabi
- salt
- pepper
- 2nd Eggs (size M)
- 4 tbsp Flour
- 80 g breadcrumbs
- 4 tbsp oil
- 1/2 bunch chives
- 6 stem (s) parsley
- Beet cress
- 150 g Whole milk yogurt
- Sprinkle of lemon juice
- sugar
- tbsp Fruit vinegar
- 1 tsp honey
- 1/2 bunch radish
- 200 g Baby leaf salad mix

Preparation

Cooking time: 35 minutes

Difficulty: light

- Peel the kohlrabis and cut it into slices about 1.5 cm thick. Season with salt and pepper. Whisk eggs. Turn the cabbage slices first in flour, then in egg, then in breadcrumbs. Heat 2 tablespoons of oil in a large pan. Fry the kohlrabi in portions for about 6 minutes, turning

- Wash herbs, shake dry. Cut the chives into small rolls. Pluck parsley leaves, chop finely. Approx. Cut 2/3 of the cress from the bed. Stir herbs into the yoghurt. Season with lemon juice, sugar, salt and pepper

- Whisk vinegar, salt, pepper and honey for the vinaigrette. Whisk in 2 tablespoons of oil. Clean, wash and quarter radishes. Wash the salad and drain well in a colander. Mix lettuce, radishes and vinaigrette. Arrange 3 cabbage schnitzel, lettuce and yoghurt dip on 4 plates. Cut the remaining cress from the bed and sprinkle over the salad

Nutritional info

1 person approx .:

- 290 kcal
- 1210 kJ
- 11 g protein
- 15 g fat
- 28 g carbohydrates

STIR-FRIED FILLET WITH SESAME VEGETABLES

Ingredients for 4 servings

- 500 g broccoli
- red bell pepper
- 200 g sugar snap
- red chili pepper
- 600 g pork tenderloin
- tbsp sesame
- tbsp oil
- 100 ml Soy sauce
- 1-2 tablespoons Liquid honey
- 1 tsp Asia spice
- 1 tsp food starch
- 4-5 stem (s) coriander

Preparation

Cooking time: 30 minutes

Difficulty: light

- Clean, wash and divide broccoli into florets. Clean, wash and cut the peppers into strips. Wash, clean and halve the sugar snap peas. Clean the chilli, cut lengthways, core, wash and chop.
- Pat the meat dry and cut into thin strips.
- Roast sesame seeds in a wok or a large pan without fat, remove. Heat the oil in the wok. Fry the meat in 2 portions, turning for approx. 3 minutes, remove. Fry broccoli and peppers in hot fat for 3-4 minutes, stirring constantly.
- Briefly fry the sugar snap peas.
- Add soy sauce, 100 ml water, honey and Asian spice, bring to the boil. Mix the starch and 1 tablespoon of water until smooth. Tie the sauce with it. Reheat the meat in it. Wash the coriander, shake dry and pluck the leaves.
- Sprinkle coriander and sesame over it. In addition: rice.

Nutritional info

1 person approx.:

- 360 kcal
- 39 g protein
- 11 g fat
- 23 g carbohydrates

SPICY MANGO SALAD WITH SHEEP'S CHEESE

Ingredients for 1 serving

Finished in 25 min

- 300 g small, ripe mango (1 small, ripe mango)
- 4th culms of chives
- 1 stem
- basil
- ½ organic lemon
- pepper from the mill
- 10 g sheep cheese (9% absolute fat)

Preparation

Cooking time: 25 minutes

Difficulty: light

- Wash the mango, rub dry and peel with a peeler. Cut the flesh from the stone in thick slices, dice and place in a bowl.
- Wash herbs and shake dry. Cut the chives into rolls. Pluck the basil leaves, put some aside and cut the rest into fine strips.
- Squeeze the lemon, add the juice with chives and basil strips to the mango cubes. Season with pepper and let steep for 10 minutes.

- Arrange the mango salad. Dab the sheep cheese dry with kitchen paper and crumble it over the salad with your fingers. Garnish with basil leaves.

Nutritional info

1 person approx.

- ❖ 270 kcal1130 kJ
- ❖ 18 g protein
- ❖ 4 g fat
- ❖ 20 g carbohydrates

TROPICAL FRUIT SALAD WITH COCONUT

Ingredients for 4 servings

- 200 g half papaya (1 half papaya)
- 300 g small mango (1 small mango)
- 125 g physalis
- 700 g medium pineapple (1 medium pineapple)
- 1 kiwi
- 1 lime
- 3 tbsp broad grated coconut
- 150 g coconut yogurt
- 2 tbsp milk (1.5% fat)

Preparation

Cooking time: 40 minutes

Difficulty: light

- Peel and core the papaya, peel the mango and cut the flesh from the stone. Cut both fruits into bite-size pieces.
- Detach, wash and halve physalis from the parchment skins.
- Peel and quarter the pineapple, cut out the stalk. Cut the pulp into bite-size pieces.
- Peel and cut the kiwi into pieces. Halve the lime, squeeze and measure 2-3 tablespoons of juice. Mix all pieces of fruit with lime juice, leave for 20 minutes.
- Roast grated coconut in a pan without fat until light brown.
- Whisk coconut yogurt and milk with the whisk of a hand mixer or a whisk just before serving.
- Spread coconut sauce over the salad and sprinkle with the toasted coconut flakes.

Nutritional info

1 serving approx.:

- ❖ 390 kcal
- ❖ 15 g protein
- ❖ 16 g fat
- ❖ 44 g carbohydrates

EXOTIC MUESLI WITH TROPICAL FRUITS

Ingredients for 2 servings

- ❖ 1 small papaya
- ❖ 1 kiwi
- ❖ 1 persimmon not too ripe
- ❖ 100 g coconut muesli (finished product)
- ❖ 200 ml coconut water (tetra-pak)

Preparation

Cooking time: 10 minutes

Difficulty: light

- Halve the papaya, remove the seeds with a spoon and peel the papaya. Finely dice the pulp.
- Peel the kiwi with the peeler and dice the pulp.
- Wash the persimmon, cut out the stem and dice the pulp. Put the cereal and fruit in bowls and pour the coconut water over them.

Nutritional info

1 serving approx.:

- ❖ 280 kcal
- ❖ 14 g protein
- ❖ 16 g fat
- ❖ 16 g carbohydrates

ABOUT THE AUTHOR

Ashley Gosling is a Californian chef and mom based in Los Angeles. After the studies in culinary arts at the San Diego Culinary Institute, she began working in San Diego for a couple years then she had the opportunity to move to Los Angeles to dedicate her career and personal life to her passion for a healthy and sustainable relationship with food.

During the last 15 years she travelled across the world, doing important life experiences especially in Africa, Asia and Europe, visiting the best restaurants and discovering the most unique recipes.
She decided to research and share informations related to healthy food, diets and recipes with as many people as possible, including the most relevant, iconic and promising trends in the culinary and nutrition business.

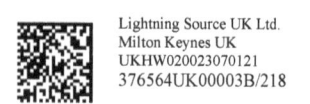

Lightning Source UK Ltd.
Milton Keynes UK
UKHW020023070121
376564UK00003B/218

9 781801 549844